Practical Handbook of
NUTRITION
in
CLINICAL
PRACTICE

Edited by
Donald F. Kirby, M.D.
Associate Professor of Medicine
Chief, Section of Nutrition
Division of Gastroenterology
Virginia Commonwealth University/Medical College of Virginia
and
Director, Nutrition Support Services
McGuire Veterans Affairs Medical Center
Richmond, Virginia

Stanley J. Dudrick, M.D.
Surgeon-in-Chief
Hermann Hospital
Houston, Texas
and
Clinical Professor of Surgery
The University of Texas Medical School at Houston

CRC Press
Boca Raton   Ann Arbor   London   Tokyo

Library of Congress Cataloging-in-Publication Data

Practical handbook of nutrition in clinical practice/co-editors,
  Donald F. Kirby, Stanley J. Dudrick.
      p.   cm. — (Modern nutrition series)
  Includes bibliographical references and index.
  ISBN 0-8493-7847-8
  1. Diet therapy. 2. Nutrition. I. Kirby, Donald F. II. Dudrick,
Stanley J. III. Series.
  [DNLM: 1. Diet Therapy. 2. Nutrition. WB 400 P895 1994]
RM216.P776 1994
615.8′54—dc20
DNLM/DLC
for Library of Congress   93–45906
                                                                                 CIP

© 1994 by CRC Press, Inc.

No claim to original U.S. Government works
International Standard Book Number 0-8493-7847-8
Library of Congress Card Number 93–45906
Printed in the United States of America   2 3 4 5 6 7 8 9 0
Printed on acid-free paper

MODERN NUTRITION

Edited by Ira Wolinsky and James F. Hickson, Jr.

Published Titles

Manganese in Health and Disease, Dorothy Klimis-Tavantzis

Forthcoming Titles

Calcium and Phosphorus in Health and Disease, John B. Anderson and Sanford Garner
Nutrition and AIDS: Effects and Treatment, Ronald R. Watson
Nutrition Care for HIV Positive Persons: A Manual for Individuals and Their Caregivers,
 Saroj Bahl and James F. Hickson, Jr.
Nutrition and Health: An International Perspective, Saroj M. Bahl
Zinc in Health and Disease, Mary E. Mohs

Edited by Ira Wolinsky

Forthcoming Titles

Advanced Nutrition: Macronutrients, Carolyn D. Berdanier
Childhood Nutrition, Fima Lifshitz
Nutrition and Cancer Prevention, Ronald R. Watson and Siraj I. Mufti
Nutrition and Health: Topics and Controversies, Felix Bronner
Nutrition and Hypertension, Michael B. Zemel
Nutrition: Chemistry and Biology, 2nd Edition, Julian E. Spallholz
 and L. Mallory Boylan
Nutritional Concerns of Women, Ira Wolinsky and Dorothy Klimis-Tavantzis

CONTENTS

SERIES PREFACE FOR MODERN NUTRITION

The CRC Series in Modern Nutrition is dedicated to producing the widest possible coverage to topics in nutrition, in all its diversity, both basic and applied.

Published for an advanced or scholarly audience, the volumes of the Series in Modern Nutrition are designed to explain, review, and explore present knowledge and recent trends, developments, and advances across the field. As such, they will also appeal to the dedicated layman. Volumes in this series will reflect the broad scope of information available as well as the interests of authors. The diversity of topics will appeal to an equally diverse readership from volume to volume. The format for the series will vary with the needs of the author and the topic, including but not limited to, edited volumes, monographs, handbooks, and texts.

Contributors from any bona fide area of nutrition, including the controversial, are welcome.

Ira Wolinsky, Ph.D.
Series Editor

PREFACE

Throughout the aeons human beings have been choosing their diets by gathering, hunting, and growing the food required for sustenance of life without determining precisely the quality and quantity of the foodstuffs ingested. With the origin and development of the sciences and scientific methods of investigation, techniques for analyzing and defining nutrient requirements became increasingly available and accurate, especially during the past century. More recently, nutrition education, research, and technology have gained greater importance to health care professionals as data and knowledge have accrued and the relevance of nutritional status to quality of life has been established. It is known that most Americans are overnourished with one third of men and two thirds of women weighing 20% or more above their ideal body weight. In addition, cigarette smoking, alcohol ingestion, drug abuse, and sexual irresponsibility add to the risk factors that can adversely affect health status and medical care. However, serious problems with malnutrition also exist in the U.S., especially among pregnant teenagers, low-birth-weight infants, families of migrant workers, the homeless, geriatric nursing home residents, and many hospitalized patients.

Most health care professionals are ill-equipped to handle complex nutritional problems and the intricate inter-relationships between malnutrition and other pathological processes. Therefore, it is vital that concerted efforts be made to impart nutritional knowledge to all those involved in health care and to encourage the team approach to patients with regard to nutritional management.

Nutrition education for physicians is grossly inadequate in virtually all medical schools, and attempts to rectify this deplorable situation have been protracted and frustrating. Curricula are directed strongly toward diagnosis and therapy of diseases and disorders with little or no emphasis on preventive medicine, nutrition, fitness, and the maintenance of optimal health. Housestaff education is equally deficient as residents and fellows are indoctrinated overwhelmingly with pharmacological and technical aspects of patient care, while nutrition education is neglected in large part because it is broad and general in nature and ostensibly does not fit in readily with highly specific specialty and sub-specialty training. Moreover, most program directors and their faculty are not only poorly qualified themselves to teach nutrition, but also are apparently more interested in tailoring the composition of their education programs to incorporate material more likely to be included in certifying board examinations. As a result, physicians having an interest in nutrition or having gained enlightenment as to its importance from personal clinical experience usually must educate themselves by reading appropriate literature and textbooks or attending nutrition-oriented continuing medical education courses.

Nutrition education in nursing schools has also been subjected to changes in curriculum emphasis, often losing the competition for the students' time and interest to newer high technology areas and thereby demeaning the importance of nutritional support. Thus, nurses, who ordinarily represent the final common pathway in the delivery of optimal patient care, risk having inadequate training and skills to carry out their responsibilities for competently obtaining an initial dietary history and nutritional assessment, reliably ensuring and documenting an adequate dietary intake, and safely and capably administering various tube feeding and parenteral nutrition regimens.

Pharmacists are trained in the essentials of compounding multiple and varied parenteral nutrition solutions, but often are not taught the theory or the practice of clinical nutrition or the means to complement the efforts of well-intentioned physicians who might have limited skills and experience in parenteral nutrition. Pharmacy schools must be encouraged to impart more comprehensive nutritional knowledge to their students and doctoral candidates that will allow them to assist physicians in the area of nutritional support and in the formulation and delivery of cost-effective and safe parenteral nutrition. Finally, pharmacists must be competent not only in the techniques of mixing the components of nutrient solutions, but in mastering the increasingly vast knowledge of nutrient/drug/patient interactions in addition to nutrient/drug incompatibilities.

While dietitians are taught all the fundamentals of nutrition, they are often not given appropriate opportunity or responsibility to apply their skills maximally as important members of the health care team. They should be used more frequently and effectively by the medical community as nutrition consultants. Physicians, in particular, must be taught early in their professional careers that dietitians have the training and capability of taking the physician's general suggestions for a particular patient's dietary goals from which to outline, implement, and supervise a specific detailed plan that the patient can follow efficaciously both as an inpatient and outpatient.

This handbook is not intended to supplant the excellent nutrition textbooks that are currently available, but rather to supplement them practically in clinical areas that might not have been covered in depth or at all. We hope that it will be an additional resource to students of nutritional support regardless of their primary interest, specialty, or educational background. Chapters include a comprehensive review of nutritional assessment techniques currently available and the judicious application of information derived from metabolic carts. There follows an examination of the body's physiological adaptation to malnutrition and the problems sometimes encountered in initiating refeeding regimens. Overnutrition, a major national health problem, is discussed, and the surgical and nonsurgical options available for its management are presented. Additional chapters cover enteral and parenteral nutrition including many new techniques and applications. Finally, several chapters explore more eclectic areas such as nutrition and cancer, nutritional fraud, and the future of food products, and ethical issues in nutritional support.

We hope that you will enjoy this handbook and use it as "food for thought" as you apply its concepts and techniques to patient care. We also hope that your interest in its contents will stimulate us to update the enclosed subject matter and add newly acquired nutritional knowledge for the upcoming century, hailed by many as the century of nutrition education, research, and support.

Donald F. Kirby, M.D.
Richmond, Virginia
Stanley J. Dudrick, M.D.
Houston, Texas

THE EDITORS

Donald F. Kirby, M.D., FACP, FACN, FACG, is an Associate Professor of Medicine, Chief of the Section of Nutrition in the Division of Gastroenterology, and the Medical Director of Nutrition Support Services at the Medical College of Virginia Hospitals in Richmond, Virginia. He is also the Director of Nutrition Support Services at the McGuire VA Medical Center in Richmond.

Dr. Kirby graduated from George Washington University in 1975 with a B.S. degree with Special Honors in Zoology and in 1979 with an M.D. degree. He completed a fellowship in both gastroenterology and nutrition between 1982 and 1985 at Northwestern Memorial Hospital in Chicago, Illinois.

Dr. Kirby is a member of the American College of Physicians, American College of Nutrition, American College of Gastroenterology, American Gastroenterological Association, American Society of Parenteral and Enteral Nutrition (Virginia Chapter: President 1988–1990, Director at Large 1991–1993), American Society for Clinical Nutrition, American Institute of Nutrition, Sigma Xi, The North American Research Society, Crohn's and Colitis Foundation of America, and the Richmond Academy of Medicine.

Dr. Kirby has written 34 articles, 25 abstracts, and 9 book chapters and has presented 57 invited lectures. His current major research includes Percutaneous Endoscopic Gastrostomies (PEGs) in the treatment of brain-injured and spinal cord patients, nutrition in short bowel syndrome patients, and new techniques in PEG and Jejunostomy (PEG/J) placement.

Stanley J. Dudrick, M.D., FACS, FACN, is a Clinical Professor of Surgery at The University of Texas Medical School at Houston and Surgeon-in-Chief at the Hermann Hospital, Texas Medical Center, Houston, Texas.

Dr. Dudrick graduated from Franklin and Marshall College in Lancaster, Pennsylvania, with a B.S. degree *cum laude,* with Honors in Biology, in 1957, and received his M.D. degree in 1961 from the University of Pennsylvania in Philadelphia. He obtained his training in general surgery at the Hospital of the University of Pennsylvania between 1961 and 1967 while also serving as a Fellow in the Harrison Department of Surgical Research in the School of Medicine at the University of Pennsylvania.

Dr. Dudrick is a member of more than 80 academic, honorary, professional, and scientific societies including the American College of Surgeons, American College of Nutrition, American Board of Surgery, American Gastroenterological Association, American Institute of Nutrition, American Society for Clinical Nutrition, American Society of Clinical Investigation, American Federation for Clinical Research, American Society of Parenteral and Enteral Nutrition (founding President), American Surgical Association, Society of University Surgeons, Sigma Xi, and the American Medical Association.

The more than 60 awards and honors he has received include the AMA Joseph B. Goldberger Award in Clinical Nutrition, the Seale Harris Medal of the Southern Medical Association, the AMA Brookdale Award in Medicine, the Grace A. Goldsmith Award of the American College of Nutrition, the Veterans Administration Commendation, and the Ladd Medal of the American Academy of Pediatrics.

Dr. Dudrick has presented more than 300 lectures at national and international meetings and more than 100 guest lectures as Visiting Professor at universities and medical schools. He also has 380 publications including research articles and chapters. He has published more than 100 abstracts and is a member of several editorial boards. His current major research interests include the interrelationships of nutrient substrates with human performance and cellular response in health and disease and the nutritional and biochemical modification of cholesterol and fat metabolism to arrest, reverse, and prevent atherosclerosis.

CONTRIBUTORS

Caroline M. Apovian, M.D.
Associate Physician
Department of Gastroenterology and
  Nutrition
Geisinger Medical Center
Danville, Pennsylvania

William L. Banks, Jr., Ph.D.
Professor of Biochemistry/Molecular
  Biophysics and Preventive Medicine
Department of Biochemistry and
  Molecular Biophysics and
  Director of Nutritional Sciences Center
Medical College of Virginia
Virginia Commonwealth University
Richmond, Virginia

Joseph F. Borzelleca, Ph.D.
Professor of Pharmacology and
  Toxicology
Department of Pharmacology and
  Toxicology
Medical College of Virginia
Virginia Commonwealth University
Richmond, Virginia

Richard B. Brandt, Ph.D.
Professor of Biochemistry/Molecular
  Biophysics and Preventive Medicine
Department of Biochemistry and
  Preventive Medicine
Medical College of Virginia
Virginia Commonwealth University
Richmond, Virginia

Mark H. DeLegge, M.D.
Assistant Professor of Medicine
Department of Gastroenterology and
  Nutrition
Medical College of Virginia
Virginia Commonwealth University
Richmond, Virginia

Daniel L. Dent, M.D.
Department of Surgery
University of Tennessee
Memphis, Tennessee

Stanley J. Dudrick, M.D.
Surgeon-in-Chief
Hermann Hospital and
  Clinical Professor of Surgery
The University of Texas
  Medical School at Houston
Houston, Texas

Amy Foxx-Orenstein, D.O.
Instructor in Medicine
Medical College of Virginia
Virginia Commonwealth University
Richmond, Virginia

Gregory G. Ginsberg, M.D.
Assistant Professor of Medicine
Gastrointestinal Division
Hospital of the University of Pennsylvania
Philadelphia, Pennsylvania

Gordon L. Jensen, M.D., Ph.D.
Director of Nutritional Support and
  Associate Physician
Department of Gastroenterology and
  Nutrition
Geisinger Medical Center
Danville, Pennsylvania

Donald F. Kirby, M.D.
Associate Professor of Medicine
Chief, Section of Nutrition
Division of Gastroenterology
Medical College of Virginia
Virginia Commonwealth University and
  Director, Nutrition Support Services
McGuire Veterans Affairs Medical Center
Richmond, Virginia

Kenneth A. Kudsk, M.D.
Department of Surgery
University of Tennessee
Memphis, Tennessee

Bobbi Langkamp-Henken, R.D., Ph.D.
Department of Microbiology and
  Immunology
University of Tennessee
Memphis, Tennessee

Rifat Latifi, M.D.
Resident in General Surgery
The Cleveland Clinic Foundation
Cleveland, Ohio

Timothy O. Lipman, M.D.
Assistant Chief, GI-Hepatology-Nutrition
  Section
Department of Veterans Affairs
  Medical Center and
  Associate Professor of Medicine
Georgetown University
Washington, DC

Kathy B. Miller, M.S., R.N.
Clinical Nurse Specialist, Nutrition
Department of Nursing
Medical College of Virginia
Virginia Commonwealth University
Richmond, Virginia

Randall S. Moore, M.D.
Vice President, Medical Director
Caremark Healthcare Services
Northbrook, Illinois

Janet V. Starkey, R.D.
Nutrition Clinic Director
Department of Food and Nutrition
  Services
Nutrition Clinic
Medical College of Virginia
Virginia Commonwealth University
Richmond, Virginia

Karen N. Swisher, M.S., J.D.
Associate Professor of Law and Ethics
Department of Health Administration
Medical College of Virginia
Virginia Commonwealth University
Richmond, Virginia

DEDICATION

To our families—whose patience and devotion have allowed us to produce this work.

To our students—whose constant hunger for useful knowledge has challenged and inspired us to sustain our own quest for knowledge and better ways to impart it.

To our colleagues—whose pursuit of excellence in the nutritional care of their patients has provided the stimulus for this handbook.

Special thanks to Ms. Sheryl Miller who shared her literary expertise in assisting with the preparation of many of the chapters.

Chapter 1

NUTRITIONAL ASSESSMENT: THE HIGH TECH AND LOW TECH TOUR

Donald F. Kirby and Mark H. DeLegge

TABLE OF CONTENTS

0-8493-7847-8/94/$0.00+$.50
© 1994 by CRC Press, Inc.

I. INTRODUCTION

It has been almost 20 years since Butterworth brought physician-induced malnutrition to national attention.[1] With simple nutrition assessment principles, including height, weight, and time from last meal, he showed that physicians needed to focus on the nutritional impact of their care. Many patients were shown to become overtly malnourished and to exhibit vitamin and mineral deficiencies while in the hospital.

Since that time many techniques have been used to assess nutritional status, and the provision of enteral and parenteral nutrition is more widely practiced. The goal is to determine which patients are at greatest risk and require urgent nutritional intervention, as well as to estimate energy reserves and function. While there is more science in the process known as Nutrition Assessment, there is still no currently accepted "Nutrition Marker". There is no single test that can be done that is sensitive or specific enough under all conditions to be considered a gold standard. The purpose of this chapter is to explore what is commonly done in most hospitals and other techniques that are presently available, but only to a few hospitals due to the expense or the continued investigational nature of the tool.

II. BODY COMPOSITION

The study of human composition has been an active area of research for over 100 years. While recent information has been accumulating quickly, there has not been an organized approach to classification. Wang and colleagues have recently published a comprehensive five-level model of body composition which will be reviewed here briefly.[2] Each level has an increasingly complex classification to define the components of total body weight (Table 1). In this schema the differences between "fat" and lipid are more clearly defined. Triglyceride, a simple lipid, is synonomous with fat and is a subset of total lipid. An adult has approximately 90% of the total body lipid as fat. Lipid can be further classified into essential and nonessential. The essential lipids are important in forming cell membranes, whereas the nonessential lipids, mostly triglycerides, are the energy stores and also provide insulation for the body.[2]

As this schema progresses to the tissue-system level (IV), fat becomes incorporated into adipose tissue in concert with elastic and collagenous fiber, fibroblasts, and capillaries. Based on its distribution, adipose tissue can be classified as subcutaneous, interstitial, visceral, and yellow marrow. Muscle tissue is still classically divided into smooth, cardiac, and skeletal tissues. Common nutrition assessment techniques often focus on this level and the whole body level (V).[2]

Methods of assessing the tissue-system level have come mostly from tissue biopsies and cadaver studies, but there are a few *in vivo* direct methods such as computerized axial tomography that can estimate the major compartments of this level. Other indirect methods include neutron-activation analysis for nitrogen content and 24-h urinary creatinine excretion to estimate skeletal muscle mass.[2]

It is more practical to study and compare measurements related to the whole body level (V). Table 2 lists 10 common dimensions at this level.[2] Some of these measures will be discussed further under nutrition assessment techniques. It is important to understand that significant changes in one level will be manifested in the other levels whether or not we currently have adequate technology to recognize these changes.

TABLE 1
The Five-Level Model of Body Composition

    I. Atomic
        a. Oxygen
        b. Carbon
        c. Hydrogen
        d. Other
    II. Molecular
        a. Water
        b. Lipid
        c. Protein
        d. Other
    III. Cellular
        a. Cell mass
        b. Extracellular fluid
        c. Extracellular solids
    IV. Tissue-system
        a. Skeletal muscle
        b. Adipose tissue
        c. Bone
        d. Blood
        e. Other
    V. Whole body

Modified from Wang, ZM, et al., *Am J Clin Nutr,* 56:19–28, 1992. With permission.

TABLE 2
Ten Dimensions of the Whole Body Level (Level V)

    1. Stature
    2. Segment lengths
    3. Body breadths
    4. Circumferences
    5. Skinfold thicknesses
    6. Body surface area
    7. Body volume
    8. Body weight
    9. Body mass index
    10. Body density

Modified from Wang, ZM, et al., *Am J Clin Nutr,* 56:19–28, 1992. With permission.

III. METABOLISM AND FUELS

The main fuels of the body consist of carbohydrates, lipids, and proteins. The final pathway for carbohydrates is to glucose, which can be metabolized or stored as glycogen or fat. While all cells of the body share the capability of storing some glycogen, liver cells can store 5 to 8% of their weight as glycogen and muscles cells 1 to 3%. Glycogen is preferentially stored in the liver and muscle until capacity is reached (glycogenesis) and then converted into fat, specifically triglycerides, in the liver (lipogenesis) and stored

TABLE 3
Effect of Starvation on Selected Organ Systems

Heart	Bradycardia, reduced venous pressure and cardiac output, mild arterial hypotension, and decreased oxygen consumption
Lungs	Weakness of muscles of respiration—decreased effectiveness in clearing secretions, decreased vital capacity, respiratory rate, minute ventilation, and tidal volume
GI tract	Decreased gastric acid secretion and gastric motility, mucosal atrophy and reduction in intestinal mass
Pancreas	Possible pancreatic cell atrophy and even fibrosis
Liver	Dependent on substrate withheld *Classic marasmus*—liver shrinks as fat and protein are lost. *Protein malnutrition (Kwashiorkor)*—liver enlarges with glycogen deposition.
Kidney	Reduced glomerular filtration rate, decreased concentrating ability of kidney
Musculoskeletal	Decrease in muscle mass, increased fatigability, possible bone loss

Modified from Silberman, H. Consequences of malnutrition. In: *Parenteral and Enteral Nutrition.* Silberman, H, Ed., 2nd ed., Appleton and Lange, Norwalk, 1989, 1–17. With permission.

in adipose tissue. At maximal glycogen storage capacity there is only enough stored energy to meet the body's need for 12 to 24 h.[3] Both glycogen and protein are inefficient methods to store energy because they require an aqueous environment. Lipid, stored as triglyceride, is a calorie-dense fuel which excludes water.

If we examine the fuel composition of an idealized 70-kg man, then fat stores account for 85% of the energy reserves in tissue, while protein and glycogen account for 14.5 and 0.5%, respectively.[4] It should be clear that survival is dependent mostly on man's fat stores and to a lesser degree protein stores, but most importantly the ability to mobilize them.[5] While the average person can tolerate 5 to 7 days without food fairly easily, longer periods are detrimental. Also, if access to water is limited, or the person is already malnourished, then bodily functions and survival can be further compromised.

While protein can be burned for energy, it must be noted that the body has no storage form of protein. Proteins function as carriers, enzymes, immunoglobulins, and in the structure and function of the body as muscle. It is muscle, a slow-turning over protein, that is sacrificed to provide part of the body's needs when calories are not available from other sources. In the early phases of fasting, infusion of 100 to 150 g of glucose as 5 to 10% dextrose and water has a protein-sparing effect. As the body adapts to starvation, 15 to 18% of calories are derived from protein, but after fat stores are depleted, then protein catabolism escalates.[6]

Studies of starvation have outlined the effect on various organs. Table 3 lists the effects of starvation on the function of several major organs. Chapter 2 will discuss issues of malnutrition and refeeding in more detail.

IV. IDEAL AND STANDARD NUTRITIONAL ASSESSMENT

Why do we perform nutrition assessments? Most clinicians* agree that malnutrition can adversely affect outcome for either hospitalized patients or those about to undergo surgery. As we have previously mentioned, weight loss and malnutrition can affect organ function in man. Thus, knowledge of a patient's nutritional status might help to predict and to prepare the clinician for complications for a patient about to undergo surgery or during hospitalization in general.

*Clinician, in this chapter, refers to any member of the medical team that has some responsibility for the nutritional care of the patient including physicians, nurses, dietitians, pharmacists, and so on.

TABLE 4
Standard Nutritional Assessment

  I. Medical history and physical exam
     A. Weight history
     B. Medication history
  II. Diet history
  III. Anthropometric measurements
     A. Triceps skinfold
     B. Midarm circumference
     C. Midarm muscle circumference
  IV. Biochemical measurements
     A. Plasma proteins
       1. Albumin
       2. Transferrin
       3. Prealbumin[a]
       4. Retinol binding protein[a]
     B. Urinary measurements
       1. Creatinine height index[a]
       2. 3-Methylhistidine[a]
  V. Immunologic markers
     A. Total lymphocyte count
     B. Assessment of delayed hypersensitivity

[a] Less readily available or performed as
routine nutrition assessment tests.

Nutritional assessment is an imperfect exercise. There is no single test that is presently able to predict a patient's nutritional status under all clinical situations. The ideal test would not be influenced by nonnutritional parameters, and it would provide clinically important information. Also, it would be inexpensive and readily available to all clinicians.[7]

When most clinicians talk about nutrition assessment, they focus on available energy reserves which are generally manifested by changes in body composition (Level V). A more useful approach also examines the patient in terms of body function and assessment of the stress factors affecting the body. Table 4 lists the components of what most clinicians perform during a nutritional assessment. Each item has potential limitations which may detract from its usefulness.

A. MEDICAL HISTORY AND PHYSICAL EXAMINATION

Either primarily performing or reviewing a patient's medical history and physical condition are important so that the clinician will have a better understanding of a patient's pathophysiologic response to the stress of the present illness. A good understanding of the medical history can lead to more disease-specific nutritional intervention.

Inquiry as to the patient's usual body weight (UBW) combined with measurement of the present body weight (PBW) and comparison to ideal body weight (IBW) can be extremely valuable. In the U.S. approximately one third of men and two thirds of women are more than 20% over their IBW so that the combination of recent weight loss and IBW may be misleading when the UBW is not considered. Calculations of % UBW (% UBW = PBW/UBW × 100) and % IBW (% IBW = PBW/IBW × 100) can be very informative. Medical students and housestaff should be taught assessment techniques so that they have an appreciation of nutrition assessment early in their careers.[8] It is also important to assess if the present weight is affected by dehydration or fluid overload. The latter is manifested by signs such as peripheral edema or ascites and can significantly alter nutritional requirement calculations.

Height is a measurement that is often not measured or inaccurately reported. It is best to have a patient's height measured on admission to the hospital, and if the patient is bedridden, then other measurements such as knee height or total arm length can be used.[9-11]

A general knowledge of a patient's medications is important so that drug side effects and interactions can be assessed. Also, this can be helpful in determining potential drug-nutrient interactions that might affect the delivery of certain medications or lead to clogging of enteral tubes.

B. DIET HISTORY

Physicians would be wise to elicit their patient's diet history. Unfortunately, most physicians are not trained to do this and so delegate this important function to dietitians. While today's hospital dietitians are extremely well trained, they are often not utilized in their best potential role as nutrition consultants. A physician may suggest that a patient follow a low-salt, low-fat diet, but it is the dietitian who has the role of taking the physician's global nutritional plan and making it practical for the average patient. This can be quite a challenge for patients on fixed or limited budgets or those who do not have access to refrigeration or proper cooking facilities.

C. ANTHROPOMETRIC MEASUREMENTS

Anthropometric measurements provide a rough estimation of body stores of energy. While some may disagree with the methodology or "normal" values, simple measurements of triceps skinfolds (TSF), midarm circumference (MAC), and midarm muscle circumference (MAMC) can be particularly useful to a patient who is followed longitudinally. The midarm muscle circumference is actually a calculated value after the TSF is measured with a special calipers and MAC is measured with a tape measure.[12] The formula is as follows: MAMC (cm) = MAC (cm) − [0.314 × TSF (mm)].

There are approximately 13 locations that have been used as measurement locations for subcutaneous fat.[13] However, for reasons of patient acceptability, ease, and reproducibility, the triceps skinfold is generally used for fat stores and midarm muscle circumference for protein stores. One limitation of the upper arm is that it is difficult to estimate bone size in different individuals, and this can introduce some error into this technique. Advantages of this technique are that it can be taught quickly, is cheap to perform, and can be performed by any member of the nutrition support team. While measurements by tape measure and calipers are generally employed, newer technologies have been introduced that can also be sensitive and specific and will be discussed later in this chapter.

D. BIOCHEMICAL MEASUREMENTS
1. Plasma Proteins

Table 4 lists the most commonly cited tests used as biochemical markers. Of the visceral protein markers, albumin is the most frequently abused "marker of nutrition." Comments like "the albumin is normal so the patient couldn't possibly be malnourished" or "the albumin is low so we had better feed the patient more protein and calories" only reinforce that we have not successfully taught our colleagues the pathophysiologic basis of malnutrition. Also, it is unrealistic to see a significant change—good or bad—in serum albumin after 1 week of nutrition support. Albumin has a half-life of 21 days and is produced only in the liver. Intrinsic liver disease can alter this production as well as the pathway being modulated by interleukin-1 (IL-1) and other lymphokines during times of stress.[14,15] However, it is a very cost-effective test since it is usually available on standard blood chemistry panels. Statistically, it can be very useful when looking at a patient's risk for surgery. Mullen et al. showed that patients with a serum albumin concentration less than 3 g/dl and transferrin levels less than 220 mg/dl were predictive of postoperative morbidity and mortality in a series of patients undergoing elective surgery.[16]

Transferrin has also been used to assess the response to feeding, since its half-life is 7 to 10 days. While it may be more sensitive to changes in protein synthesis of the liver, it may be affected by iron deficiency or overload, pregnancy, pernicious anemia, and chronic infection. Due to the added expense, some centers have discontinued following this parameter.

Prealbumin has been suggested as a good "nutrition" marker, since its half-life is 2 days.[17,18] However, it is generally more expensive than obtaining an albumin or transferrin, is not available at every institution, and may take more time to obtain results. It can be affected by infection or trauma. Prealbumin can be used more accurately than albumin when albumin has been infused exogenously into the patient for clinical reasons.[19] Many nutrition support teams follow the prealbumin, but the true cost effectiveness of this has not been evaluated.

Fibronectin was looked at briefly as a marker. It is an opsonic glycoprotein which is not dependent on liver synthesis like the previous proteins. Plasma levels were seen to correlate well with nonstressed starvation and repletion.[20] Kirby et al. showed that, with the provision of calories in malnourished patients, fibronectin levels increased to normal levels, but were not predictive after the first week.[21] Its expense, lack of specificity, and availability also limit its usefulness.[22]

Somatomedins are growth hormone-dependent growth factors that have anabolic insulin-like functions. Somatomedin activity is highly determined by nutrient intake. While Unterman et al. suggested that somatomedin-C might be a sensitive marker of nutritional depletion and repletion, this marker has never been widely used.[23]

2. Urinary Measurements

The creatinine-height index (CHI) has been used as a measure of lean body mass based on the knowledge that creatinine production from creatine is correlated in a patient without conditions that favor rapid skeletal muscle breakdown.[24] However, the index is limited by injuries to muscle that increase breakdown, certain medications, inadequate renal function or urine collections, dietary meat intake, inaccuracies of height measurements, and changes in the height-weight tables. This index is not frequently used at present.

It was hoped that urinary 3-methylhistidine (3-MH) would be a more reliable marker of total muscle mass since methylhistidine is present only in myofibrillar protein. 3-MH is released during protein catabolism and excreted unchanged into the urine. While in control patients there is a significant correlation between skeletal muscle mass and excretion of 3-MH, there are conditions that both increase and decrease 3-MH excretion, thereby limiting its usefulness in a hospitalized population.[25,26]

E. IMMUNOLOGIC TESTS
1. Total Lymphocyte Count

A total lymphocyte count (TLC), like serum albumin, is readily available on most hospitalized patients. It has been correlated with cellular immune function, and low counts reflect changes in nutritional status, especially protein depletion.[12,27] The calculation of the TLC is as follows: TLC = White Blood Count × % lymphocytes. While many non-nutritional factors can alter this count, counts of less than 1200 lymphocytes/mm^3 reflect a mild deficiency and counts less than 800 cells/mm^3, a severe deficiency. While the absolute predictive value of this parameter may not be high, several studies have noted a correlation between lymphopenia and increased morbidity or mortality in hospitalized patients which make this a useful screening test, but not necessarily a confirmatory test.[16,28,29]

2. Delayed Hypersensitivity via Skin Tests

While evaluating a patient's reaction to recall antigens can provide information on the body's cellular immunity by testing delayed hypersensitivity. Many nonnutritional factors can affect the response. These tests were performed fairly routinely in the early years of nutrition support, but many teams have deleted them from their routine due to lack of specificity and expense. However, before dismissing the utility of skin tests, it should be noted that multiple studies have noted a marked correlation between impairment of skin test reactivity and morbidity and mortality of surgical patients.[30–32]

F. SUMMARY OF STANDARD NUTRITION ASSESSMENT TECHNIQUES

While this compilation of factors is not perfect, it is very useful when the whole patient is considered and abnormal tests explained rather than taking one test separately and placing too much emphasis on it. These assessment techniques are generally adequate to determine if a patient is undernourished, adequately nourished, or overnourished. Further categorization of malnutrition will be discussed in more detail in the next chapter. These standard assessment techniques do not look at "function," and this issue as well as newer assessment techniques will subsequently be reviewed.

The search for better techniques and a true nutritional marker continues. However, the standard assessment does offer a framework for nutrition support specialists to communicate in a common language and to look for better methods to aid in understanding nutrition-related physiology.

V. ADDITIONAL NUTRITIONAL ASSESSMENT TECHNIQUES

Other assessment techniques for determining body composition are becoming increasingly available to assist in our understanding of the effects of malnutrition on body composition and to monitor the effects of nutritional intervention. While total body weight may be preserved, proportions of body fat to protein may decrease as total body water increases. Obviously, nutritional interventions that do not protect lean body mass would be less likely to positively affect outcome from a specific disease state. This was apparent in a study by Kotler, where aggressive home total parenteral nutrition in malnourished patients with AIDS preserved body weight by increasing fat stores in the face of decreasing body protein stores.[33] Direct measurements of body composition by chemical analysis is not possible; however, indirect individual laboratory measurements are available which can accurately and reproducibly assess body composition (Table 5).

The five-level model of body composition has been previously discussed. Examination of Level IV allows us to evaluate important compartments of body composition, specifically adipose tissue, or body fat, and the fat-free mass or body muscle mass. Fat-free mass has a water content of approximately 74%, a potassium content of approximately 69 mM/kg, and a protein content of approximately 20%.[34,35] Body fat has a constant water density of approximately 900 kg/m^3. By measuring total body water, total body potassium, or total body nitrogen, the quantity of fat-free mass can be determined. By measuring body density, the total quantity of body fat can be determined. Additionally, by knowing either compartment's weight, the weight of the other compartment can be determined by simple subtraction as:

$$\text{Total body fat (kg)} = \text{Body weight (kg)} - [\text{Fat-free mass (kg)}]$$

or

$$\text{Fat-free mass (kg)} = \text{Body weight (kg)} - \text{Total body fat (kg)}$$

TABLE 5
Body Composition Methodologies

Methodology	Compartment Assessed
Isotope measurements	
Total body potassium	Fat-free mass
Total body water	Fat-free mass
Absorptiometry	Fat-free mass
Total body nitrogen	Total body protein
Total body electrical conductivity	Fat-free mass
Densitometry	Body fat
Bioelectrical impedence	Body fat
Infrared interactance	Body fat
Radiographic evaluation	
Ultrasound	Body fat
Arm radiographs	Body fat/fat-free mass
Computerized axial tomography	Body fat/fat-free mass
Muscle function	
Handgrip dynamometry	Muscle mass
Muscle contraction with stimulation	Muscle mass
Indirect calorimetry	Caloric assessment
	Substrate utilization

A. FAT-FREE MASS MEASUREMENTS
1. Isotope Measurements

Potassium is an intracellular ion contained in muscle and other viscera. Total body potassium (TBK) is used as an index of fat-free mass. There is a constant fraction of ^{40}K in the body (.012% of TBK) emitting gamma radiation. Utilizing a whole body gamma spectrometer, the ^{40}K is counted and the proportionate amount of TBK is calculated. To protect from background noise, the whole body counter is lead shielded. Using the following formulas, the fat-free mass is subsequently determined as:

$$mMK = \frac{TBK(g)}{\text{Atomic weight of K (39.098)}} \qquad (1)$$

$$\frac{mMK}{69} = \text{Fat-free mass} \qquad (2)$$

The potassium content of fat-free tissue diminishes with age and obesity and increases with muscular development.[36] These variations need to be considered in each individual patient in substantiating the accuracy of this methodology. This cumbersome technique requires specialized instruments and is not practical for the critically ill patient.

Body fat contains no water. By measuring total body water, fat-free mass can be determined. Most measurements of total body water are based on the dilution technique. This technique is based on knowing the amount and concentration of a compound (isotope) and being able to calculate the amount of solvent (water) utilizing these values. The most common tracers (isotopes) used are deuterium (^{2}H), tritium (^{3}H), and a stable isotope of oxygen (^{18}O). These tracers are nonmetabolized, nontoxic, and are evenly distributed in total body water.[37]

The isotope is administered orally or intravenously. Equilibration times of 2 to 6 h are required. At the end of equilibration a sample of urine, saliva, or serum is collected. If

^{18}O is utilized, breath samples can be captured and carbon dioxide fractions analyzed for ^{18}O. Total body water can be calculated as follows:

$$\text{Total body water} = \frac{(\text{Volume of isotope}) \times (\text{Concentration of isotope})}{\text{Concentration of isotope in serum/urine/breath sample}}$$

The volume calculated from isotope dilution is approximate to body water volume. Isotope exchange with nonaqueous material can affect results. Although this error is small for most commonly used isotopes, the use of ^{18}O minimizes this problem.[38]

Isotope dilution methods can also estimate other important body compartments. The fat-free mass is made up of two smaller compartments, the extracellular mass (ECM) and the body cell mass (BCM). The ECM is the component which lies outside of the cell, such as plasma fluid and support structures (cartilage, tendons, and bones). This tissue is not metabolically active. The BCM is the metabolically active protein muscle mass. Calculating fat-free mass alone may not be an adequate indication of nutritional status in the ill patient. Although fat-free mass may remain constant, BCM may fall as ECM increases, yielding a net loss of metabolically active tissue. Utilization of ^{22}Na provides a measurement of the fluid component of ECM.[39] By calculating the fat-free mass via total body water, the actual BCM may be determined as:

$$\text{BCM (kg)} = \text{FFM (kg)} - \text{ECM (kg)}$$

Total body nitrogen (TBN) calculation provides a good measurement of total body protein. This is a result of the constant ratio of nitrogen mass to protein mass as 1 g N:6.25 g protein. Total body neutron activation has been developed to measure total body nitrogen. The patient is bombarded with a neutron flux exciting a proportion of body ^{14}N to ^{15}N. The ^{15}N decays rapidly, emitting a gamma ray which is calculated in a whole body counter. The reproducibility of this system has been validated by Knight and co-workers, who demonstrated comparable results of total body nitrogen by neutron activation and direct chemical analysis on cadavers.[40] Further studies have shown a constant relationship between TBN/TBK of 13.5% in the normal adult, which increases to 14.2% in the elderly.[41] Calculating TBK also allows one to calculate and predict TBN. However, it is interesting to note that in the malnourished cancer patient, the TBN/TBK ratio actually increases. This is most likely due to the fact that TBK is greater in skeletal muscle than TBN, and the rapid reduction of soft tissue in this malnourished patient group is primarily from skeletal muscle mass. It is obvious that further work on stable radioisotopes, as a measurement of fat-free mass, BCM, and total body nitrogen, will need to be performed in a sick patient population. These direct measurements of body compartments will allow us a much better approach to both the assessment and evaluation of nutritional therapy in complicated patient populations.

B. BODY FAT MEASUREMENTS
1. Densitometry
Underwater weighing is the most common method of determining body density. It is based on Archimede's principle which states that the volume of an object placed in water can be calculated from the apparent loss in weight. Brozek created an equation which subsequently described a relationship between body density and percentage of body fat. In this method the subject is first weighed in the laboratory in air and then after total immersion in a tank of water.[42] The underwater weight is recorded after complete expiration. Body volume is calculated from the apparent loss of weight upon total immersion

(change in weight from weighing in air) in a tank of water. This allows calculation of body density as:

$$\text{Body density} = \frac{\text{Body weight (dry weight)}}{\text{(Volume of water displaced with underwater weighing)}}$$

Using Brozek's formula:

$$\% \text{ Fat} = \left(\frac{4.570}{D} - 4.142 \right) \times 100\%$$

The reproducibility of underwater weighing has been shown by Durnin and Rahaman who were able to demonstrate a very low standard deviation in patients who had serial body fat measurements over a 3-year period.[43] Plethysmography is a modification of the underwater weighing technique. The subject is placed in a chamber that is filled with water to his or her neck. Although both of these systems are valid in determining fat mass, their requirement for body immersion places some restriction upon usage, especially in the critically ill patient.

2. Electrical Impedence Methods

Hydrated lean body tissue and extracellular fluid conduct electricity much better than fat.[44] Total body electrical conductivity (TOBEC) takes advantage of this fact. This instrument consists of a large cylindrical coil. When an electrical current is passed through the coil, an electromagnetic field is formed. The patient is placed within this electromagnetic field. A current is formed within the patient, depending on his/her inherent conductivity. A second measurement of electrical conduction is performed with the coil empty. The difference between these values is related to the body's impedance of electrical conduction. The conductivity value is proportional to the body's fat-free mass. Unfortunately, changes in body fluid status (edema, dehydration, ascites) can interfere with the readings.[45]

Body composition can also be determined by impedence to flow measured through an electrical stimulus applied to one extremity (arm) and measured in a separate and distinct extremity (leg). This methodology is known as bioelectric impedence. The human body consists of intra- and extracellular fluids, which behave as electrical conductors, and cell membranes which act as electrical condensors. A localized 50 Hz current is applied to an extremity. The impedence to the electrical flow is based on the volume of the conductor (human body) and the square of the conductor's length (height). The resistance component, to the nearest ohm, is measured. This resistance value is used to calculate the conductivity and, subsequently, the fat-free mass. Validation studies of measurement of fat-free mass and, ultimately, body fat have been clearly demonstrated utilizing densitometry as the gold standard.[46] Linear relationships have been demonstrated between bioelectric impedence, fat-free mass, TBW, and TBK.[47]

C. RADIOGRAPHIC EVALUATION

The arm radiograph technique has been used to evaluate skin, subcutaneous fat, muscle, and bone in the upper arm. The conversion of X-ray widths to body fat was based on relationships developed in the 1920s, where:

$$\% \text{ Body fat} = \frac{\text{External fat thickness}}{\text{Expression of surface area} \times k}$$

The k value expressed in this equation was determined by studying a control group, and solving for k in the above equation based on previous knowledge of % body fat determined by densitometry or isotope dilution techniques. The k value was determined to be 0.0471 by Behnke and Wilmore.[48] There is some question of reliability of this k value between men and women and between different age groups. Measurements of body fat made on separate days and repeated measurements from the same X-ray by multiple observers have been validated.[49]

Computerized axial tomography (CT) is based on the relationship between the attenuation of an X-ray beam and the density of tissue through which it is passed. Fat, lean body mass, and bone each have their own density frequency. CT scanning can be used in body composition analysis. This is done by either establishing cross-sectional areas of specific body tissues, which are measured, or by creating pixels, or picture elements, of specific tissue densities which can then be placed into a histogram form, separating fat tissue from lean body mass.[50] This technique is limited by its exposure to ionizing radiation and cost.

Magnetic resonance imaging (MRI) is based on a magnetic field created by interaction of nuclei and is dependent on their specific density. It is not dependent on ionizing radiation, and it may be applicable to specific patient populations, such as children or pregnant women, in whom nutritional assessment may be warranted. However, studies to evaluate this modality and its reproducibility are currently unavailable.

Sound waves (ultrasonography) can be utilized in delineating echogenic patterns from various body structures and recorded. Subcutaneous fat of 100 mm or more in thickness can be measured with an accuracy of 1 mm.[51] It has been compared favorably to TOBEC and standard caliper techniques.[52] In addition, mid-arm muscle mass measured by ultrasonography was found to correlate well with lean muscle mass, using the creatinine-height index as a reference measurement.[53] Ultrasonography has also been utilized to measure muscle tissue thickness. Unfortunately, many of the ultrasound machines and their software designed today were not developed with the intent to assess body composition; thus, this technique is not in wide use.

D. ABSORPTIOMETRY

Monoenergetic radiation from radionuclide sources was the basis behind the development of absorptiometric principles. Originally a collimated beam of iodine-125 was passed through a limb bone. The changes in beam intensity were analyzed and found to be proportional to mineral content in the beam path. Dual beam absorptiometry allows for the measurement of bone mineral content and lean body mass. This method utilizes a whole-body rectilinear scanner and a high activity source of gadalinium-153 that emits energy at two peaks (44 and 100 keV). The attenuation measurement at two distinct photon energies allows a quantification of both bone mineral and lean body mass.[54] Significant correlation of body composition between dual beam absorptiometry and densitometry has been documented.[55] This methodology provides accurate estimation of body composition utilizing low-dose radiation. However, the high cost of the instrument limits its usefulness in clinical practice.

E. INFRARED INTERACTANCE

This technique involves the irradiating of human tissue with a spectrum of infrared radiation. The absorptive and reflective properties of the tissue examined depend upon its chemical composition. Interactance (I) is calculated as the ratio of energy reflected from a subject as compared to a reference standard. A linear logarithm of 1/I plotted against wavelength allows an interactance spectrum to be graphed allowing for a quantitative analysis of tissue water and fat.[56] Conway et al. compared infrared interactance to ultrasound, anthropometry, and deuterium oxide at five common skinfold sites to estimate fat

TABLE 6
Activity and Stress Factors for Measured Resting Energy Expenditure

Factor	Adjustment
Fever	Reduce MREE 7% for each degree Fahrenheit >100° F
Diet	Increase 10% if receiving an oral or intravenous diet
Critically ill	Increase 10%
Critically ill with major stress	Increase 15%
Ambulatory	Increase 20%

Respiratory Quotient Values

Substrate	Net RQ
Pure carbohydrate oxidation	1.00
Pure fat oxidation	.70
Pure protein oxidation	.80
Mixed fuel oxidation	.85
Lipogenesis	1.00–1.20
Lipolysis	.70

content.[57] There was a high correlation between all methods. Elia and colleagues also confirmed a high correlation between infrared interactance, densitometry, and anthropometry in evaluating the percentage of body fat.[58]

F. CALORIC ASSESSMENT
1. Indirect Calorimetry

The energy expenditure of a patient can be measured by direct or indirect calorimetry. Direct calorimetry measures heat dissipated by the body, while indirect calorimetry measures heat produced by oxidation processes. In the method of indirect calorimetry, a ventilated hood is placed over the patient's head or attached in-line with a ventilator-dependent patient. Air is continuously drawn through a ventilated outlet tube and is sampled for both oxygen and carbon dioxide content. These measurements are taken in a thermoneutral environment, with the patient at bed rest and without nutritional intake for at least 2 h prior to the procedure. The gas analyzer is thus able to calculate resting energy expenditure (REE) via the Weir formulas.[59] Basal metabolic rate (BMR) is the energy expended by the body in the resting state under basal conditions. It varies with the size and surface area of the body and is proportional to the fat-free mass. Thermogenesis is the energy expenditure above and beyond the BMR. It includes effects of sepsis, trauma, fever, cold exposure, food intake, and other entities known to increase energy expenditure. The REE of an individual is, therefore, a combination of the BMR and thermogenic energy expenditure. True caloric needs of the patient often need to be adjusted for level of activity by multiplying the measured REE by an activity or stress factor (Table 6). This allows an adjustment from the measured resting energy expenditure (MREE) to calculate the true resting energy expenditure (TREE).

The respiratory quotient (RQ) is derived from the measurements of volume of oxygen inhalation ($\dot{V}O_2$) and volume of carbon dioxide exhalation ($\dot{V}CO_2$) of an individual. RQ is equal to $\dot{V}CO_2/\dot{V}O_2$ (Table 6). The RQ reflects substrate utilization. Pure glucose oxidation produces an RQ of 1.0; protein oxidation, an RQ of 0.8; and fat oxidation, an RQ of 0.7. The non-protein RQ (NpRQ) is normally 0.85. As the NpRQ decreases toward 0.7, it approaches 100% fat utilization and evidence of lipolysis consistent with underfeeding. As the NpRQ trends toward 1.0, there is 100% carbohydrate utilization and evidence of lipogenesis consistent with overfeeding. Although the RQ can be influenced by alcohol, ketoacidosis, hypothermia, hyperventilation, acidosis, and counterregulatory hormones, this calculation provides a yardstick in appropriate nutrient utilization and calculation of caloric needs.

Clinical efficacy of the metabolic cart is still undergoing scrutiny. Makk and colleagues demonstrated that only 32% of critically ill patients were being appropriately fed, as assessed by standard nutrition assessment equations of caloric needs and as compared to an indirect calorimetry reference standard.[60] A randomized study of enteral feedings based on the Curreri formula of calorie assessment compared to indirect calorimetry resulted in a cumulative caloric intake in the Curreri group which was 43% above measured caloric needs of the patient.[61] Additionally, Mullen demonstrated a 22% reduction in number of TPN liters utilized at a medical center based on the caloric needs calculated via the metabolic cart.[62] There is a high level of frustration with the use of the metabolic cart. McClave and Snider noted that 40% of nutrition support teams that had a metabolic cart never utilized it.[63] The majority of nutrition support teams that did utilize this instrument performed less than ten studies per month.[63] Dissatisfaction was based on expense, frequent repairs, calibration difficulties, and technical difficulties in attempting to assess critically ill patients. Further studies will be necessary to corroborate the utility of the metabolic cart and its appropriate utilization. Clearly, in our ill, complex, and elderly hospital population, this nutritional assessment tool becomes increasingly important.

G. MUSCLE FUNCTION

The majority of nutritional assessment techniques depend upon static measurements of an individual patient. These measurements provide a snapshot of a patient's current nutritional status, but may not provide a valid overall assessment. The patient's functional status or ability to perform tasks is a direct measure of muscle strength and endurance. Muscle function provides a directly measurable quantification of the patient's nutritional status over a period of time and may provide a more accurate statement of current nutritional status.

Muscle tissue is the composite of seven major chemical components, but water and protein constitute over 90% of the muscle mass. Most adults have 20 to 30 kg of muscle which contains a potential energy supply of 20,000 to 30,000 kcal.[64] Generally in the face of starvation, the body uses those proteins needed the least (muscle protein) while attempting to maintain critical proteins for last (heart, brain, kidney, and serum proteins). Skeletal muscle weight gains and losses serve as a barometer of current nutritional status. Muscle function, as a direct marker of body protein stores, or body cell mass, correlates with muscle bulk and often provides additional information about the current nutritional status.

Anthropometry, as previously described, allows the gross measurement of one muscle group, generally in the upper extremity. Interobserver variation, pendulous skinfolds, the presence of edema, and variation in measuring equipment can affect results dramatically. Muscle function is a measurable marker of muscle mass and provides a more reliable indicator of a patient's current protein status and state of nutrition. The two most common modalities in evaluating muscle function are isometric contraction of the abductor pollicus longus and handgrip dynamometry.

The force of contraction of the abductor pollicus longus following electrical stimulation of the ulnar nerve can be measured by a strain gauge looped around the interphalangeal joint of the thumb. Electrical stimulation of the ulnar nerve at the wrist is performed, and the force of contraction of the abductor pollicus is recorded with a force transducer. Lopes and colleagues demonstrated that the maximal muscle relaxation rate was reduced and muscle force was diminished with prolonged tetanic stimulation in malnourished patients as compared to controls.[65] However, the initial force of contraction to stimulation was actually higher in the malnourished patients. Newham additionally found that the maximal relaxation rate and fatigability in muscles of malnourished patients were less than normal controls.[66] This trend was not found in obese patients who were fed a hypocaloric diet.

Handgrip strength is a measure of assessing grip strength utilizing a handgrip dynamometer. Generally, patients are placed in the recumbent or semi-recumbent position. The arm is outstretched from the body, and the dynamometer is placed within the palm of the dominant hand. The handgrip is squeezed, and strength is measured on the instrument's self-contained calibration system. Grip strength has been found proportional to forearm muscle area and lean body mass.[67] Efthimiou demonstrated a reduced grip strength in poorly nourished patients with chronic obstructive pulmonary disease which improved with dietary supplementation and decreased again after dietary supplementation was stopped.[68] This instrument is relatively inexpensive and does not depend on observer technique for interpretation. It is effort dependent, unlike electrical stimulation, and this can be a source of significant error.

VI. THE EFFECT OF STRESS ON NUTRITIONAL ASSESSMENT

Severe stress and hypercatabolic disease states increase the rate of protein loss and body cell mass depletion. Many chronic disease states, such as liver failure or renal failure, are associated with an increased basal metabolic rate and, coupled with chronic undernutrition, result in chronic catabolism. The hormonal status, with high glucagon, epinephrine, and cortisol levels and reduced insulin levels, further adds to this catabolic picture. When major trauma, sepsis, or neoplasms are superimposed upon this system, protein catabolism occurs at a much higher rate.

Chronic nutritional deprivation in the face of no physical stress will ultimately result in a reduction of subcutaneous fat tissue and muscle mass. Basal metabolic rates will decline, and urinary losses will be marginal as the body attempts to preserve protein stores. Often these patients will have normal serum albumin levels. However, as the patient is physically stressed, the entire cascade of protein depletion, and its increased morbidity and mortality, is accelerated. Attempts at refeeding this type of patient may only serve to replete fat stores, without repleting protein stores. Often a patient with chronic underfeeding and acute physical stress may have a normal-appearing body habitus secondary to preservation of fat stores or generalized edema. Obviously, appropriate nutritional assessment is vital in uncovering those patients who are at nutritional risk prior to exposure to severe physical stress.

Conversely, patients often enter a hospital with normal nutritional status, but are placed under extreme physical stress from either sepsis or surgery. Serum albumin levels may rapidly fall, perhaps giving credence to its ability to define current physical state rather than act as a marker of nutritional state. These patients, unless appropriately fed, will enter a cascade of severe protein catabolism with ultimate muscle wasting. It is not unusual for these patients to lose between 15 to 30 g of nitrogen/day. Their clinically normal body habitus often precludes rapid attention to nutritional needs, ultimately compounding their primary disease state. Again, systematic, appropriate nutritional assessment may help to prevent major consequences.

Physical stress may be readily visible on inspection of the patient. However, it is often necessary to evaluate the whole clinical picture, including laboratory evaluation, to determine the degree of physical stress, and the impact it will have on the nutritional status of the patient. Tachycardia, tachypnea, hypotension, fever, and altered mental status are clinical indicators of the critically ill patient. Laboratory examination will confirm this with evidence of a rising white blood cell count with a left shift or, conversely, severe neutropenia, a fall in the serum albumin level, a drop in the hemoglobin, a drop in the platelet count, severe hyperglycemia or hypoglycemia, a rise in acute phase reactants (ferritin, transferrin, etc.) and systemic acidosis. Physical stress may worsen the precarious nutritional status of the critically ill patient as it accelerates the presence of both hypermetabolism and hypercatabolism.

VII. SUMMARY

The evaluation of nutritional status is an important step in initiating nutritional care. The interrelationship between nutritional status, morbidity, and mortality has been recognized for years. Recently, nutritional assessment has developed from a simple visual inspection to a more comprehensive evaluation. It is realized that a combination of tools may be necessary to define the nutritional state of a given patient appropriately. These tools must be utilized correctly, with a knowledgeable nutrition support team available to assist in interpreting the results. In this era of changing health care funding, the cost effectiveness of nutritional assessment is becoming more crucial. The ultimate demonstration of a functional nutritional assessment program, capable of specifically delineating those patients who would benefit from nutrition support, would prove a major health and economic advance.

After assessing a patient's nutritional state, it is important to categorize the patient as malnourished, overnourished, or normal. The subcategories of malnutrition will be discussed in detail in the next chapter. It should be noted that a patient who is overnourished can rapidly become a nutritional problem under the appropriate level of stress and by alteration of cytokines. Thus, global opinions about the nutritional status of overweight or underweight patients based on visual appearance are not likely to be accurate and should be discouraged. Many factors must be considered if nutritional assessment is to have an impact on health care.

REFERENCES

1. **Butterworth, CE, Jr.** The skeleton in the hospital closet. *Nutr Today,* 9:4–8, 1974.
2. **Wang, ZM, Pierson, RN, Jr., and Heymsfield, SB.** The five-level model: a new approach to organizing body-composition research. *Am J Clin Nutr,* 56:19–28, 1992.
3. **Guyton, AL, Ed.,** Metabolism of carbohydrates and formation of adenosine triphosphate. In: *Textbook of Medical Physiology.* 8th ed., W. B. Saunders, Philadelphia, 1991, 744.
4. **Cahill, GF, Jr.** Starvation in man. *N Engl J Med,* 282:668–675, 1970.
5. **Leiter, LA and Marliss, EB.** Survival during fasting may depend on fat as well as protein stores. *JAMA,* 248:2306–7, 1982.
6. **Levenson, SM, Crowley, LV, and Seif̌er, E.** Starvation. In: *Manual of Surgical Nutrition.* Ballinger, WF, Collins, JA, Drucker, WR, et al. Eds., W. B. Saunders, Philadelphia, 1975, 236.
7. **Silberman, H.** Evaluation of nutritional status. In: *Parenteral and Enteral Nutrition.* 2nd ed., Appleton and Lange, Norwalk, 1989, 19.
8. **Roubenoff, R, Roubenoff, RA, Preto, J, and Balke, CW.** Malnutrition among hospitalized patients: a problem of physician awareness. *Arch Intern Med,* 147:1462–5, 1987.
9. **Chumlea, WC, Roche, AF, and Mukherjee, D.** *Nutritional Assessment of the Elderly Through Anthropometry.* Ross Laboratories, Columbus, OH, 1984.
10. **Chumlea, WC, Roche, AF, and Steinbaugh, ML.** Estimating stature from knee height for persons 60–90 years of age. *J Am Geriatr Soc,* 33:116–8, 1985.
11. **Mitchell, CO and Lipschitz, DA.** Arm length measurement as an alternative to height in nutritional assessment of the elderly. *JPEN,* 6:226–9, 1982.
12. **Blackburn, GL, Bistrian, BR, Maini, BS, et al.** Nutritional and metabolic assessment of the hospitalized patient. *JPEN,* 1:11–22, 1977.

13. **Roche, AF, Abdel-Malek, AK, and Mukherjee, D.** New approaches to clinical assessment of adipose tissue. In: *Body-Composition Assessments in Youth and Adults.* Roche, AF, Ed., Report of the Sixth Ross Conference on Medical Research. Ross Laboratories, Columbus, OH, 1985, 14.

14. **Sganga, G, Siegel, JH, Brown, G, et al.** Reprioritization of hepatic plasma release in trauma and sepsis. *Arch Surg,* 120:187–99, 1985.

15. **Dinarello, CA and Mier, JW.** Lymphokines. *N Engl J Med,* 317:940–5, 1987.

16. **Mullen, JL, Gertner, MH, Buzby, GP, et al.** Implications of malnutrition in the surgical patient. *Arch Surg,* 114:121–25, 1979.

17. **Tuten, MB, Wogt, S, Dasse, F, and Leider, Z.** Utilization of prealbumin as a nutritional parameter. *JPEN,* 9:709–11, 1985.

18. **Katz, MD, Lor, E, and McGhan, WF.** Comparison of serum prealbumin and transferrin for nutritional assessment of TPN patients: a preliminary study. *Nutr Supp Serv,* 6:22–4, 1986.

19. **Vanlandingham, S, Spiekerman, AM, and Newmark, SR.** Prealbumin: a parameter of visceral protein levels during albumin infusion. *JPEN,* 6:230–1, 1982.

20. **Scott, RL, Sohmer, PR, and MacDonald, MG.** Effect of starvation and repletion on plasma fibronectin in man. *JAMA,* 248:2025–7, 1982.

21. **Kirby, DF, Craig, RM, Marder, R, et al.** The clinical evaluation of plasma fibronectin as a marker for nutritional depletion and repletion and as a measure of nitrogen balance. *JPEN,* 9:705–8, 1985.

22. **Saba, TM, Dillon, BC, and Lanser, ME.** Fibronectin and phagocytic host defense: relationship to nutritional support. *JPEN,* 7:62–8, 1983.

23. **Unterman, TG, Vasquez, RM, Slas, AJ, et al.** Nutrition and somatomedin. XIII. Usefulness of somatomedin-C in nutritional assessment. *Am J Med,* 78:228–34, 1985.

24. **Blackburn, GL and Thornton, PA.** Nutritional assessment of the hospitalized patient. *Med Clin Am,* 63:1103–15, 1979.

25. **Buskirk, ER and Mendez, J.** Lean body tissue assessment with emphasis on skeletal mass. In: *Body-Composition Assessments in Youth and Adults.* Roche, AF, Ed., Report of the Sixth Ross Conference on Medical Research. Ross Laboratories, Columbus, OH, 1985, 59.

26. **Lowry, SF, Horowitz, GD, Jeevanandam, M, et al.** Whole-body protein breakdown and 3-methylhistidine excretion during brief fasting, starvation, and intravenous repletion in man. *Ann Surg,* 202:21–7, 1985.

27. **Forse, RA, Rompre, C, Crosilla, P, et al.** Reliability of the total lymphocyte count as a parameter of nutrition. *Can J Surg,* 28:216–9, 1985.

28. **Lewis, RT and Klein, H.** Risk factors in postoperative sepsis: significance of preoperative lymphocytopenia. *J Surg Res,* 26:365–71, 1979.

29. **Seltzer, MH, Bastidas, AJ, Cooper, DM, et al.** Instant nutritional assessment. *JPEN,* 3:157–9, 1979.

30. **Meakins, JL, Pietsch, JB, Bubenick, O, et al.** Delayed hypersensitivity: indicator of acquired failure of host defenses in sepsis and trauma. *Ann Surg,* 186:241–50, 1977.

31. **Pietsch, JB, Meakins, JL, and MacLean, LD.** The delayed hypersensitivity response. Application in clinical surgery. *Surgery,* 82:349–55, 1977.

32. **Johnson, WC, Ulrich, F, Meguid, MM, et al.** Role of delayed hypersensitivity in predicting postoperative morbidity and mortality. *Am J Surg,* 137:536–42, 1979.

33. **Kotler, DP, Tierney, AR, Culpepper-Morgan, JA, and Wang, J.** Effect of total parenteral nutrition on body composition in patients with acquired immunodeficiency syndrome. *JPEN,* 14:454–8, 1990.

34. **Sheng, HP and Huggins, RA.** A review of body composition studies with emphasis on total body water and fat. *Am J Clin Nutr,* 32:630–47, 1979.

35. **Womersely, J, Durnin, JVGA, Boddy, K, and Mahaffy, M.** Influence of muscular development, obesity and age on the fat-free mass of adults. *J Appl Physiol,* 41:223–9, 1976.

36. **Pierson, RN, Lin, DHY, and Phillips, RA.** Total-body potassium in health: effects of age, sex, height and fat. *Am J Physiol,* 226:206–12, 1974.

37. **Edelman, IS, Olney, JM, James, AH, et al.** Body composition: studies in the human being by the dilution principal. *Science,* 115:447–55, 1952.

38. **Schoeller, DA, van Santen, E, Peterson, DW, et al.** Total body water measurements in humans with ^{18}O and ^{2}H labeled water. *Am J Clin Nutr,* 33:2686–94, 1980.

39. **Shizgall, HM.** Nutritional assessment with body composition measurements. *JPEN,* 11:42S–47S, 1987.

40. **Knight, GS, Beddoe, AH, Streat, SJ, and Hill, GL.** Body composition of two human cadavers by neutron activation and chemical analysis. *Am J Physiol,* 250:E179–E185,1986.

41. **Cohn, SH, Vaswani, AN, Vartsky, D, and Yasumura, S.** In vivo quantification of body nitrogen for nutritional assessment. *Am J Clin Nutr,* 35:1186–91, 1982.

42. **Brozek, JF, Grande, F, Anderson, JT, and Keys, A.** Densitometric analysis of body composition: revision of some quantitative assumptions. *Ann NY Acad Sci,* 110:113–40, 1963.

43. **Durnin, JVGA and Rahaman, MM.** The assessment of the amount of fat in the human body from the measurements of skinfold thickness. *Br J Nutr,* 21:681–9, 1967.
44. **Pethig, R.** Biologcal membranes and tissues. In: *Dielectric and Electronic Properties of Biological Materials.* Pethig, R, Ed., Wiley, Chichester, England, 1979, 225.
45. **Harrison, CG and Van Itallie, TB.** Estimation of body composition: a new approach based on electromagnetic principles. *Am J Clin Nutr,* 35:1176–9,1982.
46. **Lukaski, HC, Bolonchuk, WW, Hall, CA, and Siders, WP.** Estimation of fat-free mass in humans using bioelectric impedence method: a validation study. *J Appl Physiol,* 60:1327–32, 1986.
47. **Lukaski, HF, Johnson, PE, Bolonchuk, WW, and Lykken, GI.** Assessment of fat-free mass using bioelectric impedence of the human body. *Am J Clin Nutr,* 41:810–7, 1985.
48. **Behnke, AR and Wilmore, JH.** Analysis of radiogrammetric data. In: *Evaluation and Regulation of Body Build and Composition.* Behnke, AR, and Wilmore, JH, Eds., Prentice-Hall, Englewood Cliffs, 1974, 174.
49. **Katch, FI and Behnke, AR.** Arm X-ray assessment of percent body fat in men and women. *Med Sci Sports Exerc,* 16:316–21, 1984.
50. **Hemysfield, SB, Olafson, RP, Kutner, MH, and Nixon, DW.** A radiographic method of quantifying protein-calorie malnutrition. *Am J Clin Nutr,* 32:693–702, 1979.
51. **Fanelli, MT and Kuczmarki, RJ.** Ultrasound as an approach to assessing body composition. *Am J Clin Nutr,* 39:703–9, 1984.
52. **Booth, RAD, Goddard, BA, and Paton, A.** Measurement of fat thickness in man: a comparison of ultrasound, Harpaden calipers and electrical conductivity. *Br J Nutr,* 20:719–25, 1966.
53. **Chiba, T, Lloyd, DA, Bowen, A, and Condon-Meyers, A.** Ultrasonography as a method of nutritional assessment. *JPEN,* 13:529–34, 1989.
54. **Lukaski, H.** Methods for assessment of human body composition: traditional and new. *Am J Clin Nutr,* 46:537–56, 1987.
55. **Mazess, RB, Peppler, WW, Chestnut, CH, and Nelp, WB.** Total body composition by dual photon (153-Gd) absorptiometry. *Am J Clin Nutr,* 40:834–9, 1984.
56. **Hemysfield, SB, Rolandelli, R, Casper, K, and Settle, RG.** Application of electromagnetic and sound waves in nutritional assessment. *JPEN,* 11:64S–69S, 1987.
57. **Conway, JM, Norris, KH, and Bodwell, CE.** A new approach for the estimation of body composition: infrared interactance. *Am J Clin Nutr,* 40:1123–30, 1984.
58. **Elia, M, Parkinson, SA, and Diaz, E.** Evaluation of near infrared-interactance as a method of predicting body composition. *Eur J Clin Nutr,* 44:113–21, 1990.
59. **Weir, JB de V.** New methods for calculating metabolic rate with special reference to protein metabolism. *J Physiol,* 109:1–9, 1949.
60. **Makk, LJ, McClave, SA, Creech, PW, and Johnson, DR.** Clinical application of the metabolic cart to the delivery of total parenteral nutrition. *Crit Care Med,* 18:1320–7, 1990.
61. **Saffle, JR, Larson, CM, and Sullivan, J.** A randomized trial of indirect calorimetry based feedings in thermal injury. *J Trauma,* 30:776–83, 1990.
62. **Mullen, JL.** Indirect calorimetry in critical care. *Proc Nutr Soc,* 50:239–44, 1991.
63. **McClave, SA and Snider, HL.** Use of indirect calorimetry in clinical nutrition. *Nutr Clin Pract,* 7:207–21, 1992.
64. **Heymsfield, S, McMannus, C, Stevens, V, and Smith, J.** Muscle mass: reliable indicator of protein-energy malnutrition. *Am J Clin Nutr,* 35:1192–9, 1982.
65. **Lopes, J, Russell, DM, Whitwell, J, and Jeejeebhoy, KN.** Skeletal muscle function in malnutrition. *Am J Clin Nutr,* 36:602–10, 1982.
66. **Newham, DJ, Tomkins, AM, and Clark, CG.** Contractile properties of the adductor pollicus in obese patients on a hypocaloric diet for two weeks. *Am J Clin Nutr,* 44:756–60, 1986.
67. **Martin, S, Neale, G, and Elia, M.** Factors affecting maximal momentary grip strength. *Clin Nutr,* 39:137–47, 1985.
68. **Efthimiou, J, Fleming, J, Gomes, C, and Spiro, SG.** The effect of supplementary oral nutrition in poorly nourished patients with chronic obstructive pulmonary disease. *Am Rev Resp Dis,* 137:1075–82, 1988.

Chapter 2

UNDERSTANDING MALNUTRITION AND REFEEDING SYNDROME

Amy Foxx-Orenstein and Donald F. Kirby

TABLE OF CONTENTS

0-8493-7847-8/94/$0.00+$.50
© 1994 by CRC Press, Inc.

19

I. INTRODUCTION

Understanding the metabolic differences between the major categories of malnutrition is important in the management of the malnourished patient. Serum protein markers currently used for nutritional assessment are inadequate, as discussed in the previous chapter. However, the reliance on some of these markers is widespread. You may have heard the comment, "this patient cannot be malnourished because the albumin is normal." This conclusion may lead to inappropriate management and to miscommunication to our medical students and other health professionals. While the last chapter focused on the methods of nutrition assessment, this chapter will explore the differences in the major categories of malnutrition and their implications on the refeeding of patients.

II. CATEGORIES OF MALNUTRITION

In this chapter we shall discuss three broad categories of protein-calorie malnutrition (PCM): marasmus (or simple starvation), kwashiorkor or hypoalbuminemic malnutrition (immunorepressive malnutrition), and mixed malnutrition. Table 1 illustrates the main differences between these categories. Some of the classic terms have become modified over the past few years as our understanding of the biochemistry and pathophysiology of these conditions has improved.

A. MARASMUS

Marasmus means simple starvation; it is the body's adaptation to insufficient caloric intake to meet an individual's needs. Marasmus develops insidiously over months to years and may result from anorexia related to an illness such as alcoholism, a central nervous system event, or as a catabolic response to disease. Individuals with multiple medical problems are at increased risk for developing marasmus, particularly the elderly who may have limited access to resources. Patients appear cachectic, wasted, and may have evidence of specific nutrient deficiencies. Peripheral edema is not usually a component of this disease, but can be seen during aggressive fluid resuscitation due to fluid shifts, sodium retention, and hormonal responses associated with the refeeding syndrome, which will be discussed later.[1]

B. NUTRITIONAL BIOCHEMISTRY IN MARASMUS

Familiarity with substrate utilization in early starvation helps explain the body's response. Individuals can tolerate extended periods of semi-starvation because the body will respond to decreased energy intake by lowering the metabolism.[2–4] During an acutely stressful event such as infection or surgery, protein catabolism increases markedly, and if calories are not supplied by the diet, they will come from stores of body fat and protein, including skeletal and eventually visceral muscle.[4]

Endogenous energy stores in the form of free glucose, stored glycogen, fat, and protein are available to fuel the body in response to acute stress, but are called upon to do so at different times and at different rates. If a severely marasmic individual experiences a stressor, then the hypermetabolic, hypercatabolic response may be unable to be fueled adequately by existing stores. Visceral muscle may be broken down and used to supply energy, a situation which is associated with high morbidity and mortality.[5] This injury response in the face of pre-existing marasmus is called mixed malnutrition; this is the combination of marasmus-hypoalbuminemic malnutrition, or alternatively marasmus-immunorepressive malnutrition, and will be discussed later in more detail.

TABLE 1
Nutrition Assessment Classification in Malnutrition

	Marasmus	Kwashiorkor/ immunorepressive malnutrition	Mixed malnutrition
Nutritional intake	Decreased calorie intake	Decreased protein intake and stress	Decreased calorie and protein intakes plus stress
Time course to develop	Months to years	Weeks to months	Weeks
Physical exam	Cachetic, fat depletion, muscle wasting	May look well nourished	Cachetic, may have edema, giving more normal appearance
Anthropometric measurements			
TSF	Depressed	Relatively preserved	Variable
MAC	Depressed	Relatively preserved	Variable
Weight for height	Depressed	Relatively preserved	Variable
Skin test responses	Normal or depressed	Depressed	Depressed
Visceral proteins			
Albumin	Relatively normal	Low	Low
Transferrin	Relatively normal	Low	Low
Total lymphocyte count	Relatively normal	Low	Low

Modified from Silberman, H. *Parenteral and Enteral Nutrition.* 2nd ed., Appleton & Lange, Norwalk, CT, 1989, 55. With permission.

Glucose is the principal fuel for hematopoietic cells and the brain. After an overnight fast, glucose is produced almost entirely by the liver (glycogenolysis). Beyond 24 h, depletion of hepatic glycogen results in an increase in hepatic gluconeogenesis to produce more glucose for the brain. The liver will also remove amino acids (primarily alanine and glutamine), glycerol, lactate, pyruvate, and free fatty acids (FFA) from the blood to form newly synthesized glucose and ketone bodies. The caloric equivalents of these fuels are approximately equal.

After fasting for 48 to 72 h, plasma glucose concentrations fall, and plasma insulin levels drop as well. This fall in plasma insulin is a major hormonal cue which acts to stimulate lipolysis, ketogenesis, amino acid (AA) metabolism, gluconeogenesis, and a decrease in protein synthesis. The result is increased concentrations of FFA and ketone bodies, which serve as alternate fuels and thereby decrease the need for glucose formation.

Summarizing the events in early starvation, the body attempts to use its primary fuel, glucose, until the brain shifts to ketone bodies and FFA in an effort to minimize visceral protein breakdown. A decrease in plasma insulin concentration is the principal hormonal signal that stimulates lipolysis, ketogenesis, AA metabolism, and gluconeogenesis. An increase in serum glucagon is also an important modulator of hepatic metabolism.

The decrease in energy intake in early starvation is followed quickly by a decrease in basal energy expenditure.[2,3] This protective decrease is primarily regulated by a decrease in thyroid and sympathetic nervous system activity. Fasting causes a decrease in the activity of type 1,5'-diodinase, which converts T_4 to T_3, the biologically active form of the hormone. The net effect of the hormonal changes of starvation are to prolong survival by reducing the metabolic rate, to conserve protein, and to prolong organ function.

C. KWASHIORKOR OR HYPOALBUMINEMIC OR IMMUNOREPRESSIVE
MALNUTRITION

Classic kwashiorkor is a term used to describe the body's response to inadequate protein intake even when there are sufficient calories for energy. Clinical manifestations may include fatty liver, edema, marked hypoalbuminemia, hyponatremia, and dermatosis ("flaky-paint").[6] It is commonly seen in Third World countries and occasionally in industrialized regions. Unfortunately, we have seen this type of malnutrition again in this decade because of the severe famine in Somalia.[7]

Hypoalbuminemic malnutrition was an alternate term popularized by Blackburn and colleagues to reinforce the presence of hypoalbuminemia in patients who often appeared well nourished, but had deficits in visceral protein stores and immune function.[8] The etiology of this hypoalbuminemia has been found to relate to the body's response to inflammation or injury, thus the metabolic response to disease. It results in serious changes in the immune system, and we have coined an alternative term, *immunorepressive malnutrition,* to describe this population. It involves a series of host responses which are designed to enhance recovery and decrease the extent of injury. Hormones and monokines are the key modulators of this process.

D. NUTRITIONAL BIOCHEMISTRY IN IMMUNOREPRESSIVE
MALNUTRITION

Directly or indirectly, stress-induced hormonal changes can result in many responses, including stimulation of catecholamines resulting in an increased metabolic rate, antidiuretic hormone (ADH) and aldosterone release, and sympathoadrenal axis stimulation helping to maintain blood pressure.[2] Stimulation of counterregulatory hormones (glucagon, epinephrine, cortisol, growth hormone) can cause hyperglycemia and a breakdown in skeletal muscle, which provides precursors for synthesis of glucose and protein and stimulates lipolysis, which also provides energy.

Cytokines are protein hormones that mediate host immune responses and are activated at times of stress. Cytokines that are produced by mononuclear phagocytes are termed monokines, and those activated by lymphocytes are called lymphokines. Cytokines are biologically active in small quantities and often influence the synthesis, release, and activity of other cytokines.

The role of monokines on serum albumin is important to the understanding of albumin levels during injury. It is the balance of synthesis and catabolism and the equilibrium of albumin between the intra- and extravascular spaces that determines the serum concentration. The daily synthesis rate of albumin is about 15 g in a 70 kg individual.[9] After synthesis, it is distributed approximately 40% intravascularly and 60% extravascularly. About 10% undergoes catabolism daily in the gastrointestinal tract and vascular endothelium. During injury the liver produces acute phase proteins rather than albumin. Tumor necrosis factor-α (TNF) and interleukin-1 (IL-1) can down-regulate the albumin gene and decrease the rate of mRNA translation. The hypoalbuminemia seen with injury is, therefore, a result of decreased production, increased catabolism and extravasation. During injury albumin acts as an excellent marker for the injury response rather than as an indicator of nutritional status. As long as there are ongoing stress and suppression of albumin synthesis, the serum albumin level should not be expected to improve, despite nutritional supplementation via enteral or parenteral means.

TNF (or cachectin) is a monokine produced by monocytes, pulmonary and peritoneal macrophages, and hepatic Kupffer cells.[10,11] Synthesis of TNF can be stimulated by bacterial endotoxins, exotoxins, fungi, and viruses. TNF acts as an endogenous pyrogen with immune-stimulating capabilities, which can combat invading pathogens and can induce production and release of another monokine, IL-1.[12]

IL-1 is derived primarily from monocytes and tissue macrophages. It acts to increase the proliferation of T cells, increasing the release of immature cells from the bone marrow, and enhances the delivery of granulocytes to sites of inflammation.[13,14] Experimental evidence suggests infusion of IL-1 and TNF is associated with anorexia and weight loss. This action appears to be related to a direct effect on the satiety center of the brain.[15] IL-1 also acts as an endogenous pyrogen, inducing a febrile response by stimulating release of prostaglandins in the anterior hypothalamus, similar to TNF.[16]

IL-1 has effects on the balance of hepatic and peripheral tissue proteins. Infusion can result in depressed levels of iron and zinc, by increasing the release of proteins which bind them and by stimulating their uptake into the reticuloendothelial system.[17] IL-1 is involved in remodeling bone and tissue during injury, stimulating activity of osteoclasts in bone and degradation of collagenase and proteoglycan in connective tissue.[13] Release of IL-1 can lead to increased permeability of endothelial cells. Increased permeability of cells allows for leukocyte migration to sites of inflammation, but is also associated with leakage of circulating proteins such as albumin.[18] Elevated serum trigylceride concentrations, seen during IL-1 and TNF infusion, appear to be related to a pronounced increase in hepatic lipoprotein synthesis.[19]

IL-2 is produced by T-lymphocytes in response to mitogen or antigen stimulation. Infusion has been associated with rapid development of fever, flu-like symptoms, tachycardia, and the release of counter-regulatory hormones. These effects can be attenuated with ibuprofen, which suggests an etiologic role for prostaglandins in this setting.

Maturation and commitment of bone marrow stem cells are highly cytokine-dependent. Cytokines which stimulate marrow progenitors are collectively termed colony-stimulating factors (CFSs). IL-3 is the earliest acting factor stimulating the most immature progenitors to grow into lineages (including T and B cells), whereas GM, G, and M-CFSs (granulocytes, macrophage) act selectively during development into such cells as neutrophils, monocytes, basophils, eosinophils and platelets. IL-3 and GM-CFS are produced by the T-helper cells, whereas G-CFS and M-CFS are produced by monocytes/macrophages, endothelial cells, and fibroblasts.

IL-4 is secreted by T-helper cells, mast cells, and basophils. It is induced by antigen binding to cross-linking IgE present on the surface of mast cells and basophils. IL-4 can block the increase of citrate concentrations induced by IL-1, TNF, and IL-6, which is associated with increased activity of hepatic acetyl co-enzyme A carboxylases. Blocking the increase in citrate results in inhibition of the stimulation of hepatic lipogenesis.

IL-5 is secreted by T-helper and mast cells and is induced in a similar manner as IL-4. It acts as a growth and differentiation factor for eosinophils and can induce inflammatory mediators, such as histamine and leukotrienes, from eosinophils and mast cells.

IL-6 is secreted by T-helper cells, monocytes, macrophages, fibroblasts, B cells, and endothelial cells. It is induced by antigen stimulation, IL-1, TNF, and by bacterial products. IL-6 increases hepatocyte production of acute phase proteins and can stimulate fatty acid synthesis in the liver by increasing hepatic citrate.[20]

IL-7 is secreted by bone marrow stromal cells. It acts on lymphocyte progenitors to cause development of the B-cell lineage and serves to stimulate growth of the T-cell precursors.

IL-8 is secreted by monocytes. It can be induced by bacterial products and cytokines, IL-1 and TNF. Neutrophilic activation induced by IL-1 and TNF may be due to IL-8 induction, and in this way IL-8 may serve as a principal secondary mediator of inflammation.

IL-10 is secreted by T-helper cells, some B cells, and stromal cells. It is induced by antigen presentation and by bacterial products. The action of IL-10 is down-regulation of interferon gamma production and up-regulation of IL-4 and IL-5 production by the T-helper cells. IL-10 acts to suppress secretion of inflammatory cytokines IL-1, IL-6, IL-8, and TNF.

E. MIXED MALNUTRITION

The classifications of malnutrition are not always independent. One form of malnutrition may be predominant when an injury occurs. The event may lead to metabolic compromise characteristic of the other major form of malnutrition. The combination of both marasmus and immunorepressive malnutrition is termed mixed malnutrition. An example would be a person who has suffered gradual weight loss from altered dietary intake from an esophageal cancer. This individual might have initially presented with pure marasmus. If he then suffers a severe metabolic insult, which can alter liver protein synthesis and the immune system, then this person may have metabolic features that on standard nutritional assessment appear to be consistent with immunorepressive malnutrition (hypoalbuminemic malnutrition). Taken all together, this person would now be assessed as having mixed malnutrition. This type of patient is likely to experience a higher morbidity and mortality from these combined features.

III. MALNUTRITION AND THE BODY'S RESPONSE

The effect of malnutrition on organ structure and function can be significant. Generally, it is related to the duration and severity of the deficiency. Infection and injury affect the metabolic response in a malnourished patient much differently than in a well-nourished person. An acutely stressful event can lead to rapid metabolic decompensation in an individual with PCM.

A. WEIGHT LOSS

Weight loss is one of the most obvious consequences of poor nutrition. Most people can tolerate a loss of 5 to 10% of body weight with minimal consequence. When weight loss exceeds 20 to 25%, metabolism is stressed, and when weight loss exceeds 40%, survival is unusual.[21] Survival during starvation correlates with the quantity of fat stores that exist at the onset of the fast.[22] In marasmus, when the body adapts to starvation, the proportion of calories obtained from protein becomes constant at 15 to 18% until fat stores are depleted. When fat stores are depleted or when an acutely stressful event occurs, protein catabolism will increase. Overall changes in body composition that occur in starvation include a relative increase in the extracellular water compartment, loss of adipose stores, and, to a lesser degree, a loss of lean body tissue.

B. RESPIRATORY SYSTEM

Malnutrition affects the structure and function of the respiratory system, and pneumonia is a significant cause of mortality in patients suffering from PCM.[23–25] The reasons for this are the decrease in the following: diaphragmatic muscle mass, maximum voluntary ventilation, and respiratory muscle strength in a progressively diminishing capacity. Starvation impairs ventilatory drive and affects the pulmonary parenchyma by causing impaired ability to clear secretions, which ultimately results in emphysema-like changes. The metabolic rate affects the ventilatory response to hypoxia and hypercapnia. In starvation the metabolic rate decreases, as does minute ventilation and the ventilatory response to hypoxia.[25] During periods of stress, the response can be even further impaired, but these respiratory changes revert toward normal with refeeding. If patients receive an excess of carbohydrate, it can result in increased carbon dioxide production and further compromise of function in those patients with poor pulmonary reserve.

Malnourished patients have a decrease in sigh frequency and tidal volume which predisposes to atelectasis. PCM can result in increased extracellular fluid and interstitial fluid, which can lead to decreased functional residual capacity. Parenchymal changes of the lungs associated with malnutrition include decreased lipogenesis, emphysematous changes, and biochemical changes in connective tissue components. Hypophosphatemia has been associated with skeletal muscle dysfunction as well as ventilatory failure, and correction may improve these conditions.

C. CARDIOVASCULAR SYSTEM

It was believed for many years that the heart was a protected organ during starvation, even though many autopsy studies demonstrated heart weight declining almost proportionately to body weight. It is now realized that PCM can lead to cardiac atrophy and fibrosis if starvation persists for an extended period.[26] In autopsy specimens, gross examination revealed a decreased myocardial weight, atrophy of subepicardial fat, and interstitial edema.[27-30] Echocardiographic data has showed 60% of the loss in cardiac volume was due to a decrease in internal chamber volume and 40% to a decrease in cardiac muscle mass, especially the left ventricle.[26] When malnutrition leads to structural changes, there are often associated electrocardiographic abnormalities including sinus bradycardia, low voltage of the QRS complex, reduction in T-wave amplitude, and prolongation of the Q-Tc interval.[31-33] Associated hemodynamic responses include arterial hypotension and reduced central venous pressure, O_2 consumption, stroke volume, and cardiac output. These adaptive changes, which occur during prolonged starvation, may facilitate myocardial function at lower oxygen consumption, thus placing less demands on the body for energy.[26,34]

Refeeding can alter this adaptive state. In a study by Heymsfield et al., patients who received rapid nutritional resuscitation showed more rapid correction of ventricular volume and cardiac output than left ventricular mass.[26] The combination of increased output, excessive retention of sodium and fluid, and altered metabolic demands may promote cardiac decompensation. Cardiac failure can lead to elevated systemic venous pressures with congestion of intestinal lymphatics, compromised nutrient absorption, and further deterioration in nutritional status.

D. GASTROINTESTINAL SYSTEM

Malnutrition can have a profound effect on intestinal mass and function. The delivery of nutrients into the gut lumen is a major stimulus for mucosal growth. Usually, the cells of the small and large colon are in a state of rapid turnover. Without enteral stimulus, as in total starvation or use of parenteral alimentation alone, intestinal epithelial cells atrophy, which leads to a decrease in intestinal mass, villus size, crypt size and number, mitotic index, and disaccharidase activity.[35] Surface epithelial cells become flattened, edematous, and infiltrated with lymphocytes, which contributes to the malabsorption of disaccharides, fats, and amino acids.[36,37] Refeeding results in a rapid return to prefasting architecture, absorptive capacity, and function.

E. HEPATIC AND PANCREATIC SYSTEMS

During periods of protein-calorie malnutrition, hepatic glycogen stores are rapidly depleted and fat deposits accumulate. As starvation progresses, fat is used as an energy source, the liver becomes smaller, and liver protein is lost, yet liver function tests are often completely normal.[38] In contrast, patients with primary protein malnutrition have enlarged, fatty livers due to triglyceride accumulation.[39,40] Transaminases are often normal or only mildly elevated in protein malnutrition. Albumin levels are usually less than 3.0 to 3.5 g/dl.

Prolonged starvation has been associated with diarrhea due to exocrine pancreatic insufficiency as well as GI malabsorption. Histology of pancreatic specimens shows evidence of fibrosis and acinar atrophy, with relative preservation of the islet cells.[23,40]

F. RENAL SYSTEM

Kidney function remains normal under most conditions of malnutrition. In some cases of severely prolonged nutritional deprivation, reduced glomerular filtration rate and renal plasma flow have been noted.[41] Urinalysis is usually unremarkable, without evidence of protein, casts, white cells, red cells, or abnormal sediment.[24] The specific gravity is often low, and a defect in concentrating ability is often present.[38]

G. HEMATOLOGIC SYSTEM

Hematologic abnormalities are seen in malnutrition and are related to the severity and duration of deprivation. Cellular abnormalities include thrompocytopenia, leukopenia, anemia, and acanthocyte formation. The anemia has the appearance of chronic disease with normocytic, normochromic indices, a normal iron level, and no evidence of significant reticulocytosis. Neutropenia can be present in the face of severe infection without shift to the left. The compromised immune system in severe malnutrition can blunt the appropriate hematologic response to infection.

H. IMMUNE SYSTEM

As previously discussed, marasmus can leave the immune mechanisms intact unless a severe stimulus converts isolated marasmus to a mixed malnutrition condition. The hallmark of kwashiorkor or immunorepressive malnutrition is the altered immune system. The effect of nutrition on the immune system will be covered in more detail in Chapter 5.

IV. REFEEDING SYNDROME

Refeeding syndrome is the cascade of physiologic and metabolic effects observed with depletion, repletion, and compartmental shifts of major electrolytes, fluids, and other substrates in response to excess nutritional resuscitation after prolonged starvation.[42] Originally it was believed that hypophosphatemia was the main etiologic agent involved in the refeeding syndrome. However, it now appears that hypokalemia, hypomagnesemia, and derangements in glucose control are also important. Alerting caretakers to the presence of nutritional deficiencies and the role of adequate supplementation underlies the importance of feeding the malnourished patient. Since overfeeding may precipitate serious consequences, an understanding of the hormonal changes of semi-starvation and the potential metabolic complications are important to understanding potentially life-threatening complications.

The Minnesota Experiment, a classic study by Keys et al. in the 1940s, studied the effects of food restriction and subsequent refeeding in previously healthy persons.[24] After 6 months the subjects showed no evidence of increased venous pressure, cardiac dilatation, or dyspnea. However, in the recovery period during refeeding, a marked decrease in cardiac reserve was noted, with some subjects developing congestive heart failure. These findings have been seen again in severely malnourished patients receiving excessive enteral and/or parenteral nutrition.

In addition to cardiac decompensation, paresthesias, seizures, myocardial infarction, and death have been attributed to overzealous nutritional resuscitation.[42] A chronically starved individual has achieved a new metabolic steady state, and sudden refeeding can represent a significant physiologic stressor. The nutritional status of the individual influences the body's metabolic response to injury. The balance between the severity of stress

TABLE 2
Avoiding the Refeeding Syndrome

1. Understand what refeeding syndrome is and the population it affects.
2. Monitor electrolytes prior to and after initiating oral, enteral, or parenteral nutrition support.
3. Vigorously replete any electrolyte deficiencies with special emphasis on potassium, phosphorous, and magnesium levels.
4. Maintain glucose control.
5. Monitor pulse rate, intake, and output carefully while judiciously restoring circulatory volume.
6. Assess caloric needs, ideally with a metabolic cart. Aim for *meeting* the measured needs first and then *slowly* increasing calories to assist in weight gain.
7. Administer vitamin and mineral supplements routinely.

and energy reserves determines whether malnutrition will present as marasmus, immunorepressive malnutrition, or mixed malnutrition.

Hormone and cytokine-induced changes are responsible for the acute phase response, which serves to limit injury and enhance healing.[43] The markers of injury include fever, leukocytosis, increase in acute phase reactive proteins, hypoalbuminemia, hyperglycemia, release of immature forms from the bone marrow, and possibly negative nitrogen balance.[2,3,21,44] Recognition of the major forms of malnutrition is important for the following reasons. First, in uncomplicated semi-starvation, mortality rates do not increase until weight loss exceeds 40%, but in the presence of injury, a 25% loss may be fatal. Second, in the well nourished, the metabolic response to injury is beneficial for 10 to 14 days, at which time the immune function becomes impaired.[2,17,45]

Refeeding with carbohydrate-containing compounds results in hyperinsulinemia. In the presence of a physiologic increase in insulin, sodium excretion falls. The increase in plasma aldosterone and ADH, which occurs during injury, further impairs sodium and water excretion in those patients who may already have fluid overload status due to cardiac, liver, or kidney disorders. In this situation, marasmic individuals may also experience refeeding edema.

Refeeding may lead to a drop in plasma phosphorous, potassium, and magnesium if supplementation is inadequate. The hypophosphatemia may be caused by depleted body stores, hyperinsulinemia, or anabolism. Potassium is stored almost entirely within lean tissue, and as muscle stores are depleted in protein-calorie malnutrition, it follows that potassium stores may also be depressed. Hyperinsulinemia can cause a fall in potassium by enhancing entry into the muscle and hepatic cells. Insulin increases the sodium permeability of skeletal muscle cells, and the increased cytosolic sodium concentration activates sodium-potassium dependent ATPase. As sodium is transported from the cell, the electronegativity generated promotes inward movement of potassium from the extracellular environment which leads to hypokalemia. Phosphorous plays an important role in intermediary metabolism. Insulin-stimulated glycolysis enhances cellular uptake and utilization of phosphorous which can lead to depressed serum levels. Magnesium also resides in lean tissues and with malnutrition or refeeding with inadequate supplementation, hypomagnesemia can develop. In 1975, Rudman et al. demonstrated in balance studies that nitrogen, sodium, potassium, phosphate, and magnesium must all be added to parenteral nutrition solutions to allow repletion of lean tissue and retention of trace minerals.[46]

Patients at particular risk for refeeding syndrome include the following: anorexia nervosa, classic marasmus or kwashiorkor, chronic alcoholism, morbid obesity with massive weight loss (usually postoperatively), and any patient who has not received nutrition for 7 to 10 days and has evidence of significant metabolic stress.[42] Nutritional support should be provided urgently to those who have lost 10 to 20% of their usual weight and are severely stressed and to those individuals who have lost more than 20% of their usual weight. If the gastrointestinal tract is functional, then it should be used for repletion.

Table 2 shows suggestions for avoiding the refeeding syndrome when initiating nutrition support.[42] It is important to monitor weight, fluid status, and serum electrolytes closely. A heart rate of 90 to 100 may be the harbinger of impending heart failure in a severely malnourished patient who previously was bradycardic. Electrocardiograms should be analyzed for characteristic changes of malnutrition including bradycardia, prolonged Q-Tc interval, depression in QRS voltage, and ST-T wave changes. A useful measure of the relative muscle mass is the creatinine-height index. Accurate recording of weights is essential, and an increase of greater than .50 lb in a 24-h period should be attributed to water weight. Edema formation may be minimized by restricting both total volume and sodium input for the first 2 to 3 days of refeeding. Electrolyte replacement should be guided by measurement of the urinary and gastrointestinal losses. Recall that depressed levels of zinc and iron may reflect sequestration rather than actual deficiency.

The caloric requirements of a well-nourished individual can be estimated by the Harris-Benedict Equation (HBE), which assumes that basal caloric requirements are related to body cell mass. This equation was formulated in 1919 using data from normal men and women.[47] The use of the HBE was discussed in Chapter 1, but it is important to note that malnourished patients have altered energy metabolism and using the HBE to determine the daily caloric needs may actually miscalculate requirements. Despite extreme stress, it is uncommon for individuals to require more than 40 kcal/kg/d. Relating resting energy to body weight is not appropriate for the malnourished because they do not have a normal body composition. A more general system of estimating values of caloric intake for individuals was derived by Jeejeebhoy.[48,49] This system assigned ranges of kcal/kg of ideal body weight to various clinical states. A normal weight person without stressors may require 25 to 30 kcal/kg/d to maintain a positive nitrogen balance. Additional stressors increase caloric requirements, yet despite extreme stress, individuals rarely require more than 40 kcal/kg/d. Delivery of calories in excess of the estimated requirements will not enhance healing. As discussed in the previous chapter, a metabolic cart determination, when available, is an ideal method of assessing the caloric requirements of this type of individual so that needs are not overestimated.

V. CONCLUSION

Categories of malnutrition have been established to define populations according to nutritional deficiencies and associated metabolic complications. The first category, marasmus, represents simple starvation. Marasmus is generally well tolerated unless a significant stressor occurs or if more than 40% of body weight is lost. Below 40% the body can no longer compensate adequately and mortality rises sharply.

The second category is immunorepressive (or hypoalbuminemic) malnutrition. This involves inadequate protein with sufficient caloric intake but is generally associated with a major stressor that causes a cascade of hormonal changes. As the name implies, the immune system may be severely compromised, while clinically a person may show few signs of overt deficiency.

Mixed malnutrition is the third major category and represents a combination of the preceding two. It is the most commonly seen form of malnutrition in a hospital setting. A careful nutritional assessment can identify an underlying nutritional disorder with acute metabolic compromise. Awareness of this co-morbid state may affect prognosis and enhance response to therapies over time.

Refeeding syndrome is a summation of the acute physiologic and metabolic effects in response to excess nutritional resuscitation in a chronically starved individual. Understanding hormonal, immunological, and biochemical responses to malnutrition can help avert complications during refeeding. Careful replenishment with evaluation of clinical response by frequent physical examinations with attention to fluid status and adequate laboratory assessment generally results in safe nutrition resuscitation.

Recognizing malnutrition and evaluating and implementing therapies can shorten hospital stays as well as reduce health care costs, enhance healing rates, help prevent co-morbidity, and avoid potential complications, such as refeeding syndrome. The assistance of a nutrition support team can be invaluable in assessment, following nutritional parameters, knowing regional and national resources, and arranging outpatient follow-up and education of the patient and the family. It is vital that medical staff intervene early in the malnourished population to effect a more positive outcome.

REFERENCES

1. **Foxx-Orenstein, A, Jensen, GL, and McMahon, MM.** Overzealous resuscitation of an extremely malnourished patient with nutritional cardiomyopathy. *Nutr Rev,* 48:406–11, 1990.
2. **McMahon, MM, and Bistrian, BR.** The physiology of nutritional assessment and therapy in protein-calorie malnutrition. *Dis Month,* 36:373–417, 1990.
3. **Love, AHG.** Metabolic response to malnutrition: its relevance to enteral feeding. *Gut,* 27(Suppl. 1): 9–13, 1986.
4. **Silberman, H.** Evaluation of nutritional status. In: *Parenteral and Enteral Nutrition,* 2nd ed., Silberman H, Ed., Appleton and Lange, 1989, 19.
5. **Bistrian, BR.** Nutritional assessment and therapy of protein-calorie malnutrition in the hospital. *J Am Diet Assoc,* 71:393–397, 1977.
6. **Viteri, FE, and Pineda, O.** Effects on body composition and body function, psychological effects, In *Famine, A Symposium Dealing with Nutrition and Relief Operations in Times of Disaster,* Blix, G, Hofvander, Y, and Vahlquist, B, Eds., Almqvist & Wiksells, Uppsala, Sweden, 1981, 25.
7. **Graham, GG.** Starvation in the modern world, *N Engl J Med,* 328, 1058–1060, 1993.
8. **Blackburn, GL, Bistrian BR, Maini, BS, et al.** Nutritional and metabolic assessment of the hospitalized patient. *JPEN,* 1:11–22, 1977.
9. **Gersovitz, M, Munro, HN, Udall, J, et al.** Albumin synthesis in young and elderly subjects using a new stable isotope methodology: response to level of protein intake. *Metabolism,* 29:1075–1086, 1980.
10. **Beutler, B, and Cerami, A.** Cachectin: more than tumor necrosis factor. *N Engl J Med,* 316:379–385, 1987.
11. **Aggarwal, BB, Kohr, WJ, Hass, PE, et al.** Human tumor necrosis factor: production, purification and characterization. *J Biol Chem,* 260:2345–2354, 1985.
12. **Long, CL, and Lowry, SF.** Hormonal regulation of protein metabolism. *JPEN,* 14:555–562, 1990.
13. **Fong, Y, Moldawer, LL, Shires, T, et al.** The biological characteristics of cytokines and their implication in surgical injury. *Surg Gynecol Obstet,* 170:363–378, 1990.
14. **Dinarello, CA.** Biology of interleukin-1. *FASEB J,* 2:108–115, 1988.
15. **Oomura, Y.** Chemical and neuronal control of feeding motivation. *Physiol Behav,* 44:555–560, 1988.
16. **Walter, JS, Meyers, P, and Krueger, JM.** Microinjection of interleukin-1 into the brain: separation of sleep and fever responses. *Physiol Behav,* 45:169–176, 1989.
17. **Hardin, T.** Cytokine mediators of malnutrition: clinical implications. *Nutr Clin Pract,* 8:55–59, 1993.
18. **Watson, ML, Lewis, GP, and Westwick, J.** Increased vascular permeability and polymorphonuclear leukocyte accumulation in vivo response to recombinant cytokines and supernatant from cultures of human synovial cells treated with interleukin-1. *Br J Exp Pathol,* 70:93–101, 1989.
19. **Price, SR, Mizel, SB, and Pekald, PH.** Regulation of lipoprotein lipase synthesis and 3T3-L1 adopocyte metabolism by recombinant interleukin. *J Biochem Biophys Acta,* 374–81, 1986.
20. **Grunfeld, C, Verdier, JA, Neese, R, et al.** Mechanisms by which tumor necrosis factor stimulates hepatic fatty acid synthesis. *J Lipid Res,* 29:1327–1335, 1988.
21. **Bistrian, BR.** Nutritional assessment in the hospitalized patient: a practical approach, In *Nutritional Assessment.* Wright, RA, and Heymsfield, S, Eds., Blackwell Scientific Publications, Boston, 1984, 183.
22. **Bistrian, BR, Blackburn, GL, Vitale, J, et al.** Prevalence of malnutrition in general medical patients. *JAMA,* 235:1567–1570, 1976.
23. **Windsor, JA, and Hill, GL.** Risk factors for postoperative pneumonia: the importance of protein depletion. *Ann Surg,* 208:209–214, 1988.

24. **Keys, A, Brozek, J, Henshel, A, et al.** *The Biology of Human Starvation. Vol. 1 & 2, University of Minnesota Press, Minneapolis, 1950.*

25. **Sheldon, GF, and Peterson, SR.** Malnutrition and cardiopulmonary function: relation to oxygen transport. *JPEN,* 4:376–383, 1980.

26. **Heymsfield, SB, Bethel, RA, Ansley, JD, et al.** Cardiac abnormalities in cachetic patients before and during nutritional repletion. *Am Heart J,* 95:584–594 1978.

27. **Chauhan, S, Nayak, NC, and Ramalengswami, V.** The heart and skeletal muscle in experimental protein malnutrition in rhesus monkeys. *J Pathol Bacteriol,* 90:301–309, 1969.

28. **Wharton, BA, Balmer, SE, Somers, K, and Templeton, AC.** The myocardium in kwashiorkor. *Q J Med,* 38:7–16, 1969.

29. **Keys, A, Henshel, A, and Taylor, HL.** The size and function of the human heart at rest in semi-starvation and in subsequent rehabilitation. *Am J Physiol,* 150:153–169, 1947.

30. **Garnett, ES, Barnard, DL, Ford, J, et al.** Gross fragmentation of cardiac myofibrils after therapeutic starvation for obesity. *Lancet,* 1:914–916, 1969.

31. **Sonis, HE, Fratelli, VP, Brand, CD, et al.** Sudden death associated with very low caloric weight reduction regimens. *Am J Clin Nutr,* 34:453–461, 1981.

32. **Isner, JM, Roberts, WC, Heymsfield, SB, and Yojer, J.** Anorexia nervosa and sudden death. *Ann Intern Med,* 102:49–52, 1985.

33. **Ellis, LB.** Electrocardiographic abnormalities in severe malnutrition. *Br Heart J,* 8:53–63, 1946.

34. **Schocken, DD, Holloway, JD, and Powers, PS.** Weight loss and the heart: effects of anorexia nervosa and starvation. *Arch Intern Med,* 149:877–881, 1989.

35. **Levine, GM, Deren, JJ, Steiger, E, and Zinno, R.** Role of oral nitrate in maintenance of gut mass and disaccharide activity. *Gastroenterology,* 67:975–982, 1974.

36. **Maxton, DG, Menzies, IS, Slavin, B, and Thompson, RP.** Small intestinal function during enteral feeding and starvation in man. *Clin Sci,* 77:401–406, 1989.

37. **Herskovic, T.** Protein malnutrition and the small intestine. *Am J Clin Nutr,* 22:300–4, 1969.

38. **Levenson, SM, Crowley, LV, and Seifter, E.** Starvation, In *Manual of Surgical Nutrition,* Bullinger, WF, Collins, JA, and Drucker, WR, et al., Eds, W.B. Saunders, Philadelphia, 1975, 236–264.

39. **Blanchard, J, Steiger, E, O'Neil, M, et al.** Effect of protein depletion and repletion on liver structures, nitrogen content and serum proteins. *Ann Surg,* 190:144–150, 1979.

40. **Madi, K, Jervis, HR, Anderson, PR, and Zimmerman, MR.** A protein deficient diet: effect on liver, pancreas, stomach and small intestine of the rat. *Arch Pathol,* 89:38–52, 1970.

41. **Ichikawa, I, Purkerson, ML, Klahr, S, et al.** Mechanism of reduced glomerular filtration rate in chronic malnutrition. *J Clin Invest,* 65:982–988, 1980.

42. **Solomon, SM, and Kirby, DF.** The refeeding syndrome: a review. *JPEN,* 14:90–97, 1990.

43. **Long, CL, and Lowry, SF.** Hormonal regulation of protein metabolism. *JPEN,* 14:555–562, 1990.

44. **Apovian, CM, McMahon, MM, and Bistran, BR.** Guidelines for refeeding the marasmic patient. *Crit Care Med,* 18:1030–1033, 1990.

45. **Nimmanwudipong, T, Cheadle, WG, Appel, SH, and Polk, HC.** Effect of protein malnutrition and immunomodulation on immune cell populations. *J Surg Res,* 52:233–238, 1992.

46. **Rudman, D, Millikan, WJ, Richardson, TJ, et al.** Elemental balances during intravenous hyperalimentation of underweight adult subject. *J Clin Invest,* 55:94–104, 1975.

47. **Harris, JA, and Benedict, FG.** A biometric study of basal metabolism in man. Carnegie Institution of Washington, Washington, DC, publication no. 279, 1919.

48. **Jeejeebhoy, KN.** Total parenteral nutrition. *Ann R Coll Phys Surg Can,* 9:287–300, 1976.

49. **Lemoyne, M, and Jeejeebhoy, KN.** Total parenteral nutrition in the acutely ill patient. *Chest,* 89: 568–575, 1986.

50. **Goldblaum, SEA, Cohen, DA, Jay, M, et al.** Interleukin-1 induced depression of iron and zinc: role of granulocytes and lactoferrin. *Am J Physiol,* 252: E27–32, 1987.

Chapter 3

OVERNUTRITION AND OBESITY MANAGEMENT

Caroline M. Apovian and Gordon L. Jensen

TABLE OF CONTENTS

0-8493-7847-8/94/$0.00+$.50
© 1994 by CRC Press, Inc.

I. INTRODUCTION

Obesity, defined as body weight 20% or more above ideal body weight, affects about 26% of adults in the U.S., making it a national health problem. In addition, approximately 5% of men and 7% of women in the U.S. meet the criteria for morbid obesity, which is defined as body weight in excess of 100% or more greater than ideal.[1]

Obesity is a disease that is associated with profound medical morbidities as well as psychological and social afflictions. The co-morbid diseases associated with obesity (Table 1)[2] probably account for the increased mortality observed as body weight increases beyond the mean.

The psychological and social problems associated with obesity can be devastating as well. Factors that may contribute to overeating include impulsive or compulsive behaviors, depression, anxiety, ready availability of calorically dense foods, and sedentary lifestyle. These contributing factors combined with discrimination the obese suffer in our society can create a "vicious cycle" that is difficult to overcome. Evidence suggests that the etiology of obesity is multifactorial and that some of the origins are inherited, environmental, socioeconomic, and psychological. Obesity is not simply caused by lack of willpower, but is a complex disorder of appetite regulation and energy metabolism.[3]

Although the problems associated with increased body weight are well recognized, obesity is notoriously difficult to treat. Many persons have a chronic tendency to become overweight, which requires lifelong attention. Recidivism is high and may also contribute to morbidity.

Analysis of data from the Framingham study has shown that persons whose body weight fluctuates frequently or greatly (yo-yo dieting) have a higher risk of coronary heart disease and a higher risk of mortality than do persons with stable body weights.[4] The basis of this association is not known, but it has been suggested that large and rapid weight gain after a weight loss regimen could cause peaks in serum cholesterol concentration that could accelerate atherogenesis.[5] There have also been suggestions that "yo-yo" dieting causes a permanent loss of lean body mass because regained weight is primarily fat. A recent study of "yo-yo" dieting, however, revealed no evidence of an excessive loss of lean tissue in moderately obese women who underwent three cycles of weight loss and relapse.[6]

This chapter will examine the causes of obesity, the medical consequences of obesity, the medical and surgical options currently available for treatment of moderate to morbid obesity, and the factors common to successful weight loss therapy.

II. DEFINITIONS AND ASSESSMENT

Obesity and overweight are often used interchangeably; however, they are not synonymous. Overweight is defined as body weight above a standard defined in relation to height. It may not reflect an increase in body fat. Obesity is defined as an increase in body adipose tissue. In men, the normal percentage of body fat is between 15 and 22%, and in women between 18 and 32%. Obesity is defined as body fat greater than 22% for young men less than 35 years of age and greater than 25% for older men greater than 35 years; in women these numbers are 32% and 35%, respectively.[7]

Overweight has been defined traditionally in relation to desirable weight for height as determined by the Metropolitan Life Insurance Company tables.[8] More recently, overweight has been defined in relation to data from the second National Health and Nutrition Examination Survey (NHANES II)[9] conducted between 1976 and 1980. Body mass index (BMI), the ratio of body weight in kilograms to height in meters squared, was utilized as a measure (Table 2).[10] Overweight is defined as BMI greater than or equal to the 85th

TABLE 1
Medical Complications Associated with Obesity

Gastrointestinal
    Cholecystitis
    Cholelithiasis
    Hepatic steatosis
    Delayed orocecal transit time
Endocrine/reproductive
    Type II diabetes mellitus
    Hirsutism
    Dyslipidemias
    Menstrual disorders
    Preeclampsia
    Endometrial disorders
Respiratory
    Sleep apnea
    Obesity hypoventilation syndrome
    Erythrocytosis
    Respiratory tract infections
Cardiovascular
    Coronary artery disease
    Congestive heart failure
    Systemic hypertension
Malignancy
    Colon
    Prostate
    Endometrium
    Gallbladder
    Cervical
    Ovarian
Musculoskeletal
    Osteoarthritis
    Gout

percentile. The cut-off points for BMIs at the 85th percentile for 20- to 29-year-old men and women were 27.8 and 27.3 kg/m^2, respectively. Severely overweight was defined as BMI at or above the 95th percentile, which was 31.1 for men and 32.3 kg/m^2 for women. Morbidly obese was defined as BMI greater than or equal to 39.0 kg/m^2.[11] The BMI is gaining popularity as a reference standard because of its practicality, and it is more highly correlated with total body fat than other indices of height and weight.[10] More sophisticated techniques are described below.

III. TECHNIQUES OF OBESITY ASSESSMENT: ANTHROPOMETRY

There are a number of methods in which body fat can be measured. Anthropometric measures are the most widely used for office assessment. Height and weight are easily obtained and are used to assess BMI. There are height and weight nomograms available for BMI that obviate the need for calculation as well. Circumferences are popular because of the tendency for abdominal obesity to be a stronger predictor of medical risk than other parameters. The waist to hip circumference ratio evaluates the tendency to deposit fat on the abdomen. Skinfold assessment is more poorly correlated with fat mass than weight, height, BMI, and circumferences. Skinfolds can be obtained by caliper measurements of the trunk and extremities. The ratio of skinfolds on the trunk to those on the extremities

TABLE 2
Clinical Use of the Body Mass Index (BMI)

Definitions:

$$BMI = \frac{\text{Weight in kilograms}}{(\text{Height in meters})^2}$$

Obesity is defined as BMI >27.8 (men) and >27.3 (women). If risk factors such as heart disease, hypertension, diabetes, or elevated serum cholesterol are present, then intervention may be warranted for BMI between 23 and 27.

Example 1: A 30-year-old asymptomatic woman desires weight loss. Weight 48 kg, height 157 cm, small frame.

$$BMI = \frac{48}{(1.57 \text{ m})^2} = 19.5 \text{ kg/m}^2$$

The patient is at ideal body weight and is not an appropriate candidate for weight loss.

Example 2: A 43-year-old man presents with hypertension and adult-onset diabetes mellitus. Weight 100.5 kg, height 183 cm, large frame.

$$BMI = \frac{100.5 \text{ kg}}{(1.83 \text{ m})^2} = 30 \text{ kg/m}^2$$

The patient is obese and should be considered for a weight reduction diet.

can be used to assess regional fat distribution. However, these measurements require the availability of trained operators. Also, there are high interobserver variations and limited reference standards available. Nonetheless, skinfolds remain an easily obtainable estimate of body fat.[12,13]

IV. INSTRUMENTAL METHODS

Precise assessment of body fat requires the use of instrumental techniques not readily available in a physician's office. The "gold standard" of body composition measurements is underwater weighing to determine body density, by which weight under water and out of water is used to calculate density, which is then converted into body fat and fat-free mass using the Siri equation.[14] Other methods, including dual photon absorptiometry (DPA) and dual energy X-ray absorptiometry (DEXA), are also reliable. These instruments provide estimates of a three-compartment model of fat, lean mineral mass, and bone mineral.[12,15] Bioelectrical impedance analysis can also provide estimates of body water and fat contents. Isotope dilution can be used as another method of obtaining a two-compartment model of body composition. Total body water and body potassium are measured with stable isotopes. The most accurate assessment of visceral fat is currently obtained by computed tomography or nuclear magnetic resonance at the level of L4 to L5. Ultrasound may also be useful for subcutaneous fat thickness and visceral fat estimation.[12]

V. CLASSIFICATION OF OBESITY

There are three anatomic methods to classify obesity in current use (Table 3).[13] The first is classification according to size and number of fat cells. Hypertrophic obesity refers to enlarged fat cells, and hyperplastic obesity refers to an increased number of cells. This classification is useful in defining obesity in a temporal manner. When one overeats, fat cells grow larger. At a certain point, the formation of new fat cells is initiated, and these

TABLE 3
Classification of Obesity

Anatomic Methods
    Size and number of adipocytes—hypertrophic, hyperplastic
    Percent body fat
    Distribution of body fat—gynoid, android
Etiologic Methods
    Neuroendocrine disorders
    Excessive dietary intake
    Obesity syndromes
    Pharmacologic agents

cells are permanent. In weight loss, fat cells size decreases, but the number remains the same. The second method with which to classify obesity is based on total amount of body fat, as determined using methods of body composition assessment outlined above. The third classification involves distribution of body fat. Adipose tissue forms in a predominantly peripheral (gynoid) fashion or in a predominantly central (android) fashion on the human body. This classification has become increasingly important as studies continue to show that, in both men and women, a central or android body fat distribution conveys an increased risk of morbidity and mortality over a peripheral fat distribution pattern.[7,13]

VI. ETIOLOGY AND PATHOPHYSIOLOGY OF OBESITY

Etiologic factors provide another way of classifying obesity. There are four etiologic groups that can be identified.[13] The first group encompasses the neuroendocrine disorders including injury to the hypothalamus, Cushing's syndrome, polycystic ovary syndrome, and gonadal failure. In these syndromes, a defect in energy metabolism is generally found. The second group includes dietary intake in excess of metabolic needs. While overeating and sedentary life-style favor positive energy balance and obesity, genetic factors do seem to play a significant role in the development of weight excess. Studies with monozygotic twins have suggested that resting metabolic rage, thermogenesis, energy storage, and energy expenditure and BMI may have significant genetic components.[16] The third group are the characterized syndromes of obesity including Prader-Willi syndrome, the Cohen syndrome, the Carpenter syndrome, and the Bardet-Biedl syndrome, which are all rare (Appendix I).[17] The fourth etiologic group includes drugs which cause obesity. These drugs encompass the phenothiazines, antidepressants, antiepileptics, steroids, and certain antihypertensives.

VII. MEDICAL CONSEQUENCES OF OBESITY

It is clear that the prevalence of morbidity and premature mortality among those with morbid obesity ($\geq 100\%$ ideal body weight) is substantial. However, most medical complications of obesity manifest at considerably lower degrees of overweight than that of morbid obesity, and their prevalences are correlated with body weight. The most important health risks of obesity, namely diabetes, hypertension, coronary artery disease, cancer, and sudden death, are curvilinearly related to overweight. Their prevalence increase progressively and disproportionately with increasing weight.[18] Although obesity is associated with many risk factors for diseases, the mechanisms are not as yet fully understood. Perhaps, weight excess produces clinical disease only in those who harbor a defective gene mechanism. The major complications associated with obesity are discussed later.

VIII. DIGESTIVE DISEASES

A. CHOLELITHIASIS

A strong association between obesity and gallbladder disease has been documented in many studies. The incidence of gallbladder disease is three to four times as great in obese as in non-obese individuals. Also, gallbladder disease increases in prevalence with greater age and weight excess. There is a full threefold rise in the morbidly obese.[18,19]

The most probable explanation for the increased risk of gallbladder disease is increased cholesterol production and secretion. It has been found that about 20 mg/d of cholesterol is produced for each additional kilogram of adipose tissue. Bennion and Grundy, in a study of obese persons, have found that bile was more saturated with cholesterol in the obese as compared to non-obese controls.[20]

There have been reports of increased bile saturation and gallstone formation in obese individuals who have participated in aggressive weight reduction plans, such as liquid fasts and extremely low-calorie diets. Also with weight reduction, there is a reduction in bile secretion, causing more lithogenic bile.[21] This is a particular problem for those obese patients who go through frequent episodes of weight loss and regain.

B. HEPATIC STEATOSIS

Steatosis occurs in 68 to 94% of obese patients. Fatty infiltration of more than one half of the hepatocytes occurs in 25 to 35%. This is not usually accompanied, however, by elevations of liver function tests.[18] There are reports in the literature of obese individuals with steatosis accompanied by hepatic necrosis with Mallory bodies (steatohepatitis) and progression to cirrhosis. A study of 351 patients at autopsy found steatohepatitis in 18.5% of obese patients and 2.7% of lean patients. An abnormality in free fatty acid metabolism was postulated because there was a trend toward increased prevalence of steatohepatitis among type II diabetes requiring insulin. It is known that insulin inhibits fatty acid oxidation, which may lead to increased cellular levels of toxic free fatty acids. Obese individuals have abundant fatty acid stores in adipose tissue, and they are insulin resistant as well. These factors, combined with diabetes, cause further insulin resistance with elevation of plasma insulin levels, thus favoring free fatty acid accumulation in hepatocytes.[22]

C. DIABETES MELLITUS

The association of obesity and type II diabetes mellitus (NIDDM) has been known for many years. The NHANES II data revealed that the relative risk of developing diabetes was 2.9 times greater for obese persons 20 to 75 years of age. The relative risk for those 2 to 45 years was 3.8, and that for the 45- to 75-year-old group was 2.1 The risk of diabetes also increases with greater waist-hip ratio or android obesity. Also, 70 to 80% of NIDDM patients are obese, and about 40 to 60% of obese individuals eventually develop NIDDM.[23]

The potential pathophysiology of this association bears mention. Most feel that there is a genetic predisposition to NIDDM and that the overnutrition of obesity is enough to precipitate overt diabetes. Obese individuals exhibit insulin resistance, which is common in NIDDM. The insulin resistance could be due to high levels of free fatty acids in the obese state, which are used by muscle at the expense of glucose. This is called the Randle effect. Alternately, overnutrition may cause peripheral insulin resistance and downregulate peripheral insulin receptors, promoting insulin resistance.[23]

D. PULMONARY FUNCTION

It is well established that obesity alters respiratory function. Altered chest wall mechanics may lead to restrictive impairment. Usually seen are a decreased functional residual capacity (FRC) and expiratory reserve volume (ERV), probably the result of splinting of the diaphragm.[24] Oxygen consumption ($\dot{V}O_2$) is increased during passive ventilation because of the extra work required to move the obese chest wall.[18,24] Ventilation-perfusion mismatch is a common finding in gas-exchange determinations of the morbidly obese patient. This leads to variable decreases in arterial oxygenation, worse in the supine position.[18,24,25]

In patients with morbid obesity, a severe respiratory insufficiency may develop, commonly known as the Pickwickian syndrome. This syndrome encompasses two primary breathing disorders, which can occur alone or in combination: obstructive sleep apnea syndrome and obesity hypoventilation syndrome. There are two types of sleep apnea, central and obstructive. Central apnea is associated with the transient impairment of neural signals from the central nervous system to the lung musculature during sleep. Obstructive sleep apnea occurs when the tongue obstructs the glottis during sleep, preventing air from entering the trachea. Only 5% of sleep apnea patients have Pickwickian syndrome; however, the symptoms of Pickwickian syndrome are largely due to sleep apnea.[26] The end result is severe hypoxemia during sleep, which can often produce periodic respirations called Cheyne-Stokes breathing. This interferes with Stage III, IV, and REM sleep and can produce severe daytime somnolence.[27]

Obesity hypoventilation syndrome is associated with hypoxemia and hypercarbia while awake and is due to decreased lung volumes probably from an elevated diaphragm and heavy chest wall. Obesity hypoventilation syndrome often leads to cardiac dysfunction with either right or biventricular failure.[28] Arterial blood gases often show an arterial oxygen tension (PaO_2) ≤55 mmHg and/or a $PaCO_2$ ≥47 mmHg.[29]

Pickwickian syndrome can become a medical emergency, sometimes requiring tracheostomy. In less acute settings, progestational agents may help. Studies have shown that arterial pCO_2 will return to normal in 90% of cases after treatment with 20 mg/d medroxyprogesterone.[30] A tricyclic antidepressant, protriptyline, has also been shown to reduce the number and duration of apneic episodes in these patients.[31] More recently, moderate weight loss from very low calorie diets has been shown to improve oxygenation and sleep apnea in obese subjects. The amount of improvement is, however, highly variable. The mechanism of improvement after modest weight loss is unknown, but most likely results from an increase in airway size or from changes in ventilatory drive which increase upper airway muscle activity.[32]

Gastric surgery-induced weight loss has also been shown to be beneficial in reducing the respiratory insufficiency of morbidly obese patients.[29,33,34] Although patients with Pickwickian syndrome have a higher operative risk than patients without pulmonary dysfunction, weight loss after gastric bypass is associated with improvements in arterial blood gases, lung volumes, polycythemia, cardiac dysfunction, and sleep apnea.[29]

E. CARDIOVASCULAR DISEASE

The prevalence of cardiovascular disease may be related to the presence of hypertension (HTN) and elevated blood lipids. Obese persons are more likely to be hypertensive than the non-obese, and 30 to 50% of hypertension in the U.S. is attributed to obesity. The obesity related risk for HTN decreases with age. In adults 20 to 45 years of age, obesity adds a four- to sixfold increase in HTN risk; and in people 45 to 75 years of age, the risk is doubled with obesity. NHANES II showed that the link between BMI and HTN rises in the 25 to 54-year-old age group and drops in the 65 to 74-year-old age group. Obesity exerts greater effect on risk for HTN in whites than in blacks, although HTN is more prevalent in the black population.[1]

Blood lipids are generally elevated in obese patients. According to NHANES II, the relative risk of hypercholesterolemia is 1.5 times greater in obese than in lean patients. If the data is broken down into two age groups, the younger group (20 to 45 years) has a relative risk of 2.1, and the older group (45 to 75 years) has no elevated risk of hypercholesterolemia. HDL concentrations are lower in obese individuals, and low HDL concentrations are a risk for coronary artery disease, independent of LDL cholesterol concentration.[1]

Despite the well-established association between obesity and unfavorable coronary risk factors (elevated blood lipids, HTN, and diabetes), the influence of weight excess independently on the risk of CAD still remains controversial. It seems plausible that there should be a link between obesity and atherogenic heart disease. Studies that have been done conflict, but the majority of evidence suggests that obesity is indeed an independent, long-term risk factor for cardiovascular disease. Obese individuals are at even greater risk when other factors are present, namely HTN, elevated LDL cholesterol, decreased HDL cholesterol, diabetes mellitus, and elevated serum triglycerides.

The Framingham study and the Los Angeles Heart Study found a stronger independent link between adiposity and cardiovascular disease in men in more recent reports than in their earlier studies. It may be that body weight is a long-term independent risk factor for cardiovascular disease which requires time to develop a threshold amount of atherosclerosis to manifest an effect.[35,36]

In a prospective study of 115,886 women, Manson et al. found a strong association between obesity and coronary disease. Controlling for HTN, diabetes and elevated blood lipids reduced the magnitude of the association; however, obesity retained a moderate residual effect. The researchers postulated that obesity may increase coronary risk by an additional mechanism as yet undocumented. Postulated mechanisms included increased intravascular volume and cardiac workload as well as altered fibrinogen levels and fibrinolytic activity.[37]

An increase in body weight in adulthood may be more important than obesity in early adulthood in determination of risk for cardiovascular disease. Heyden et al. and Abraham et al. have suggested that the presence of cardiovascular disease and HTN is greater in those who have become overweight as adults than in those who have been overweight since childhood.[38,39]

F. REGIONAL FAT DISTRIBUTION

Body fat distribution in relation to morbidity and mortality has been studied by numerous researchers. Individuals with upper body obesity, as assessed by the waist-to-hip ratio (WHR), are at greater risk for developing diabetes mellitus, cardiovascular disease, and breast, ovarian, and endometrial carcinomas. The etiology seems to be both genetic and environmental. Smoking, lack of exercise, and stress are factors associated with upper body fat distribution. Upper body obesity is also associated with overall body weight. Efforts to reduce weight may also reduce WHR with presumed risk benefit.[25,40–42]

Because excess upper body fat and especially visceral fat are most highly correlated with the metabolic complications of obesity, there has been interest in the regional metabolism of adipocytes. Preliminary studies suggest that upper body adipose cells seem to have a higher rate of lipolysis than lower body fat cells. This causes an excess of free fatty acid availability which, in turn, would impair metabolism of glucose and insulin in the liver, contributing to the development of diabetes mellitus. In addition, increased VLDL production by the liver would contribute to hyperlipoproteinemia and ischemic heart disease.[43]

G. CANCER

A study of 750,000 men and women followed for 12 years found a significant relationship between obesity and cancer.[44] It was found that the mortality ratio for cancer in men who were ≥40% obese was 1.33 and for women 1.55. Obese men had significantly higher mortality ratios for colorectal and prostate cancers, and obese women had high rates of endometrial, gallbladder, cervical, ovarian, and breast cancers. There is some evidence in the literature that relates certain dietary factors to cancer. One theory is that overnutrition, regardless of type of diet, promotes tumor growth. It has been noted that breast cancer patients are more overweight than the general population,[45] and studies have revealed that there is a correlation between increased body weight and decreased disease-free interval and decreased overall survival in breast cancer. A study of over 8000 breast cancer patients found that women who were in the highest percentile of body mass had a death rate 1.7 times higher than women in the lowest percentile of body mass.[46] Another study evaluating both body weight and cholesterol levels in breast cancer patients found that the shortest 5-year disease-free survival was found in patients of higher weight (>68 kg) or with higher serum cholesterol levels (above the median). The combination of elevated weight and cholesterol was associated with an extremely poor 5-year disease-free survival (32%) compared with that observed for those in whom either or both values were low (68%).[47] The typical American diet, high in fat, low in carbohydrates and fiber, has been implicated in increasing breast tumor size and altering hormone receptor content as a possible explanation for the association between overweight and breast cancer.[48]

It has been noticed that breast cancer patients on adjuvant chemotherapy, including tamoxifen, frequently gain weight. Chlebowski reviewed 10 such reports and noted an increased tendency to disease relapse in patients who gained substantial amounts of weight during adjuvant therapy.[49] Thus, for breast cancer, being overweight at onset and weight gain during adjuvant treatments have been found to be adverse prognostic factors. Trials testing the postulate that weight loss might improve treatment results and survival are now in progress. Specific components of diet have been implicated in the association of overnutrition with cancer, specifically protein, total fat, and polyunsaturated fatty acids. Studies have associated these factors with cancer in laboratory animals, but whether or not these are punitive dietary factors in humans remains to be determined.[23]

H. DESTRUCTIVE JOINT DISEASE (OSTEOARTHRITIS)

Data from the Framingham study covering a 35-year period demonstrates that both men and women in the highest percentile of body mass had increased risk for osteoarthritis of the knees. Several other studies have shown an increased prevalence of osteoarthritis with obesity.[18] The knee seems to be the most frequently involved joint, most likely due to its weight-bearing function.

I. GOUT

Obesity is also associated with an increased risk of gout. Rimm et al.[49] found that the relative risk for obese women is 2.56. In the Framingham study, there was a significant correlation between uric acid concentrations and weight,[50] and gout was found to be more common in the obese.[18]

TABLE 4
Contraindications for Very Low-Energy Diets

Recent myocardial infarction
Unstable angina
Malignant arrhythmias
Cerebrovascular disease
Serious underlying disease—malignancy, liver or renal failure
Type I diabetes mellitus
Pregnancy
Certain drug therapies[a]—steroids, antineoplastics
Untreated metabolic cause of obesity
Hypothyroidism and other disorders
Cosmetic motivation—body weight less than 20% above ideal

[a] Medications such as insulin, oral hypoglycemics, and antihypertensives must be carefully monitored and often tapered
for patients enrolled in very low-energy diets.

IX. OBESITY: MEDICAL THERAPY

The treatment of obesity is very difficult, with a resultant high recidivism rate. Very low calorie diets (VLCDs) became popular in the 1970s because of the modest weight loss usually observed with conventional hypocaloric diets. Because VLCDs are severely limited in energy (1675 to 3350 kJ/d or 400 to 800 kcal/d), a large caloric deficit results in weight losses of 18 to 22 kg in 12 to 15 weeks and 30 to 35 kg in 25 weeks. Now that the formulas contain high-quality protein and the necessary vitamins and minerals, they are relatively safe.

Only moderate and severely obese patients should be placed on these diets because obese persons can protect their lean body mass much better than leaner persons. Obese persons lose predominantly fat, while leaner persons lose predominately lean body mass. Thus, some researchers feel that VLCDs should be contraindicated for anyone less than 40% overweight or at a BMI ≤30.[52] Other contraindications are summarized in Table 4.[10]

The medical management of patients on VLCDs requires knowledge of the physiology of starvation. Alternative sources of energy are utilized for preservation of brain activity, and, thus, ketone bodies are used from lipolysis of fat stores and glucose from gluconeogenesis.[53] It is necessary to ensure adequate protein intake so that lean muscle mass, cardiac muscle contractility, hair growth, and immune system function are maintained. Ketone body production causes an osmotic diuresis which may lead to dehydration, electrolyte disturbances, and loss of water-soluble vitamins and trace minerals. Therefore, a very low calorie diet plan requires the supplementation of high biologic quality protein, vitamins, minerals, and water. Medical supervision should include weekly clinic visits with monitoring of serum electrolytes, magnesium, calcium, phosphate, and urine samples for ketones. Blood pressure and cardiac function should be assessed. Medications, such as insulin, oral hypoglycemic agents, and antihypertensives, need to be adjusted as weight loss progresses. The complications of VLCDs are summarized in Table 5.[54] One of the more publicized complications of severely restricted diets has been increased incidence of cholecystitis, presumably by enhanced crystallization of cholesterol stones. Obese patients are at greater baseline risk of developing gallstones and cholecystitis, even without VLCD. An obese patient who has a history of gallstones or cholecystitis should be considered to have a relative contraindication to VLCD.[52]

TABLE 5
Complications of Very Low-Calorie Diets

Cardiovascular
    Postural hypotension, arrhythmias, myocardial atrophy, cardiomyopathy, sudden death
Gastrointestinal
    Constipation, diarrhea, abdominal discomfort, biliary stasis, cholelithiasis/cholecystitis
Genitourinary
    Menstrual abnormalities, uric acid nephrolithiasis, loss of libido
Other
    General malaise, fatigue, cold sensitivity, xerosis, hair loss, halitosis, hunger, loss of lean body mass,
        vitamin and mineral deficiencies, electrolyte derangements, acute gout, cramps, paresthesias

Two kinds of VLCDs are widely used in a medical setting. The protein-sparing modified fast (PSMF) provides 1.5 g/kg of ideal body weight as lean meat, fish, or poultry. Fat and carbohydrate sources are largely eliminated. At least 1500 ml of water is required per day, and vitamin, calcium, magnesium, and potassium supplements are provided daily. In recent years, liquid formula diets have gained popularity. They contain 33 to 70 g protein, 30 to 45 g carbohydrate, and 1 to 2 g fat. In semistarvation, there is a protein-sparing effect with the small amounts of glucose found in the liquid diet preparations. As in the PSMF, vitamin supplements and water are required daily. Weight loss is dramatic and substantial with either approach, but the gradual reintroduction of food over several weeks may produce greater recidivism with the liquid diets. This is expected since subsistence on a liquid preparation does not provide an opportunity for the patient to alter fundamental eating and life-style behaviors to ensure that weight loss remains permanent. Therefore, a strong weight maintenance program should be continued for 6 to 12 months after the patient is off any VLCD. Limited follow-up has been one of the failures of many VLCD programs. Many patients regain 50% or more of lost weight in the year following treatment.[55] Success in VLCD programs demands a multidisciplinary approach, and physicians prescribing VLCDs should have a thorough training in clinical nutrition.[56]

X. EXERCISE

It seems that neither diet nor exercise alone is effective in the treatment of obesity.[57] Limited studies show, however, that although VLCDs can preserve physical function over major weight loss, long-term maintenance of weight loss is favorably influenced by a regular exercise regimen beyond the post-diet period. In fact, continued exercise was the best predictor of long-term weight loss maintenance in a study of 35 moderately obese males.[58] Exercise has beneficial effects independent of weight loss, and these include increased high-density lipoprotein cholesterol and an increase in lean body mass.[3]

XI. BEHAVIOR MODIFICATION

Behavior modification techniques are often used in conjunction with dietary weight loss programs. The goal of behavior modification is to modify eating and physical activity habits to patterns that induce or maintain weight loss. When used alone, behavior modification programs available are typically 18 weeks long, and patients usually lose 1 to 15 pounds per week. However, follow-up studies show that most of the weight is regained in 1 to 5 years. Studies suggest that better long-term weight loss can be achieved with intensive behavioral programs involving long-term ongoing care combined with structured diet and exercise interventions.[3,59]

TABLE 6
Anorectic Drugs

Generic name	Trade name	Schedule
Noradrenergic		
Phenylpropanolamine	Dexatrim®	Over-the-counter
Diethylpropion	Tenuate®, Propion	IV
Mazindol	Sanorex®, Mazanor®	IV
Phentermine	Ionamin®, Adipex-P®	IV
Phendimetrazine	Plegine®, Bontril®, Prelu-2®	III
Benzphetamine	Didrex®	III
Amphetamine	Dexedrine®	II
Methamphetamine	Desoxyn®	II
Serotonergic		
Fluoxetine	Prozac®[a]	Not a controlled substance
d-Fenfluramine	Pondimin®	IV

[a] Not FDA-approved as an anorectic drug at the time of this publication.

From Silverstone, T. and Goodall, E. *Am Clin Nutr,* 55:2115–45, 1992. With permission.

XII. DRUG TREATMENT

The currently available drugs used in the treatment of obesity have an anorectic mode of action, i.e., they reduce hunger and food intake. The centrally acting drugs are shown in Table 6.[60,61] They have all been shown to be effective in producing weight loss in obesity over the short term (2 to 3 months). There have been relatively few long-term studies, but these have shown that these drugs at least limit weight gain. Both d-amphetamine and phenmetrazine are potent stimulants and have been drugs of abuse. They are, therefore, not recommended any longer as treatment for obesity. The other adrenergic compounds have less stimulants and, therefore, less abusive properties. The compounds that act via the serotoninergic system have no stimulant action and are, thus, more advisable in the treatment of obesity. Clinical studies have shown no adverse effects in treatment up to 1 year. Withdrawal from treatment seems to cause considerable weight gain; therefore, a maintenance dose alternating with treatments such as intensive behavior modification could prove beneficial.[61] Given as 15 mg twice daily, d-Fenfluramine has been shown to increase adherence to diet, to enhance diet efficacy, and to prevent regain when continued over 1 year.[62] Fluoxetine, used at a dose of 60 mg daily, was deemed to be effective, safe, and well tolerated for the treatment of obesity and obese diabetics, in particular.[63]

XIII. SURGICAL THERAPY OF OBESITY

Obese patients who manifest serious co-morbidity and have failed medical therapy may be candidates for surgical treatment. Surgical procedures have evolved over nearly 4 decades because of the limited success of medical therapies. Early procedures like the jejunal bypass were associated with serious complications that have resulted in abandon-
    ~t Only two procedures were recommended at the recent NIH Consensus Conference
        the vertical banded gastroplasty and the Roux-en-Y gastric bypass operation.[64]
            banded gastroplasty, as developed and perfected by Mason,[65] is an oper-
            controls weight by restricting intake and delaying gastric emptying. The
            eates a 15 ml stapled proximal stomach reservoir to limit the amount of food

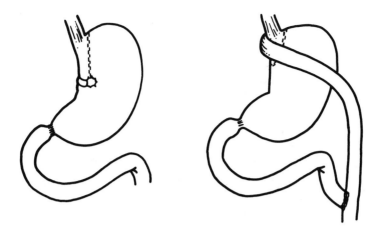

FIGURE 1. Gastric surgical techniques that have been clinically useful include the vertical banded gastroplasty (left) and the Roux-en-Y gastric bypass (right).

taken in. The opening between this reservoir and the rest of the stomach is banded externally to a diameter of 1 cm to delay emptying (Figure 1).[10]

Failures include distention of the wall of the pouch, rupture of the staple line, or erosion of the band into the stomach. Other complications include subsequent consumption of soft, calorically dense foods and vomiting from inadequate mastication and inappropriate intake.[66]

Mason also developed the gastric bypass, which resembles the gastroplasty in its formation of a small pouch and limited outlet, but which also bypasses the stomach, duodenum, and first portion of the jejunum (Figure 1). This operation is more likely to cause iron, calcium, and vitamin B_{12} deficiencies because there is interference with digestion and absorption. Marginal ulceration may also occur at the anastomosis.

Overall mortality with gastroplasty and gastric bypass is less than 2%, but the gastric bypass is superior in terms of the amount of weight loss achieved.[67] Surgery for obesity reduces diabetes mellitus, hypertension, hyperlipidemia, respiratory failure, and other co-morbidities in the majority of those patients with a maintenance of weight loss of 5 years or more. There is a resultant increase in life expectancy that may approach that of the general population.[66] With the continuing refinement of surgical procedures for obesity and increased sophistication of perioperative care, surgery is a reasonable therapeutic option for carefully selected morbidly obese patients who have failed other modalities. The contraindications are listed in Table 7.[10]

XIV. SUMMARY

Obesity is a significant national health problem associated with serious co-morbidities: hypertension, diabetes mellitus, hyperlipidemia and cardiovascular disease, pulmonary failure, osteoarthritis, and gallbladder disease. The complex factors involved in producing obesity necessitate a multidisciplinary approach to treatment that includes dietary programs, clinical support, behavior modification, and exercise.

A well-balanced, low calorie diet (1000 to 1800 kcal) is the recommended initial approach for most moderately obese patients with mild co-morbidity. Selected morbidly obese patients may benefit from very low-calorie diets (400 to 800 kcal), but the metabolic changes of semistarvation associated with VLCDs warrant close supervision by physicians well trained in clinical nutrition.

TABLE 7
Contraindications for Bariatric Surgery[a]

1. Less than 100 lb (45 kg) overweight
2. Organic cause for obesity
3. Age over 50 years
4. Serious underlying disease—cardiac, liver, or renal
5. Psychiatric disorder
6. Alcoholism or substance abuse
7. Endogenous depression
8. Misguided or ill-conceived motivation for surgery
9. Lack of support systems for follow-up and care
10. Has not failed conventional medical therapy for obesity
11. History of gallstones or cholecystitis

[a] Many surgeons require proven medical complications of obesity prior to consideration of surgery, so their absence would be a relative contraindication.

Bariatric surgery is a viable option for carefully screened morbidly obese patients who have failed an exhaustive trial of medical therapy. Improvements in gastric bypass and gastroplasty have made these procedures safer for the morbidly obese patient who has life-threatening co-morbidities associated with his/her obesity.

Although weight loss can be safely achieved through a variety of techniques, weight loss is still difficult to maintain for many patients. Successful patients generally take advantage of behavior modification techniques designed to help relearn eating behaviors with a goal of achieving a balanced diet and regular exercise.

REFERENCES

1. **Van Itallie, TB.** Health implications of overweight and obesity in the United States. *Ann Intern Med,* 103(6, Pt. 2):983–988, 1985.
2. **Prasad, N.** Very-low-calorie diets. Safe treatment for moderate and morbid obesity. *Postgrad Med,* 88:179–182, 187–188, 1990.
3. **NIH Technology Assessment Conference Panel.** Methods for voluntary weight loss and control. *Ann Intern Med,* 116:942–949, 1992.
4. **Lissner, L, Odell, PM, D'Aqostino, RB, et al.** Variability of body weight and health outcomes in the Framingham population. *N Engl J Med,* 324:1839–44, 1991.
5. **Hamm P, Shekelle, RB, and Stamler, J.** Large fluctuations in body weight during young adulthood and twenty-five year risk of coronary death in men. *Am J Epidemiol,* 129:312–8, 1989.
6. **Prentice, AM, Jebb, SA, and Goldberg, GR, et al.** Effects of weight cycling on body composition. *Am J Clin Nutr,* 56:209S–16S, 1992.
7. **Bray, GA.** Pathophysiology of obesity. *Am J Clin Nutr,* 55:488S–94S, 1992.
8. **1983 Metropolitan Height and Weight Tables.** *Stat Bull Metrop Life Insur Co,* 64:2–9, 1984.
9. **National Center for Health Statistics.** *Plan and Operation of the National Health and Nutrition Examination Survey, 1976–80,*DHHS publication no. (PHS) 81–1317 (Vital and Health Statistics, Ser. 1, No. 15), U.S. Public Health Service, Washington, DC, 1981.
10. **Taraszewski, R and Jensen, GL.** Nutrition and obesity management. *Pract Gastroenterol,* 16:9–16, 1992.
11. **Kuczmarski, RJ.** Prevalence of overweight and weight gain in the United States. *Am J Clin Nutr,* 55:495S–502S, 1992.

12. **Lukaski, H.** Methods for the assessment of human body composition: traditional and new. *Am J Clin Nutr,* 46:537–56, 1987.
13. **Bray, G and Gray, D.** Obesity part 1—pathogenesis. *West J Med,* 149:429–441, 1988.
14. **Garrow, JS.** *Treat Obesity Seriously.* Churchill Livingstone, London, 1981.
15. **Heymsfield, SM, and Waki, M.** Body composition in humans: advances in the development of multicompartment chemical models. *Nutr Rev,* 49(4):97–108, 1991.
16. **Wilber, JF.** Neuropeptides, appetite regulation, and human obesity. *JAMA,* 266:257–259, 1991.
17. **Buyse, ML, Ed.** *Birth Defects Encyclopedia.* Center for Birth Defects Information Services, Dover, 1990.
18. **Bray, GA.** Complications of obesity. *Ann Intern Med,* 103 (6, Pt. 2):1052–1062, 1985.
19. **Bennion, LJ and Grundy, SM.** Risk factors for the development of cholelithiasis in man (Pts. 1 & 2). *N Engl J Med,* 299:1221–1227, 1161–1167, 1978.
20. **Bennion, LJ and Grundy, SM.** Effects of obesity and caloric intake on biliary lipid metabolism in man. *J Clin Invest,* 56:996–1011, 1975.
21. **Anderson, T.** Liver and gallbladder disease before and after very-low-calorie diets. *Am J Clin Nutr,* 56:235S–9S, 1992.
22. **Wanless, IR and Lentz, JS.** Fatty liver hepatitis (steatohepatitis) and obesity: an autopsy study with analysis of risk factors. *Hepatology,* 12:1106–1110, 1990.
23. **Grundy, SM and Barnett, JP.** Metabolic and health complications of obesity. *Dis Month,* 36:641–731, 1990.
24. **Rubenstein, I, Zamel, N, DuBarry, RPT, and Hoffstein, V.** Airflow limitation in morbidly obese, nonsmoking men. *Ann Intern Med,* 112:828–832, 1990.
25. **Pi-Sunyer, FX.** Health implications of obesity. *Am J Clin Nutr,* 53:1595S–1603S, 1991.
26. **Sharp, JT, Barrocas, M, and Chokroverty, S.** The cardiorespiratory effects of obesity. *Clin Chest Med,* 1:103–18, 1980.
27. **Guilleminault, C, Partinen, M, and Quera-Salva, MA, et al.** Determinants of daytime sleepiness and obstructive sleep apnea. *Chest,* 94:32–7, 1986.
28. **Rochester, DF and Enson, Y.** Current concepts in the pathogenesis of the obesity-hypoventilation syndrome: mechanical and circulatory factors. *Am J Med,* 57:402–20, 1974.
29. **Sugerman, HJ, Fairman, RP, Sood, RK, et al.** Long-term effects of gastric surgery for treating respiratory insufficiency of obesity. *Am J Clin Nutr,* 55:597S–601S, 1992.
30. **Sutton, FD, Jr., Zwillich, CW, Creagh, CE, Pierson, DJ, and Weil, JV.** Progesterone for outpatient treatment of Pickwickian syndrome. *Ann Intern Med,* 83:476–9, 1975.
31. **Whitcomb, ME, Altman, N, Clark, RW, and Ralstin, JH.** Central and obstructive sleep apnea: pulmonary disease conference at the Ohio State University, Columbus. *Chest,* 73:857–60, 1978.
32. **Suratt, PM, McTier, RF, Findley, LJ, Pohl, SL, and Wihoit, SC.** Effect of very-low-calorie diets with weight loss on obstructive sleep apnea. *Am J Clin Nutr,* 56:182S–4S, 1992.
33. **Sugerman, HJ, Baron, PL, Fairman, RP, Evans, CR, and Vetrovec, GW.** Hemodynamic dysfunction in obesity hypoventilation syndrome and the effects of treatment with surgically induced weight loss. *Ann Surg,* 207:604–613, 1988.
34. **Sugerman, HJ, Fairman, RP, Baron, PL, and Kwentus, JA.** Gastric surgery for respiratory insufficiency of obesity. *Chest,* 89:81–86, 1986.
35. **Chapman, JM, Coulson, AH, Clark, VA, et al.** The differential effect of serum cholesterol, blood pressure, and weight on the incidence of myocardial infarction and angina pectoris. *J Chronic Dis,* 23:631–45, 1971.
36. **Hubert, HB, Feinleib, M, McNamara, PM, and Castelli, WP.** Obesity as an independent risk factor for cardiovascular disease: a 26-year follow-up of participants in the Framingham Heart Study. *Circulation,* 67:968–77, 1983.
37. **Manson, JE, Colditz, GA, Stampfer, MJ, et al.** A prospective study of obesity and risk of coronary heart disease in women. *N Engl J Med,* 322:882–9, 1990.
38. **Heyden, S, Hames, CG, Bartel, S, Cassel, JC, Tynler, HA, and Cornoni, JC.** Weight and weight history in relation to cerebrovascular and ischemic heart disease. *Arch Intern Med,* 128:956–60, 1971.
39. **Abraham, S, Collins, G, and Nordsieck, M.** Relationship of childhood weight status to morbidity in adults. *HSMHA Health Rep,* 86:273–84, 1971.
40. **Higgins, M, Kannel, W, Garrison, R, Pinsky, J, and Stokes, J.** Hazards of obesity—the Framingham experience. *Acta Med Scand, Suppl,* 723:23–36, 1988.
41. **Lapidus, L and Bengtsson, C.** Regional obesity as a health hazard in women—a retrospective study. *Acta Med Scand, Suppl,* 723:53–9, 1988.
42. **Larsson, B.** Regional obesity as health hazard in men—prospective studies. *Acta Med Scand, Suppl,* 723:45–51, 1988.

43. **Seidell, JC.** Regional obesity and health. *Int J Obesity,* 16 (Suppl. 2):S31–S34, 1992.

44. **Garfinkel, L.** Overweight and cancer. *Ann Intern Med,* 103:1034–6, 1985.

45. **Schrijver, J, Alexeiva-Fiqusch, J, von Breederode, N, et al.** Investigations on the nutritional status of advanced breast cancer patients: the influence of long-term treatment with meqestrol acetate or tamoxifen. *Nutr Cancer,* 10:232–245, 1987.

46. **Tretli, S, Haldovsen, T, and Ottestad, L.** The effect of pre-morbid height and weight on the survival of breast cancer patients. *Br J Cancer,* 62:299–304, 1990.

47. **Tartter, PI, Papatestas, AF, et al.** Cholesterol and obesity as prognostic factors in breast cancer. *Cancer,* 47:2222–2227, 1981.

48. **Holm, L, Callmer, E, Hjalmar, M, et al.** Dietary habits and prognostic factors in breast cancer. *J Natl Cancer Inst,* 81:1218–1223, 1989.

49. **Chlebowski, RI, Rose, D, et al.** Dietary fat reduction in adjuvant breast cancer therapy: current rationale and feasibility issues. *Prof Clin Biol Res,* 339:201, 1990.

50. **Rimm, AA, Werner, LH, Van Yserloo, B, and Bernstein, RA.** Relationship of obesity and disease in 73,532 weight-conscious women. *Public Health Rep,* 90:44–51, 1975.

51. **Higgins, M, Kannel, W, and Garrison, R.** Hazards of obesity—the Framingham experience. *Acta Med Scand,* 723 (suppl):23–36, 1988.

52. **Pi-Sunyer, FX.** The role of very-low-calorie diets in obesity. *Am J Clin Nutr,* 56:240S–3S, 1992.

53. **Apovian, CM, McMahon, MM, and Bistrian, BR.** Guidelines for refeeding the marasmic patient. *Crit Care Med,* 18:1030–1033, 1990.

54. **Bistrian, BR.** Clinical use of a protein-sparing modified fast. *JAMA,* 240:2299–2302, 1978.

55. **Hoffer, LI and Bistrian, BR.** Dietary treatment of obesity. *Med Times Feb,* 90S–97S, 101S, 1982.

56. **Wadden, TA, Van Itallie, TB, and Blackburn, GL.** Responsible and irresponsible use of very-low-calorie diets in the treatment of obesity. *JAMA,* 263:83–85, 1990.

57. **Phinney, SD.** Exercise during and after very-low-calorie dieting. *Am J Clin Nutr,* 56:190S–4S, 1992.

58. **Pavlou, KN, Krey, S, and Steffee, WP.** Exercise as an adjunct to weight loss and maintenance in moderately obese subjects. *Am J Clin Nutr,* 49:1115–23, 1989.

59. **Wing Rena, R.** Behavioral treatment of severe obesity. *Am J Clin Nutr,* 55:545S–51S, 1992.

60. **Bray, G.** Drug treatment of obesity. *Am J Clin Nutr,* 55:538S-44S, 1992.

61. **Silverstone, T and Goodall, E.** Centrally acting anorectic drugs: a clinical perspective. *Am J Clin Nutr,* 55:211S–4S, 1992.

62. **Guy-Grand, B.** Clinical studies with d-fenfluramine. *Am J Clin Nutr,* 55:173S–6S, 1992.

63. **Wise, SD.** Clinical studies with fluoxetine in obesity. *Am J Clin Nutr,* 55:181S–4S, 1992.

64. **Summary of the NIH Consensus.** NIH Consensus Development Conference, March 25–27, National Institutes of Health, Washington, DC, 1991.

65. **Mason, EE, Scott, DH, Maher, JW, et al.** The first decade of vertical banded gastroplasty (VBG) for treatment of extreme obesity. *Obesity Surg,* 1:228, 1991.

66. **Kral, JG.** Overview of surgical techniques for treating obesity. *Am J Clin Nutr,* 55:552S–5S, 1992.

67. **Sugerman, HJ, Lundrey, GL, Kellum, J, et al.** Weight loss with vertical binded gastroplasty and roux Y gastric bypass for morbid obesity with elective versus random assignment. *Am J Surg,* 157:93–102, 1989.

APPENDIX I

CHARACTERISTICS OF THE OBESITY SYNDROMES

Prader-Willi syndrome (defective chromosome 15)
   Obesity, hypogonadism, hypotonia, mental retardation, type II diabetes mellitus
Bardet-Biedl syndrome (autosomal recessive)
   Obesity, hypogonadotropic hypogonadism, retinitis pigmentosa, polydactyly, mental retardation, renal anomalities, diabetes mellitus
Cohen syndrome (probably autosomal recessive)
   Obesity, short stature, mental retardation, hypotonia, maxillary hypoplasia, short-phittrum, micrognathia, narrow hands and feet, narrow and high-arched palate
Carpenter syndrome (autosomal recessive) (acrocephalopolysyndactyly, type II)
   Acrocephaly and facial and limb abnormalities, obesity, hypogonadism, congenital heart disease, abdominal hernias

Chapter 4

NUTRITION IN GASTROINTESTINAL DISEASE: AN OVERVIEW

Gregory G. Ginsberg and Timothy O. Lipman

TABLE OF CONTENTS

0-8493-7847-8/94/$0.00+$.50
© 1994 by CRC Press, Inc.

I. INTRODUCTION

The gastrointestinal (GI) tract is a complex organ system responsible for digestion, absorption, nutrient and drug metabolism, and elimination of waste. Ingested food is mechanically disrupted and mixed with digestive enzymes to produce readily absorbable particles. The GI tract also functions as an immunologic barrier to ingested and colonized microorganisms.

Gastrointestinal diseases are the most frequent disorders resulting in synchronous gut and nutritional compromise. Abnormalities of GI function may produce nutritional deficiencies secondary to disruption of normal nutrient delivery, digestion, or absorption. Knowledge of normal GI anatomy and physiology enables the clinician to understand nutritional deficiencies produced by GI tract dysfunction. Additionally, the clinician may be able to prevent or treat those deficiencies. In this chapter, we review the normal mechanisms of digestion and absorption with emphasis on nutritional abnormalities. The implications of acute GI tract failure are discussed. Finally, specific diseases involving the GI system are addressed with emphasis on the impact of nutritional therapy. The role of nutritional support in these disorders as both primary and adjunctive therapy is discussed. Recommendations for the use of nutritional intervention and therapy are offered as indicated. More detailed discussions will follow in subsequent chapters.

II. NORMAL DIGESTION AND ABSORPTION

Digestion can be defined as the physical and chemical processes of breaking complex nutrients into simpler forms ready for absorption. Absorption is the process by which nutrients are taken up into the intestinal cell, processed, and transferred into the portal or lymphatic circulation.

Ingested food is mechanically disrupted by mastication and mixed with oral secretions in the mouth. Coordinated muscular contraction in the oropharynx and esophagus delivers the food bolus to the stomach. Vagal-mediated gastric accommodation permits the upper body and fundus to function as a reservoir and slow the rate of gastric emptying of liquids. Muscular contraction in the antrum, in coordination with the pylorus, provides further mechanical disruption, mixes the ingested contents with gastric secretions, and allows gradual release of gastric chyme into the duodenum. Non-nutrient liquids empty most rapidly initially, with their rate of emptying slowing as volume decreases.[1] Nutrient-rich liquids empty at a relatively constant rate. Digestible solids are ground into particles <1 mm before emptying.[2] Indigestible particles are cleared subsequently by cyclic contractions. The pylorus and small bowel offer resistance to outflow, helping to control the rate of nutrient delivery to the duodenum. Gastric emptying may be slowed by increased osmolality, fat content, and acidity.

The majority of digestion and absorption takes place in the small intestine. Protein, fats, and carbohydrates are digested for absorption at the enterocyte level. In the ileum bile acids and vitamin B_{12} are absorbed. The colon's main functions are the absorption of water, sodium, and the products of colonic bacterial metabolism.

A. CARBOHYDRATES

Salivary amylase initiates starch digestion in the mouth. However, this activity is short-lived, as the enzyme is denatured by low gastric pH. In the duodenum, oligo- and disaccharidases undergo hydrolysis by pancreatic amylase. Further hydrolysis is carried out by brush border enzymes, specific disaccharides located on the enterocyte microvilli (lactase, sucrase, maltase). The resultant monosaccharides are absorbed by specific, sodium-dependent, coupled-transport carrier mechanisms.[3] Carbohydrate malabsorption occurs when there is insufficiency of any of the above processes. Clinical examples include pancreatic insufficiency, specific brush border enzyme insufficiency (e.g., lactase deficiency), disruption of the brush border (e.g., celiac disease, Crohn's disease), or loss of total intestinal mucosal surface area (e.g., extensive resection). The D-xylose test is a useful means to assess intestinal mucosal absorptive function.

B. PROTEINS

Gastric acid and pepsin initiate the digestion of dietary protein. Hydrolysis in the duodenum by proteolytic pancreatic enzymes creates oligopeptides. Intestinal brush border peptidases accomplish final digestion. Proteins are absorbed as dipeptides, tripeptides, free amino acids, and probably other short-chain peptides. Like carbohydrate malabsorption, protein malabsorption can occur with pancreatic insufficiency, diseases affecting enterocyte function, and loss of absorptive surface. Proteolytic enzymes have an optimal pH of 8. Gastric acid hypersecretion, by lowering duodenal pH, may impair protein digestion. There are no simple, direct tests of protein digestion or absorption available to the clinician.

C. FATS

Processing of dietary fat is the most complex of the digestive and absorptive processes. Fat is water insoluble; hence, the GI tract must transform large water-insoluble particles into a soluble, absorbable form.

Fat digestion begins in the mouth with secretion of lingual lipases. Muscular contractions in the stomach cause fat emulsification, dispersing fat globules into an evenly divided phase. In the intestine, pancreatic enzymes cleave triglycerides into fatty acids and monoglycerides; additionally, pancreatic enzymes hydrolyze various polyesters. These then combine with bile acids and phospholipids secreted by the liver to form micelles. The process of micellarization completes the transformation of water-insoluble fat into a water-soluble form which is absorbed in the proximal small intestine.

After absorption, fatty acids and other fats are re-esterified in the intestinal cell to form chylomicrons, which are then secreted into the lymphatic system. Medium-chain triglycerides can be absorbed directly in the jejunum without undergoing hydrolysis and micellarization. Disruption of bile synthesis or flow, pancreatic insufficiency, or enterocyte disruption can lead to fat malabsorption. Thus, biliary tract obstruction, chronic pancreatitis, Crohn's disease, celiac disease, or extensive intestinal resection may all cause fat malabsorption.

Fat malabsorption is best diagnosed by quantitative measurement of fecal fat. The patient must be eating 100 g/d of fat for at least 3 days prior for the test to be valid. Serum carotene is a useful clinical marker of fat malabsorption, since it reflects absorption of fat-soluble vitamin A.[4] Again, the clinician needs to ensure that there was sufficient carotene and vitamin A intake when interpreting this test.

D. MINERALS AND VITAMINS

The primary site for divalent cation absorption is the duodenum and proximal jejunum. Iron is actively absorbed in the duodenum. Organic (heme) iron is more rapidly absorbed than inorganic (ferrous) iron. Zinc is absorbed by facilitated diffusion throughout the small intestine. Zinc-binding ligands, found in pancreatic secretions (and human milk), facilitate zinc absorption. Zinc deficiency may be seen with other malabsorptive states. Calcium absorption is regulated by vitamin D and occurs in the duodenum. Since vitamin D is a fat-soluble vitamin, fat malabsorption may impair calcium absorption.

Absorption of water-soluble vitamins is predominantly passive and carrier-mediated. Folic polyglutamate is hydrolyzed to monoglutamate by zinc-dependent folate deconjugase in the brush border. Absorption of folic acid takes place in the jejunum. The most common cause of folate deficiency is a deficient diet. Absorption is also reduced with intestinal damage or B_{12} deficiency.

Cobalamin (vitamin B_{12}) is released from food by gastric acid and pepsin. It binds with R proteins present in saliva and gastric juice. It is then separated from R protein in the duodenum by pancreatic enzymes and binds to intrinsic factor released from gastric parietal cells. Intrinsic factor facilitates B_{12} absorption primarily in the distal ileum. The following conditions may lead to B_{12} deficiency: pernicious anemia, gastric resection, pancreatic insufficiency, bacterial overgrowth (consumption of ingested B_{12}), absent or diseased ileum (Crohn's disease, sprue).

The absorption of fat-soluble vitamins (A, D, K, E) parallels that of other fats. Thus, impaired fat absorption will lead to fat-soluble vitamin deficiency.

III. ACUTE VS. CHRONIC GI TRACT FAILURE

Acute failure of the GI tract occurs when an individual is unable to eat or when there is abrupt onset of GI tract malfunction. Examples include post-operative ileus, intestinal obstruction, acute bowel inflammation (peritonitis, diverticulitis, ischemic bowel), and acute pancreatitis. These entities usually have an abrupt onset and, with optimal therapy, have a finite course with expectations of resuming a normal diet. Unless inadequate intake is prolonged, this may not constitute a need for specific nutritional support.

Chronic GI tract failure occurs when one or more components of GI tract function are crippled over prolonged periods. Examples of chronic GI tract failure include short bowel syndrome, intestinal malabsorption, hepatic insufficiency, chronic pancreatitis, and inflammatory bowel disease. Nutritional intervention depends upon specific nutrient deficiencies involved, as well as ultimate access to, and function of, the GI tract.

Inadequate nutrient intake over days or weeks results in malnutrition and impaired intestinal function. Total absence of enteral nutrition can lead to atrophy of the small intestinal mucosa in only a few days. This, accompanied by diminished bowel motility and altered immunity, may be associated with a higher rate of sepsis, multiorgan failure, and death in critically ill patients.[5] Whereas total parenteral nutrition (TPN) provides adequate calories, protein, and micronutrients, it is associated with atrophic changes in the muscular and mucosal layers of the bowel and with decreased enterocyte enzyme activity.[6] Enteral nutrition, when instituted early and individualized to a patient's needs, preserves intestinal mucosal form and function.[7] In all instances of nutritional intervention, the dictum: "if the gut works, use it", should be heeded. In situations when enteral nutrition alone is inadequate, it might still be continued in conjunction with TPN.

IV. SHORT BOWEL SYNDROME

Short bowel syndrome occurs relatively infrequently. However, understanding underlying pathologic mechanisms will enhance the practitioner's knowledge of GI tract nutrition. Short bowel syndrome exists when extensive resection of, or damage to, the small intestine compromises the ability to digest and absorb nutrients. This most commonly results from intestinal infarction, trauma, chronic disease (e.g., Crohn's disease), radiation, or, occasionally, malignancy. The main clinical manifestations are diarrhea, weight loss, and malaise.[8] The minimum length of small bowel sufficient to allow adequate digestion and absorption is variable and dependent upon a number of factors including the location, length, functional status, and adaptive capacity of the remaining bowel, as well as the presence or absence of a functional ileocecal valve.[9]

Gastrointestinal motility is altered after intestinal resection. Proximal resection may result in loss of inhibition of gastric emptying, causing dumping. The ileum is normally a site of slowed small bowel transit. Likewise, the ileocecal valve functions to prolong intestinal transit time. Removal of these areas may cause a reduction in the time nutrients are in contact with intestinal surfaces with resultant decreased absorption.[10]

It is generally accepted that patients require a minimum of 2 ft of small intestine beyond the duodenum to survive on oral intake. Resection of short segments of small bowel is normally well tolerated, especially if the ileocecal valve is left intact.[11] There is a great degree of functional reserve in the normal gut, and adaptation of the remaining bowel allows for increased absorption. In patients who have had 50% or more of their small bowel resected, adaptation to full or partial diet is possible, but may take months to years. Patients with short bowel syndrome require a broad range of nutritional support depending on length and location of bowel removed. Nutritional support in this group is non-static and requires changes as adaptation of the bowel proceeds.

A. SITE-DEPENDENT PATHOLOGY

Specific nutritional requirements are site dependent. If the duodenum is removed, malabsorption of iron, calcium, and folic acid will ensue.[12] When large segments of jejunum are removed, remaining segments of large and small bowel can usually resorb excess fluid and electrolytes. However, intestinal lactase activity may be diminished, resulting in lactose intolerance.[13]

Ileal resection results in significant volume increase reaching the colon with resultant diarrhea. In addition, bile salts, ordinarily absorbed in the distal ileum, undergo bacterial conversion to free bile acids which stimulate colonic water and electrolyte secretion, resulting in cholorrhea. With greater than 100 cm ileal resection, enterohepatic circulation of bile salts is disrupted, resulting in fat malabsorption and steatorrhea.[14]

Most patients with an intact colon will not lose excessive amounts of fluid and electrolytes. However, with total or partial colectomy accompanying ileal resection, hypovolemia, dehydration, and electrolyte imbalance may ensue.

B. MANAGEMENT OF SHORT BOWEL SYNDROME

The nutritional considerations in patients with short bowel syndrome are based on the length and location of segments removed.[15] In the initial postoperative period, all patients will require i.v. fluids and electrolytes, monitoring especially Na, K, Ca, Mg, and PO_4 levels. Most patients are kept NPO for 10 days post-operatively to decrease osmotic load. H-2 blockers are used to decrease gastric hypersecretion.[16] Oral loperamide, paregoric, diphenoxylate, tincture of opium, or intramuscular codeine can be given to slow intestinal motility, improve ion transport, and decrease diarrhea.

Once the patient's cardiopulmonary status has stabilized, TPN can be initiated. Additional fluid and electrolyte supplementation may be needed to match GI tract losses due to diarrhea. As the patient's oral intake increases, TPN can be gradually decreased.

Once oral feedings are to begin, an isotonic feeding formula may be given progressively. If enteral feeding solutions are tolerated in patients with less than 50% small bowel resection, a dry solid meal, high in complex carbohydrates, given apart from isotonic liquids 1 to 2 hours later can be tried. The caloric intake is increased as tolerated to achieve around 30 kcal/kg ideal body weight per day. In patients who have greater than 50% bowel resection, the amount eaten should be doubled to make up for calories lost to malabsorption. Low fat diets have not been proven superior and are rather unpalatable.

After significant ileal resection, cholestyramine may reduce bile salt-induced diarrhea. Vitamin B_{12} deficiency can be expected, and levels should be monitored. Replacement vitamin B_{12} may be administered by injection of 100 µg monthly.

Patients who fail a trial of normal diet, and those with very little remaining bowel (60 to 80 cm), should be tried on constant infusion of an enteral formula. Constant flow rate helps reduce diarrhea. Full-strength isotonic solutions can be used and increased as tolerated to target rate. Predigested low residue or "elemental" diets require no digestive effort from the remaining short bowel and have been useful during early readaptive phases. However, these still require intact absorptive mechanisms, and these formulas are expensive. While elemental diets were favored originally, recent data supports the use of polymeric diets because of increased stimulation of the mucosa and lower cost.[17]

Patients with less than 60 to 80 cm of remaining bowel and those who will require prolonged gradual adaptation to enteral feeding will require long-term TPN. If gut adaptation improves with time, TPN can be gradually eliminated. In some patients, calories are provided enterally, but fluids and electrolytes require lifelong parenteral replacement.

V. INFLAMMATORY BOWEL DISEASE

The emphasis on nutrition in the management of inflammatory bowel disease (IBD) has received increasing recognition as an adjunctive therapy for both ulcerative colitis and Crohn's disease, but also as a primary therapy in Crohn's disease. Patients with IBD are often nutritionally deficient and in negative nitrogen balance.[18] This may be caused by inadequate intake, decreased absorption due to mucosal involvement or previous resection, catabolic effects of the disease, and/or the catabolic effects of corticosteroid therapy. Besides protein-calorie malnutrition, specific deficiencies of iron, vitamin B_{12}, folic acid, calcium, magnesium, zinc, and fat-soluble vitamins are seen, based upon location and extent of disease. Replacement of these vitamins and minerals should be carried out when deficiency is anticipated or identified.

There is little evidence that low-residue or high-fiber diets alter frequency of relapse or severity of disease in Crohn's disease or ulcerative colitis. Dietary restrictions are felt to be unnecessary, and patients should be allowed intake of their favorite foods to supply normal energy intake. Lactose intolerance may be present in some patients and should be treated on an individual basis.

No primary therapeutic benefit has been observed in patients with acute ulcerative colitis with either enteral or parenteral nutrition. In one study, TPN was no more likely to induce remission than a combination of bowel rest and steroid therapy.[19] Adjunctive enteral nutrition as compared to parenteral nutrition given to patients with moderate to severe acute ulcerative colitis may result in improved serum albumin;[20] no differences in clinical outcome were found. Patients receiving TPN in this study, however, did have more post-operative infectious complications than did the patients receiving enteral nutrition. Overall, the chief role of nutritional therapy in the acute and toxic setting is to maintain a positive nitrogen balance while awaiting the outcome of anti-inflammatory, antibiotic, or surgical therapy.

Controlled trials of TPN as primary therapy for acute Crohn's disease have not demonstrated any benefit over enteral formula feeding.[21] Chronic home TPN may be required in patients with Crohn's disease complicated by short bowel syndrome resulting from previous resections. A retrospective study by Galandiuk[22] reported that home TPN improved nutritional status and quality of life, but had no advantage with regard to need for surgery or hospitalization.

In patients with active Crohn's disease, there is increasing evidence that, in addition to maintaining nutritional status, elemental or polymeric diets may reduce disease activity and induce remission. Elemental diets provide nutrients in their simplest forms: protein as amino acids and carbohydrates as simple sugars. Several studies have shown that an elemental diet is as successful or even better than steroids in inducing remissions.[23] A retrospective assessment by Teahon reported that elemental diet therapy was as effective as corticosteroids for controlling active Crohn's disease.[24] In addition, at more than 5 years follow-up, patients treated with elemental diets had an annual relapse rate of only 8 to 10%, no different from those treated with corticosteroids. Patients with perirectal involvement did not respond as well. Unpalatability, however, has restricted the use of elemental diets.

While the use of polymeric diets, it was thought, might overcome the palatability problem, results have not been encouraging. First, the European Cooperative Crohn's Disease (ECCD) Study III[25] suffered from a high drop-out rate of patients on an orally administered polymeric diet, attributed to poor palatability. Second, to overcome the compliance problem, enteral feeding tubes were used in ECCD Study IV,[26] which compared one group of patients treated with 6-methylprednisolone and sulfasalazine to a second group treated with an oligopeptide diet. Significantly more patients in the drug treatment group (41 of 52) achieved remission than in the diet treated group (29 of 55).

Studies comparing the effect of polymeric vs. elemental diets for the treatment of active Crohn's disease have yielded contradictory results.[27] Further, larger, controlled trials are needed to determine whether more expensive elemental diets substantially improve outcome in patients with acute Crohn's disease. In patients without perirectal disease and in whom steroids are not a satisfactory component of therapy, elemental diet may be considered.

VI. ACUTE AND CHRONIC PANCREATITIS

Nutritional management of acute and chronic pancreatitis presents many challenges to the clinician.[28] Patients with acute pancreatitis have increased metabolic requirements similar to those seen with sepsis. The patient with alcoholic pancreatitis or acute exacerbation of chronic pancreatitis is likely to be malnourished at the onset or may rapidly develop nutritional deficiencies. Many hold that the pathogenesis of acute pancreatitis is due to autodigestion of the pancreas by its own secretory enzymes. It follows, then, that minimizing pancreatic exocrine secretion may improve outcome. Dietary manipulations to this end, however, have been disappointing. Whereas TPN has been demonstrated to decrease pancreatic juice flow, efforts to demonstrate a similar effect in response to elemental diets or intrajejunal feedings have not been convincing.[29]

Generally, acute pancreatitis is managed with "bowel rest" (NPO), i.v. fluids, and analgesia. The use of nasogastric suction is disputed, but is certainly indicated when nausea and vomiting are symptoms and when paralytic ileus is present. Most episodes of acute pancreatitis are short, self-limited, and do not require extraordinary nutritional support. However, in patients with multiple adverse prognostic factors, many advocate early use of TPN within a week of the onset of the attack.[30] Conversely, several retrospective studies and one randomized controlled study have not shown benefit from early TPN.[31] Most would agree that TPN should be reserved for those patients, in whom, due to complications (abscess, complicated pseudocyst, pancreatic ascites) or severity of attack, the resumption of enteral feeding will be delayed for several weeks.

The optimal time to resume oral diet is disputed. It is often feared that "too early" resumption may result in relapse. It is generally accepted that oral feeding can begin when the patient feels hungry. A judicious trial of water and then clear liquids should be tried before advancing the diet. Failure to tolerate oral intake may indicate development of pseudocyst, abscess, or continuing inflammation. Presence of an elevated amylase in the absence of abdominal pain or ileus should not preclude advancing to an oral diet.

The major complaints associated with chronic pancreatitis are pain, weight loss, and diarrhea. The most important nutritional recommendation is abstinence from alcohol. Nonetheless, complete abstinence may not guarantee resolution of symptoms or freedom from exacerbations. The role of elemental diets in chronic pancreatitis has not been defined. TPN is reserved for patients who cannot eat due to pain or in whom frequent recurrent exacerbations do not allow adequate sustained oral intake. Exocrine pancreatic function must be diminished by 90% before steatorrhea occurs. In most patients this can be managed by avoiding large fatty meals. A low-fat, high-protein, diet containing 50 to 100 g/d, or less than 25% of total calories, of mainly vegetable fat will avoid diarrhea and supply essential fatty acids and fat-soluble vitamins. Pancreatic enzyme supplementation has been demonstrated in some studies to reduce steatorrhea, reduce pain, and increase weight in patients with chronic pancreatitis. Deficiencies of fat-soluble vitamins (A ,D, K, E), vitamin B_{12}, zinc, and magnesium may be evident in patients with chronic pancreatitis and require replacement.

VII. LIVER DISEASE

Approximately 40% of patients with non-alcoholic chronic liver disease will have some degree of malnutrition due to poor intake, mild steatorrhea, or fat-soluble vitamin deficiency. Virtually 100% of patients with chronic alcoholic liver disease will be malnourished.[32] There is some evidence that aggressive nutritional support may result in more rapid improvement in liver function[33] and outcome.[34]

In patients with alcoholic liver disease, the reasons for malnutrition include poor intake, malabsorption, and altered metabolism. Poor intake may be the result of anorexia, nausea and vomiting due to gastritis or pancreatitis, and socioeconomic factors. Once hospitalized, patients are often made NPO for treatment of associated disorders (e.g., GI bleeding, pancreatitis) and in preparation for diagnostic tests. Malabsorption may result from the primary effect of alcohol, folate deficiency, and concomitant pancreatic insufficiency. Patients with advanced liver disease often are hypermetabolic; there is less efficient utilization of nutrients and increased substrate turnover.[35]

Anorexia often accompanies the early stages of acute hepatitis, whether due to alcohol, drug, or viral etiology. This is usually short lived and only rarely requires i.v. supplements. Most patients can, and should, assume a regular diet as soon as tolerated. When anorexia is prolonged, tube feeding may be instituted.

In alcoholic patients with chronic liver disease, specific nutrient deficiencies may be present. The clinician should be aware of possible folate, thiamin, niacin, magnesium, zinc, and vitamins A and D deficiencies. In patients who are actively drinking, thiamin and folic acid should be administered parenterally on admission to avoid precipitation of Wernicke-Korsakoff's syndrome. In most cases, a daily oral multivitamin supplement with minerals is adequate to restore other vitamin and mineral deficiencies.

Basal energy requirements of patients with acute hepatitis and cirrhosis are similar to controls, 25 to 30 kcal/kg/d. The presence of ascites or encephalopathy may increase energy expenditures. Adequate daily protein (1 g/kg) to maintain a positive nitrogen balance is important for overall care. There is no need for protein restriction in patients without encephalopathy. There is some evidence that vegetable protein is less encephalopathogenic than animal protein.[36] Fat restriction is unnecessary.

In the past, primary therapy for hepatic encephalopathy relied on protein restriction. Although there is still a role for protein restriction in some cases, the importance of maintaining positive nitrogen balance is emphasized. When correction of precipitating factors and therapy with lactulose and/or neomycin fail, special diets have been advocated. Data supporting the use of branched chain amino acid formulas in these cases is, at best, controversial. If the gut is functioning, supplementation with a ''hepatic'' formula may be tried if all other standard therapies have failed.

There is insufficient data to support the use of standard TPN solutions vs. oral diet in patients with cirrhosis or hepatic encephalopathy. However, in patients with prolonged hepatic coma or encephalopathy and a non-functioning gut, parenteral nutrition may be instituted. The use of branched-chain amino acid TPN solutions are expensive, and controlled trials do not convincingly demonstrate a benefit over standard TPN.[37,38,39] As in other disease states, enteral nutrition should be reinstituted as early as possible.

VIII. DIVERTICULAR DISEASE

Prior to 1970, diverticular disease was treated with a ''low residue'' diet to ''rest'' the bowel. It was suggested that plant matter, particularly seeds, would lodge in diverticula, leading to complications. In 1971, Painter and Burkitt[40] reported their observation on the possible relationship between reduced fiber consumption in the West and the increased incidence of diverticular disease, which is relatively rare in Asia and Africa where high-fiber diets are consumed. Applying Laplace's law (pressure = tension in bowel wall/radius of the bowel wall), it has been suggested that the increased bulk of stool produced by consumption of a high-fiber diet reduces the development of high intracolonic pressure and consequent mucosal herniation.

These hypotheses were further supported by comparisons of the low prevalence of asymptomatic colonic diverticulosis in English vegetarians compared to non-vegetarians.[41] Reduction of symptomatic diverticular disease has been demonstrated when patients consumed high-fiber diets.[42,43] Additionally, over 90% of patients previously hospitalized for complicated diverticular disease remained symptom free over the follow-up period of 5 to 7 years on a high-fiber diet.[44]

Despite sufficient evidence to support the therapeutic effect of a high-fiber diet in the management of diverticular disease, specific recommendations are less clear due to the variety of fiber sources used in studies. Diets high in lignin and whole cereal grains produce bulky stool, due to their undigested mass and water-holding qualities. It is recommended to gradually increase intake of whole wheat bran, in divided doses, over a period of 4 to 6 weeks to achieve the maximum tolerated amount, or at least 10 to 25 g/d. Similar high, insoluble fiber sources include whole wheat bread, various high-fiber breakfast cereals, bran muffins, and, at a higher cost, manufactured high-fiber supplements. It should be noted that the fiber in oat bran, currently in favor because of potential hypocholesterolemic effects, will not affect fecal bulk or diverticulosis.

IX. PEPTIC ULCER DISEASE

Peptic ulcer disease (PUD) is a manifestation of many different processes. Etiologic factors include acid, pepsin, *Helicobacter pylori,* use of nonsteroidal anti-inflammatory drugs (NSAIDs), stress, and, perhaps, diet. Until recent times, dietary restrictions were a major component of PUD management. The traditional ulcer diet was composed of bland, low-fiber, ''soft'' foods, like milk, eggs, white bread, and soups or purees. The beneficial effects of such traditional ''ulcer diets'', however, have never been documented. Conversely, comparative trials suggested that no benefit was demonstrated and patients on regular diets actually fared better than those treated with ''ulcer diets''.[45,46,47,48] Epidemiologic data now suggest that diets high in fiber, complex carbohydrates, and low in saturated fats benefit treatment and prevention of PUD.[49]

The introduction of H-2 blockers and other effective ulcer medications diminished the interest in diet as primary therapy. Nonetheless, components of traditional "ulcer diets" remain in the minds of many patients and health-care workers alike. Spicy food, alcohol, coffee, and caffeine-containing beverages are often restricted in patients with PUD, though their relationships are questionable.

While alcohol has been demonstrated to cause mucosal injury in experimental animals and human volunteers, no studies have demonstrated a direct adverse effect of alcohol on ulcer healing or relapse.[50] In fact, small amounts of alcohol (30 to 60 ml) may even promote ulcer healing and protect against mucosal injury induced by NSAIDs via prostaglandin stimulation.[51] Less data are available on beer and wine which have additives— the effects of which on PUD may act independently of the alcohol content. Nonetheless, alcohol has been associated with acute gastritis and may contribute to symptoms of abdominal discomfort. For these reasons, patients with PUD should avoid excess alcohol, though an absolute restriction is probably unnecessary.

Regular coffee stimulates gastric acid secretion, but to similar degrees, so do decaffeinated coffee, teas, colas, and some caffeine-free soft drinks.[52] Paffenbarger et al.[53] observed that drinking coffee was associated with an increased incidence of PUD later in life. However, this data was not controlled for NSAID use and other parameters that may have affected their outcome. Others[54] have failed to demonstrate a positive association. No studies have demonstrated a negative effect of coffee on ulcer healing or recurrence. Regular and decaffeinated coffee, tea, and carbonated soft drinks are associated with increased esophageal reflux symptoms and should be restricted as indicated to eliminate reflux symptoms.

Results of studies linking PUD and spicy foods are contradictory and unconvincing. While capsaicin, the active ingredient in red pepper and chilies, causes increased gastric acid output, no difference in duodenal ulcer healing or gastric mucosal abnormalities was observed after 4 weeks in patients consuming red chilies.[55] We recommend that patients avoid intake of alcohol in excess and all items identified to cause or exacerbate their abdominal discomfort.

X. DUMPING SYNDROME

Gastric surgery not infrequently results in some degree of chronic GI tract failure and malnutrition, depending on type and extent of surgery performed. B_{12} deficiency may result from partial or total gastrectomy due to inadequate intrinsic factor.[56] Iron and folate deficiencies are also observed; however, their etiologies are unclear. Inadequate or misplaced anastomosis may result in delayed gastric emptying with subsequent decreased intake secondary to nausea, vomiting, and early satiety. More commonly, symptoms result from changes in the motor function of the stomach and upper small intestine secondary to the operation.[57]

Dumping is one of the most common postgastrectomy syndromes. The disruption of the normal regulatory mechanisms in the upper GI tract results in the rapid emptying of nutrient-rich, hypertonic gastric contents into the small intestine. An early and late phase are described. Early dumping occurs in approximately 25% of patients who have ablation, bypass, or alteration of the pyloric sphincter mechanism.[58] Gastrointestinal and vasomotor symptoms of early dumping begin 10 to 30 min after a meal and are due to the swift delivery of hyperosmolar gastric chyme into the small bowel.[59] This results in the transfer of water and electrolytes—up to 25% of plasma volume—into the small bowel lumen.[60] Gastrointestinal symptoms are due to rapid distention of the small bowel lumen and consist of crampy abdominal pain, distention, nausea, vomiting, and early satiety. Vasomotor symptoms include weakness, diaphoresis, lightheadedness, flushing, and palpitations. In addition to the rapid loss of intravascular volume, several gut hormones, including serotonin, GIP, VIP, neurotensin, and enteroglucagon, contribute to the manifestations of vasomotor symptoms.

Late dumping affects <2% of patients after gastrectomy. Symptoms occur 1 to 3 h after a meal due to a reactive hypoglycemia. This results from increased insulin levels following the rapid onset of hyperglycemia occurring during early dumping.[61] Symptoms are similar to the vasomotor manifestations of early dumping.

Nutritional therapy for dumping requires lowering the volume and osmolality of gastric chyme delivered to the small intestine. Symptoms are generally benefited by frequent, small, dry, solid meals high in protein, fat, and complex carbohydrates and low in simple sugars. Fluid intake with meals should be restricted. Foods rich in the dietary fiber pectin (e.g., apple, bananas, and oranges) will contribute to a slowing of gastric output and may prevent postprandial hypoglycemia.[62] Additives such as glucomannan[63] and acarbose,[64] an alpha-glucosidase inhibitor, may also reduce the insulin response by slowing carbohydrate absorption. Milk products are to be avoided because of functional lactase deficiency. The dry meal may be followed, after 1 or 2 h, by hypotonic fluid (water or weak tea) to avoid dehydration. Octreotide, a synthetic somatostatin analogue now available in a longer-acting form, appears to be a promising new adjunctive therapy in patients severely affected. Its benefits are seen with respect to both GI transit time and hormonal changes.

XI. IRRITABLE BOWEL SYNDROME

The classic triad of abdominal pain, constipation, and/or diarrhea in the absence of organic disease describes the irritable bowel syndrome (IBS). Attention generally has been paid to motor dysfunction of the colon. More recently, the syndrome has been viewed as a visceral nocioseptive problem affecting all the hollow organs of the GI tract. In addition to antispasmodic therapy, dietary treatment has been a mainstay. Specific food intolerance may lead to symptoms of IBS. A detailed dietary history should be sought, with emphasis on identifying foods containing caffeine, lactose, sorbitol, and fructose. Caffeine may cause increased gut motility resulting in decreased transit time and subsequent diarrhea.

Lactase deficiency in small bowel mucosa leads to the delivery of poorly digested lactose-containing foods to the colon. Fermentation and digestion by colonic bacteria results in gas formation and osmotic diarrhea. Lactase deficiency can be documented by hydrogen breath testing. However, a trial on a lactose-free diet is, at once, diagnostic and therapeutic. Commercial lactase enzyme supplements (e.g., Lactaid™, Dairy Ease™) may be utilized by some patients.

Sorbitol is a natural-occurring sugar in some fruits and plants, but, more significantly, it may be found as a commercially synthesized artificial sweetener in many dietetic foods. Malabsorption of sorbitol along with fructose, a natural sugar in fruits, berries, and plants, has been implicated in contributing to the symptoms of IBS. This malabsorption may be secondary to a specific disaccharidase deficiency. Hydrogen breath testing is diagnostic, but identifying and eliminating these dietary components is more practical.

Colonic motility remains the focus of diagnosis and therapy in IBS, in part due to the availability of the left colon to clinical investigation. That patients with IBS have hyperactivity of colonic smooth muscle compared to normals to a variety of stimulants is generally accepted. The bulk of research on dietary intervention has centered on dietary fiber and its effect on colonic motility and symptoms.

Dietary fiber consists of non-starch plant polysaccharides and lignin that are resistant to hydrolysis by the digestive enzymes of man. The non-starch polysaccharides include cellulose, hemicelluloses, gums, mucilages, and pectin. Dietary fiber may be classified on the basis of solubility in water. Structural fibers (lignins, cellulose, and some hemicelluloses) are insoluble. Sources, among others, include cereals and whole grains. Insoluble fiber is largely excreted undigested in the feces. In addition to increasing the dry weight of stool, the presence of fiber particles in the colon draws water into the lumen, increasing the wet weight as well.

Pectin, gums, mucilages, and most hemicelluloses constitute soluble fiber. They have natural viscosity of gel-forming qualities which prolong GI transit time and lubricate the stool. Soluble fiber sources, among others, include legumes, beans, and psyllium. Most soluble fiber undergoes fermentation by colonic bacteria, leading to bacterial proliferation and considerably adding to fecal bulk. The high-fiber diet works to increase volume and residue of the feces, increasing GI motor function in those patients in whom it was decreased and decreasing intraluminal colonic pressure in those patients in whom it was increased.

Controlled trials of fiber in IBS have met with both failure and success. Comparative evaluations are difficult due to the variations in study design and types of fiber used. The consumption of 20 g/d of fine wheat bran, compared to a low-fiber regime, offered symptomatic improvement in one study, measured by relief of pain, reduced mucous production, and improved bowel habits.[65] Another study demonstrated favorable symptomatic improvement using psyllium hydrophilic mucilloid.[66] Generally, patients whose symptoms are dominated by constipation benefit from the bulking effects of insoluble fiber. This may then be combined with quantities of soluble fiber sources titrated to the patient's specific symptoms. It is important to emphasize intake of adequate free liquids. In patients in whom diarrhea predominates, hydrophilic mucilloids (Metamucil™, Konsyl™) may add bulk and decelerate rapid intestinal transit, thereby reducing symptoms.

The quality and combination of fiber used needs to be tailored to the individual patient's symptoms. Bacterial fermentation of soluble fiber produces short-chain fatty acids, carbon dioxide, hydrogen, and other gases. The resultant increased gas and bloating may be unacceptable to some patients. When adjusting the dose of dietary fiber, begin with a low dose and gradually increase to the highest tolerated dose, or 20 to 25 g/d. Initial symptoms of increased bloating, distention, and gas are generally overcome within 2 weeks. Allow sufficient time to evaluate response to therapy when adjusting the combination and quantity of dietary fiber or fiber supplements.

XII. FISTULAS

Enterocutaneous fistulas most commonly occur after abdominal surgery. Other causes include Crohn's disease (with or without prior surgery), malignancy, and radiation. There are no prospective, randomized trials of nutritional therapy for fistulas. Considerations in management include anatomic location of the fistula, volume of drainage, fluid and electrolyte replenishment, concurrent malnutrition, and sepsis. Retrospective studies have supported claims that TPN lowers mortality and improves spontaneous healing. However, these results may be attributed to improved perisurgical care and infection control.[67]

With the institution of TPN, a decrease in fistula output is usually noted when accompanied by complete bowel rest. It is possible to manage some enterocutaneous fistulas with an elemental diet. The theoretic benefit of the latter is that it is easier to manage, safe, less expensive, and without the risks associated with TPN (catheter-associated sepsis, pneumothorax, and metabolic abnormalities). However, use of elemental diet may be thwarted by GI tract intolerance, diarrhea, or increased fistulous output. Most authorities agree that TPN is able to achieve full caloric and nitrogen replenishment more adequately.

Besides decreasing fistula output by decreasing intestinal stimulation, secondary gains of improved nutrition are also beneficial in wound-healing and resistance to infection.

Patients often require 4 to 8 weeks nutritional therapy before spontaneous closure occurs or before surgical repair is undertaken. Once the fistula has been demonstrated to be closed by radiographic fistulogram, an additional 7 days of parenteral nutrition is recommended before challenging the patient with an oral diet. The use of somatostatin analogues to decrease fistulous output appears to have markedly improved the clinician's ability to treat fistulas.[68]

XIII. CONCLUSIONS

Optimal nutrition is important in health and disease. Appropriate diet and coordinated function of gut, liver, and pancreas are required for adequate digestion and absorption. Diseases of the GI tract may result in general or specific nutritional deficiencies. In nearly all cases, nutritional therapy plays a supportive role in maintaining or improving nutritional status to increase chances of recovery. In some cases, nutritional therapy assumes a primary role, reducing symptoms or affecting remission. Parenteral nutrition generally can be administered safely; however, it is expensive and carries a variety of risks. Its use should be reserved for specific situations. When oral intake is inadequate or not feasible, administration of enteral formulas via a feeding tube is preferred.

REFERENCES

1. **Collins, PJ, Horowitz, M, Cook, DJ, Harding, PE, and Shearman, DJC.** Gastric emptying in normal subjects—a reproducible technique using a single scintillation camera and computer system. *Gut,* 24, 1417, 1983.
2. **Meyer, JH, Ohashi, H, Jehn, D, and Thomson, JB.** Size of liver particles emptied from the human stomach. *Gastroenterology,* 80, 1489, 1981.
3. **Crane, RK, Malathi, P, and Preiser, H.** Reconstitution of specific Na-dependent D-glucose transport in liposomes by Triton X-100 extracted proteins from purified brush border membranes of hamster small intestine. *Biochem Biophys Res Commun,* 71, 1010, 1976.
4. **Kergoat, MJ, Leclere, BS, Petit Clerc, C, and Imbach, A.** Discriminant biochemical markers for evaluating the nutritional status of elderly patients in long-term care. *Am J Clin Nutr,* 46, 849, 1987.
5. **Zaloga, GP and MacGregor, DA.** What to consider when choosing enteral or parenteral nutrition. *J Crit Illness,* 5, 1180, 1990.
6. **Guedon, C, Schmitz, J, Lerebours, E, Metayer, J, Audran, E, Hemet, J, and Colin, R.** Decreased brush border hydrolase activities without gross morphologic changes in human intestinal mucosa after prolonged total parenteral nutrition in adults. *Gastroenterology,* 90, 373, 1986.
7. **Biasco, G, Callegari, C, Lami, F, Minarini, A, Miglioli, M, and Barbara, L.** Intestinal morphologic changes during oral refeeding in a patient previously treated with total parenteral nutrition for short bowel resection. *Am J Gastroenterol,* 79, 585, 1984.
8. **Starzl, TE, Rowe, MI, Todo, S, Jaffe, R, Tzakis, A, Hoffman, AL, Esquivel, C, Porter, KA, Venkataramanen, R, Makowka, L, and Duquesnoy, R.** Transplantation of multiple small bowel viscera. *JAMA,* 261, 1449, 1989.
9. **Dudrick, SJ, Latifi, R, and Fosnocht, DE.** Management of the short bowel syndrome. *Surg Clin N Am,* 71, 625, 1991.
10. **Rombeau, JL and Rolandelli, RH.** Enteral and parenteral nutrition in patients with enteric fistulas and short bowel syndrome. *Surg Clin N Am,* 67, 551, 1987.
11. **Dudrick, SJ, O'Donnell, JJ, and Englert, DM.** Ambulatory home parenteral nutrition for short-bowel syndrome and other diseases, in *Nutrition in Clinical Surgery,* Deitel, M, Ed., Williams & Wilkins, Baltimore, 1985, 276.
12. **Allard, J and Jeejeebhoy, K.** Nutritional support and therapy in the short bowel syndrome. *Gastroenterol Clin N Am,* 18, 589, 1989.

13. **Richards, AJ, Condon, JR, and Mallinson, CN.** Lactose intolerance following extensive intestinal resection. *Br J Surg,* 59, 493, 1971.
14. **Deitel, M and Wong, KH.** Short bowel syndrome, in *Nutrition in Clinical Surgery,* Deitel, M, Ed., Williams & Wilkins, Baltimore, 1980, 189.
15. **Purdum, PP, III and Kirby, DF.** Short bowel syndrome: a review of the role of nutrition support. *JPEN,* 15, 93, 1991.
16. **Cortot, A, Fleming, CR, and Malagelada, JR.** Improved nutrient absorption after cimetadine in short bowel syndrome with gastric hypersecretion. *N Engl J Med,* 300, 79, 1979.
17. **McIntyre, PB.** The short bowel. *Br J Surg,* 72, S92, 1985.
18. **Butt, JH.** Outpatient management of inflammatory bowel disease. *Postgrad Med,* 92, 69, 1992.
19. **Dickinson, RJ, Ashton, MG, Axon, HTR, Smith, RC, Yeong, CK, and Hill, GL.** Controlled trial of intravenous hyperalimentation and total bowel rest as an adjunct to routine therapy of acute colitis. *Gastroenterology,* 79, 1199, 1980.
20. **González-Huix, F, Fernández-Banares, F, Esteve-Comas, M, Abad-Lacruz, A, Cabré, E, Acero, D, Figa, M, Guilera, M, Humbert, P, de León, R, and Gassul, MA.** Enteral vs. parenteral nutrition as adjunct therapy in acute ulcerative colitis. *Am J Gastroenterol,* 88, 227, 1993.
21. **Lipman, TO.** Efficacy and safety of total parenteral nutrition. *Nutrition,* 6, 319, 1990.
22. **Galandiuk, S, O'Neill, M, McDonald, P, Fazio, VW, and Steiger, E.** A century of home parenteral nutrition for Crohn's disease. *Am J Surg,* 159, 540, 1990.
23. **O'Morain, CA.** Does nutritional therapy in inflammatory bowel disease have a primary or adjunctive role? *Scand J Gastroenterol,* 25, S29, 1990.
24. **Teahon, K, Bjarnason, I, Pearson, M, and Levi, AJ.** Ten years experience with an elemental diet in the management of Crohn's disease. *Gut,* 31, 1133, 1990.
25. **Malchow, H, Steinhardt, HJ, Lorenz-Meyer, H, Strohm, WD, Rasmussen, S, Sommer, H, Jarnum, S, Brandes, JW, Leonhardt, H, Ewe, K, and Jesdinsky, H.** Feasibility and effectiveness of a defined formula diet regime in treating active Crohn's disease: ECCD study III. *Scand J Gastroenterol,* 25, 235, 1990.
26. **Lochs, H, Steinhart, HJ, Klaus-Wents, B, Zeitz, M, Vogelsang, H, Sommer, H, Fleig, WE, Bauer, P, Schirrmeister, J, and Malchow, H.** Comparison of enteral nutrition and drug treatment in active Crohn's disease: results of the ECCD study IV. *Gastroenterology,* 101, 881, 1991.
27. **Greenberg, GR.** Nutritional support in inflammatory bowel disease: current status and future directions. *Scand J Gastroenterol,* 27, S117, 1992.
28. **Kirby, DF, and Craig, RM.** The value of intensive nutritional support in pancreatitis. *JPEN,* 9, 353, 1985.
29. **Kelly, GA, and Nahrwold, DL.** Pancreatic secretion in response to an elemental diet and intravenous hyperalimentation. *Surg Gynecol Obstet,* 143, 87, 1976.
30. **Latifi, R, McIntosh, JK, and Dudrick, SJ.** Nutritional management of acute and chronic pancreatitis. *Surg Clin N Am,* 71, 579, 1991.
31. **Sax, HC, Warner, BW, Talamini, MA, Hamilton, FN, Bell, RH, Fischer, JE, and Bower, RH.** Early total parenteral nutrition in acute pancreatitis: lack of beneficial effects. *Am J Surg,* 153, 117, 1987.
32. **Marasnao, L, and McClain, CJ.** Nutrition and alcoholic liver disease. *JPEN,* 15, 337, 1991.
33. **Kerns, PJ, Young, H, Garcia, G, Blaschke, T, O'Hanlon, G, Rinki, M, Sucher, K, and Peter, G.** Accelerated improvement of alcoholic liver disease with enteral nutrition. *Gastroenterology,* 102, 200, 1992.
34. **Mendenhall, C, Bongiovanni, G, and Goldberg, S.** VA cooperative study on alcoholic hepatitis III: changes in protein-calorie malnutrition associated with 30 days of hospitalization with and without enteral nutritional therapy. *JPEN,* 9, 590, 1985.
35. **Shanbhoge, RLK.** Resting energy expenditure in patients with end-stage liver disease and in normal population. *JPEN,* 11, 305, 1987.
36. **Greenberg, NJ, Carley, J, and Schenker, S.** Effects of vegetable and animal protein diets in chronic active encephalopathy. *Am J Dig Dis,* 22, 845, 1977.
37. **Michel, H, Pomier-Layrargues, C, and Aubin, JP.** Treatment of acute hepatic encephalopathy in cirrhotics with branched-chain amino acid enriched versus a conventional amino acid mixture: a controlled study of 70 patients. *Liver,* 5, 282, 1985.
38. **Eriksson, LS, and Conn, HO.** Branched-chain amino acids in the management of hepatic encephalopathy: an analysis of varients. *Hepatology,* 10, 228, 1989.
39. **Naylor, CD, O'Rourke, K, Detsky, AS, and Baker, JP.** Parenteral nutrition with branched-chain amino acids in hepatic encephalopathy: a meta-analysis. *Gastroenterology,* 97, 1033, 1989.
40. **Painter, NS and Burkitt, DP.** Diverticular disease of the colon: a deficiency disease of western civilization. *Br Med J,* 2, 450, 1971.

41. **Gera, JSS, Ware, A, Fursdon, P, Nolan, PJ, Mann, JI, Brodribb, AJM, and Vessey, MP.** Symptomless diverticular disease and intake of dietary fiber. *Lancet,* 1, 511, 1979.
42. **Brodribb, AJM.** Treatment of symptomatic diverticular disease with a high-fiber diet. *Lancet,* 1, 664, 1977.
43. **Plumley, PE and Francis, B.** Dietary management of diverticular disease. *J Am Diet Assoc,* 63, 527, 1973.
44. **Hylan, JD and Taylor, I.** Diverticular disease—has its natural history been altered? *Gut,* 20, 441, 1979.
45. **Nicol, BM.** Peptic ulceration. Results of modern treatment. *Lancet,* 1, 466, 1942.
46. **Lawrence, JS.** Dietetic and other methods in the treatment of peptic ulcer. *Lancet,* 1, 482, 1952.
47. **Doll, R, Freidlander, P, and Pygott, F.** Dietetic treatment of peptic ulcer. *Lancet,* 1, 5, 1956.
48. **Kumar, N, Kumar, A, Broor, SL, Viji, JC, and Anand, BS.** Effect of milk on patients with duodenal ulcers. *Br Med J,* 293, 666, 1986.
49. **Segal, I, Walker, AR, and Vorster, HH.** Dietary factors associated with duodenal ulcer. *Gut,* 32, 456, 1991.
50. **Marotta, RB and Floch, MH.** Diet and nutrition in ulcer disease. *Med Clin N Am,* 75, 967, 1991.
51. **Sonnenberg, A.** Factors which influence the incidence and course of peptic ulcer. *Scand J Gastroenterol,* 155, 119, 1988.
52. **McArthur, K, Hogan, D, and Isenberg, J.** Relative stimulatory effects of commonly ingested beverages on gastric acid secretion in humans. *Gastroenterology,* 83, 199, 1982.
53. **Paffenbarger, RS, Wing, AL, and Hyde, RT.** Chronic disease in former college students. *Am J Epidemiol,* 100, 307, 1974.
54. **Kurata, JH, Nogawa, AN, Abbey, DE, and Petersen, F.** A prospective study of risk for peptic ulcer disease in Seventh-day adventists. *Gastroenterology,* 102, 902, 1992.
55. **Kumar, N, Viji, JC, Sarin, SK, and Anand, BS.** Do chilies influence healing of duodenal ulcer? *Br Med J,* 288, 1803, 1984.
56. **Way, LW.** Stomach and duodenum, in *Current Surgical Diagnosis and Treatment,* Dunphy, JE and Way, LW, Eds., Lange Medical Publications, Los Altos, 1981, 409.
57. **Eagon, JC, Miedema, BW, and Kelly, KA.** Postgastrectomy syndromes. *Surg Clin N. Am,* 72, 445, 1992.
58. **Sawyers, JL.** Management of postgastrectomy syndromes. *Am J Surg,* 159, 8, 1990.
59. **Machella, TE.** The mechanism or the post-gastrectomy ''dumping'' syndrome. *Ann Surg,* 130, 145, 1949.
60. **Scott, HW, Weidner, MG, Shull, HJ, and Bond, AG.** The dumping syndrome. II. further investigations of etiology in patients and experimental animals. *Gastroenterology,* 37, 194, 1959.
61. **Lamers, CB, Biljlstra, AB, and Harris, AG.** Octocreotide, a long-acting somatostatin analog, in the management of postoperative dumping syndrome. *Dig Dis Sci,* 38, 359, 1993.
62. **Jenkins, DJA, Glassell, MA, and Leeds, AR.** Effects of dietary fiber on complications of gastric surgery: prevention of postprandial hypoglycemia by pectin. *Gastroenterology,* 72, 215, 1977.
63. **Hopman, WPM, Houben, PG, Speth, PA, and Lamers, CB.** Glucomannan prevents post prandial hypoglycemia in patients with previous gastrectomy. *Gut,* 29, 930, 1988.
64. **Speth, PAJ, Jansen, JB, and Lamers, CB.** Effect of acarbose, pectin, a combination of acarbose and pectin, and placebo on postprandial reactive hypoglycemia after gastric surgery. *Gut,* 24, 789, 1983.
65. **Manning, AP, Heaton, KW, Harvey, RF, and Vglow, P.** Wheat fiber and irritable bowel syndrome. *Lancet,* 2, 417, 1977.
66. **Prior, A and Whorwell, PJ.** A double blind study of ispahula in irritable bowel syndrome. *Gut,* 28, 1510, 1987.
67. **Soeters, PB, Ebeid, AM, and Fischer, JE.** Review of 404 patients with gastrointestinal fistulas. *Ann Surg,* 190, 189, 1979.
68. **Torres, AJ, Landa, JI, Moreno-Azcoita, M. Argüello, J, Silecchia, G, Castro, J, Hernandez-Merlo, F, Jover, J, Moreno-Gonzales, IE, and Balibrea, J.** Somatostatin in the management of gastrointestinal fistulas: a multicenter trial. *Arch Surg,* 127, 97, 1992.

Chapter 5

NUTRITION AND THE IMMUNE SYSTEM

Daniel L. Dent, Bobbi Langkamp-Henken, and Kenneth A. Kudsk

TABLE OF CONTENTS

Severe malnutrition and specific nutrient deficiencies predispose individuals to infection. Only recently have clinicians had techniques to provide adequate quantities of nutrients to critically ill patients. These techniques of specialized nutrition support through enteral and parenteral feeding provide tools to study the impact of nutrient supplementation on patient outcome.[1] This chapter reviews systemic and mucosal immune system dynamics, specific nutrients which alter immune system function, and the clinical data substantiating the importance of nutrition on recovery of critically ill patients.

I. THE SYSTEMIC IMMUNE SYSTEM

The immune system protects the body by warding off infectious organisms while neutralizing host malignant and autoimmune cells. Meticulously regulated interactions between immune cells and mediating molecules keep this system in check to avoid harmful autoimmune reactions. Physiochemical barriers such as skin and mucous membranes, in conjunction with nonspecific inflammation and phagocytosis, neutralize potential pathogens without eliciting a specific pathogen-directed immune response.

The immune system also provides specific immunity selectively to neutralize antigens recognized as foreign to the host. The immune system dramatically amplifies and directs the immune response to an invading pathogen and subsequently remembers the antigen it encounters for future recognition, facilitating more efficient immune responses. Although natural and specific immunity are described independently, maintenance of proper immunity requires the simultaneous function and interaction of both systems.[2]

A. NATURAL IMMUNITY

The natural immune system consists of primary and secondary defenses. Skin and mucous membranes serve as the primary defense by providing a physiochemical barrier to most microbes. Macrophages and granulocytes, the secondary defense, generate an acute inflammatory response nonspecifically to neutralize and ingest invading material.

Granulocytes are white blood cells important in inflammation and natural immunity. These cells derive their name from the staining characteristics of their abundant cytoplasmic granules. Polymorphonuclear leukocytes, or neutrophils, the most numerous of the granulocytes, characterize the acute inflammatory response and, when activated, eliminate pathogens through phagocytosis. Following local tissue damage, neutrophils respond rapidly to the release of inflammatory mediators including cytokines, complement proteins, and eicosanoids (products of fatty acid metabolism consisting of leukotrienes, thromboxanes, prostacyclins, and prostaglandins). These mediators further enhance the acute inflammatory response by increasing the local accumulation of acute-phase proteins, including albumin and C-reactive protein, and by increasing vascular permeability to facilitate neutrophil infiltration.[3] Neutrophils and macrophages then engulf, or phagocytose, necrotic debris and foreign substances, including pathogenic microorganisms. Nonspecific elimination by phagocytosis is potentiated when immunoglobulins and complement proteins coat invading microorganisms.[4,5]

In addition to neutrophils, other types of granulocytes have immune roles. Eosinophils express receptors for IgE antibodies and are important in the immune response to parasitic infections and allergic reactions. Basophils, the third type of granulocyte, also express IgE receptors and are involved in allergic reactions. Mast cells are not granulocytes, but are granule-containing cells found mainly in the skin and mucous membranes. Mast cells become active when stimulated by IgE antibodies and are, therefore, also actively involved in allergic reactions.[6,7]

The complement system, which consists of a group of at least 25 proteins, plays an important role in natural immunity. Complement proteins bind directly to the surface of a pathogen and activate the complement system. When activated, complement proteins are capable of cytolysis, further activation of inflammatory responses, and opsonization (binding and promotion of phagocytosis) of foreign particles. Complement is one of many immune components active in both natural and specific immunity. In specific immunity, antigen-antibody complexes efficiently activate the complement system.[8,9]

Like complement, macrophages function in both natural and specific immunity. These cells originate from bone marrow as monocytes and settle in all organs and connective tissues to mature into tissue-specific macrophages such as the Kupffer cells of the liver, alveolar macrophages of the lung, and epithelioid cells of the skin. Macrophages become activated as part of the nonspecific inflammatory response and serve, along with neutrophils, as phagocytic effector cells of the natural immune system.[6,7] The role of macrophages in specific immunity will be described later.

In summary, physical barriers protect the host internal environment from external pathogens. Disruption of these barriers elicits a nonspecific acute inflammatory response. This response is mediated by components of the immune system that also participate in the specific immune response when appropriately stimulated and regulated.

B. SPECIFIC IMMUNITY

The specific immune system focuses the immune response on a specific foreign substance or antigen. Antigen-specific amplification and memory are two hallmarks of a specific immune response. Once an antigen is defined, the immune system amplifies the response to facilitate efficient elimination of the specific antigenic material. As the immune response is amplified, clonal memory cells are "set aside" for future antigen recognition.

The specific immune system functions through cell-mediated or humoral (antibody-mediated) immunity depending upon the effector component of the immune response. Maintenance of cell-mediated and humoral immunity requires complex communication between cells. This communication is accomplished through direct cell-cell surface molecule interaction and through cytokines, secreted immune regulatory proteins. For example, macrophages initiate the specific immune response by presenting antigen to T cells, providing co-stimulatory activity, and secreting interleukin-1 (IL-1), a T lymphocyte stimulatory cytokine (see Figure 1).[6,7]

Macrophages present antigen and activate T cells in the context of major histocompatibility complex (MHC) proteins. After macrophage antigen presentation, T lymphocytes largely direct the immune response and enhance macrophage phagocytosis.[6,7] T lymphocytes originate in the bone marrow but mature in the thymus gland. T cells contain surface receptors which only recognize antigens presented in conjunction with MHC protein found on the surface of macrophages and other antigen-presenting cells. Like other hemopoietic cells, T lymphocytes are classified under the cluster of differentiation (CD) nomenclature. Helper or inducer T cells (CD4$^+$) are induced by antigenic stimulation and IL-1 to increase expression of interleukin-2 (IL-2) receptors and to produce IL-2 and other cell growth and differentiation cytokines. This T cell activation dramatically amplifies the immune response. Activated cytotoxic T lymphocytes (CD8$^+$) are capable of lysing cells which express foreign antigens.[3,6,10]

T cell activation of B lymphocytes is important for amplification and memory of the specific immune response. B lymphocytes undergo early maturation in the bone marrow and are characterized by surface immunoglobulin or antibodies. These cells are the only cells in the body that produce antibodies. T cell-secreted cytokines stimulate clonal proliferation among B and T lymphocytes. When the surface immunoglobulin binds an antigen, the B cell, with the help of CD4$^+$ T cells and their cytokines, differentiates into a plasma cell which actively secretes antibody. A subpopulation of B cells becomes memory

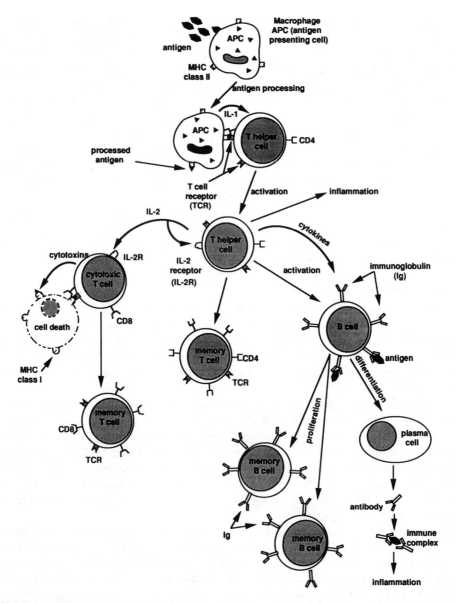

FIGURE 1. Schematic representation of cells involved in specific immunity (see text for explanation). (Adapted from Goodman J. W. *Basic and Clinical Immunology,* 7th ed. Stites, D. P. and Terr, A. I. Eds., Appleton and Lange, 1991, 36. With permission.)

cells when appropriately stimulated. These memory B cells in conjunction with memory T cells "remember" specific antigens and facilitate a more efficient immune response in repeated antigenic challenge.[6,10]

Activated B cells produce antibodies which mediate humoral immunity. Each antibody molecule possesses a specific antigen-binding site, and every human has at least 10 million different antibody molecules with unique antigen-binding sites. This diversity allows for a specific immune response to a vast number of different antigens.[11]

Antibodies are divided into classes based on structural differences which have functional significance. The five classes of antibodies in man are IgA, IgD, IgE, IgG, and IgM. IgA antibodies are dimeric, consisting of two linked antibody units, each with its own antigen-binding site. These molecules are transported to mucosal sites, including lactating breast tissue, and play a role in mucosal and neonatal immunity. IgG constitutes the majority of serum immunoglobulin. IgG crosses the placenta and is found in breast milk, thus providing fetal and neonatal immunity. IgM is usually formed in the initial response to antigenic stimulation and is found as a pentamer. IgM is the most efficient complement-activating antibody, but both IgM and IgG easily activate the complement system to enhance bacterial neutralization. IgE is largely involved in allergic or hypersensitivity reactions.[11]

While antibodies are important immune effector molecules, cytokines are the regulatory molecules of the immune response. Cytokines may stimulate distant cells in an endocrine manner, but usually act on the local immune system (paracrine effect) or directly on the cytokine-producing cell (autocrine effect). At least 17 cytokines have been identified, but the 6 most relevant to the topic of nutrition and immunity are IL-1, IL-2, tumor necrosis factor (TNF), transforming growth factor-beta (TGF-β), gamma interferon (IFN-γ), and interleukin-6 (IL-6).

IL-1 is produced by many cells, but the primary source is activated mononuclear phagocytes. In large quantities, IL-1 produces systemic effects including induction of acute-phase plasma protein synthesis by the liver, initiation of hypermetabolism, and production of fever. IL-1 enhances the proliferation of CD4$^+$ T cells and the growth and differentiation of B cells. IL-1 also augments the inflammatory response through its action on vascular endothelium and mononuclear phagocytes, thereby enhancing coagulation and further cytokine synthesis.[2,3,12,13]

IL-2 is largely produced by CD4$^+$ T cells, with CD8$^+$ T cells being a lesser source. IL-2 binds to receptors on T-cell surfaces, stimulating cell growth and further cytokine production. At high concentration IL-2 acts on natural killer (NK) cells to enhance growth and cytolytic function and on B cells to stimulate growth and antibody production. The net result of IL-2 stimulation is the production of T- and B-cell clones specific to the initiating antigen.[2,3,12,13]

Activated macrophages and a variety of other immune system cells produce TNF which is the major mediator of the host response to bacterial challenge. TNF generates local and systemic effects similar to IL-1. However, the administration of systemic TNF to animals at concentrations found in bacterial sepsis results in a septic shock-like syndrome and death from circulatory collapse. Just prior to death, myocardial contractility and vascular tone are reduced and severe metabolic disturbances are observed.[3,12,13]

The specific roles of TGF-β, IFN-γ, and IL-6 are less well understood. TGF-β is produced by many immune cells and largely inhibits lymphocyte responses but, under certain conditions, also acts as a stimulatory molecule. It appears to be important in mucosal immunity, as it stimulates B cells to produce IgA antibodies. IFN-γ is produced by T cells and, to a lesser extent, by NK cells. It is the primary macrophage-activating factor and is capable of stimulating virtually all immune cells and endothelial cells. IL-6 is produced by a variety of immune cells in response to IL-1 and TNF and is the principal growth factor for B cells late in the process of growth and differentiation. Additionally, IL-6 stimulates hepatocytes to synthesize fibrinogen and other plasma proteins that contribute to the acute-phase response.[12,13]

Two other cell types important to immune function are dendritic cells and NK cells. Dendritic cells process and present antigen; thus, they can initiate an immune response. NK cells are large granular lymphocytes which do not express T- or B-cell surface markers. The numerous cytoplasmic granules within NK cells play a role in tumor- and virus-infected cell lysis. Such target cell lysis by NK cells is part of natural immunity. However, NK cells function in specific immunity as well, by recognizing and killing IgG-coated target cells.[14]

The effector phases of natural and specific immunity are similar. However, through cytokine regulation and cell-cell stimulation, the effector phase of specific immunity is amplified and focused on elimination of the specific inciting antigen. Activated CD8[+] T cells and NK cells lyse cells with foreign surface antigens. Antibody and complement act as opsonins to enhance the elimination of foreign substances through phagocytosis by macrophages and neutrophils. Additionally, complement-mediated cell lysis is initiated in two ways. Antigen-antibody complexes activate the complement system or, as in natural immunity, foreign cells may directly activate complement proteins.[8,14]

In summary, a variety of cells and modulating proteins contribute to the specific immune response. This response is initiated by antigen presentation to CD4[+] T cells. In turn, CD4[+] T cells proliferate and aid in the activation of B cells and cytotoxic T cells. Specific antigen elimination is accomplished by cytolysis mediated by CD8[+] T cells, NK cells, or complement or by phagocytosis enhanced by opsonization. Memory T and B cells generated during the immune response facilitate future antigen recognition and elimination (see Figure 1).

II. GUT-ASSOCIATED LYMPHOID TISSUE (GALT)

The components of the systemic immune system also function locally in mucosal immunity. The rich bacterial flora of the GI tract necessitate active mucosal immunity to provide continuous protection without invoking a systemic immune response. To carry out this protective function, the GI tract contains 70 to 80% of all immunoglobulin-secreting cells and is, therefore, the richest lymphoid tissue in the body.[15]

The aggregated and non-aggregated lymphoid tissue within the intestinal wall compose the gut-associated lymphoid tissue (GALT). The aggregated components of GALT consist of organized lymphoid follicles (i.e., Peyer's patches, lymphoid aggregates in the appendix) and lymphoid nodules. Peyer's patches are found within the human small intestine, while lymphoid nodules are found scattered throughout the small and large intestine. Lamina propria lymphoid cells and intraepithelial lymphocytes compose the nonaggregated lymphoid tissue. CD4[+] T cells and IgA-secreting plasma cells populate the lamina propria, whereas CD8[+] T cells predominantly populate the intraepithelium.[16] Additionally, mucosal mast cells, intestinal macrophages, and dendritic cells are found interspersed within the vascular and lymphatic-rich lamina propria of the intestine (see Figure 2).[17]

The mucosal immune system protects the body from invading enteric microbes. The protective process is initiated by antigen uptake and presentation within the Peyer's patches. Activated T and B cells migrate from the Peyer's patches through the lymph to the systemic circulation and extravasate mainly into the intestinal mucosa. These activated cells also migrate into other mucosal tissues within the body including lactating breast tissue,[18-20] bronchial tissue, salivary glands, and the female genital tract (Figure 3).[21-24] Once within these sites, B cells differentiate into plasma cells and secrete IgA. Each process involved in mucosal antigen sampling, presentation, and processing will now be discussed in further detail.

Within the Peyer's patch, circulating B and T cells compartmentalize into three distinct regions, the follicles, the dome, and the thymus-dependent area between follicles.[25] The B cells enter the follicles, while T lymphocytes enter the interfollicular and above-dome regions.[26] The dome region is rich in plasma cells and antigen-presenting cells, i.e. macrophages and dendritic cells.[27-29] From between villi, the domed surface of the Peyer's patch protrudes into the intestinal lumen, allowing luminal contents to be sampled by specialized membranous (M) cells interspersed among the columnar epithelial cells of the dome.[27,30]

M cells, which lack regular microvilli on the luminal surface,[31] form thin bridges of cytoplasm that allow lymphocytes and macrophages in the extracellular space to approach within 0.3 μm of the intestinal lumen.[16] M cells endocytose, transport, and release antigens

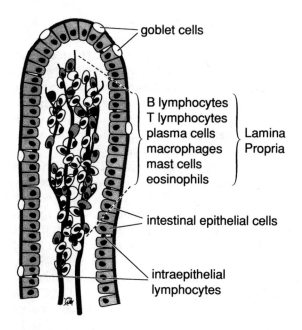

FIGURE 2. Diagrammatic representation of immunologically active cells within the intestinal villus. (From Langkamp-Henken, B., Glezer, J. A., and Kudsk, K. A., *Nutr Clin Pract*, 7, 100, 1992. With permission.)

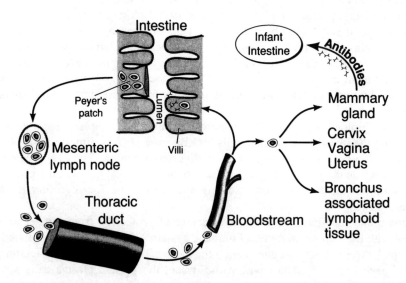

FIGURE 3. Migration pathway of GALT lymphocytes (see text for explanation). (From Langkamp-Henken, B., Glezer, J. A., and Kudsk, K. A., *Nutr Clin Pract*, 7, 100, 1992. With permission.)

into the extracellular space within the Peyer's patches.[30-33] Dendritic cells and macrophages process and present the antigen to CD4[+] T helper lymphocytes. These activated helper T cells direct the development of B cells and induce an isotype switch within the B cells, i.e., transforming IgM lymphocytes into IgA-bearing cells. TGF-β, secreted by T cells and/or macrophages, preferentially induces this switch to IgA.[34,35] Interleukin-5 acts as a maturation factor inducing the differentiation of IgA[+] B cells into IgA-secreting plasma cells.[34] Many other cytokines are nonspecifically involved in the processes of differentiation and proliferation of mucosal T and B lymphocytes.

Activated T cells and newly switched IgA-specific B cells leave the Peyer's patch via the mesenteric lymph nodes, enter the systemic circulation by way of the thoracic duct, and travel to the intestinal lamina propria (see Figure 3). This recirculation of lymphocytes is controlled by the binding of adhesion molecules on lymphocytes to specialized venules (high endothelial venules) in the mucosal lamina propria. Upregulation of lymphocyte adhesion molecules is controlled by antigenic activation.[36] After entering the mucosal lamina propria, a majority of CD8+ T cells migrate into the villous epithelium where they are thought to mediate oral tolerance to food antigens.[16] Within the lamina propria, T-cell dependent B-cell terminal differentiation occurs.[37]

The newly differentiated B lymphocytes (plasma cells) begin to secrete IgA. Although a majority of the IgA is secreted into the intestinal lumen, some enters the portal, lymphatic, and systemic circulations.[38] The dimeric form of IgA secreted into the intestinal lumen, saliva, and breast milk differs from monomeric serum IgA. These structural differences may be due to their different origins.[17] Secretory IgA (sIgA) is composed of two monomer subunits of IgA, a J chain, and a secretory component. The J chain and IgA are synthesized by the plasma cells within the lamina propria.[38] The secretory component, which serves as a membrane receptor for dimeric IgA, originates as a transmembrane protein on the basal and lateral plasma membrane of luminal epithelial cells.[39] Once IgA binds the secretory component, both are taken up into the cell and are transported to the apical surface of the epithelial cell. The dimeric IgA, still covalently coupled to the secretory component, is secreted into the lumen of the intestine as sIgA.[40] The structure of sIgA allows it to function in the proteolytic enzyme-rich intestinal lumen.[41]

Secretion of IgA is regulated by the expression of IgA receptors, i.e., secretory components.[42] Cytokines secreted by activated T cells and macrophages within the lamina propria upregulate the secretory component and, therefore, luminal secretion of IgA.[17] The physiologic role of IgA is still unclear. Unlike IgG and IgM, sIgA has limited ability to fix complement and opsonize bacteria.[38] Since the intestinal mucosa is in continual contact with luminal antigens, this relative inability to activate mucosal inflammation is an asset to the body.

The prime biologic function of sIgA is to prevent microorganisms from attaching to and invading the intestinal epithelial cells.[43,44] Because sIgA is dimeric, it has four sites available to bind luminal pathogens or undigested proteins. These aggregations are thought to impede the passage of antigens across the intestinal mucosa, thereby retaining them within the mucus coat and allowing increased time for digestion by luminal proteases.[45,46]

An additional function of sIgA is the transfer of protection from mother to nursing infant through the "common mucosal immune system". Lymphocytes stimulated by antigenic uptake from Peyer's patches within the mother's intestine home to lactating breast tissue[18–20] (see Figure 3). Once within the tissue, the primed plasma cells synthesize significant amounts of IgA.[20]

In summary, the GI tract is one of the richest lymphoid tissues in the body. Luminal antigens presented to GALT immune cells initiate a sequence of events leading to the migration of antigen-specific B and T cells to mucosal surfaces. Within the lamina propria, plasma cells produce sIgA, the primary antibody of mucosal secretions. These processes maintain optimal host defense against enteric pathogens without activating the powerful mediators involved in systemic immune responses.

III. NUTRIENT DEFICIENCIES AND IMMUNITY

The association between malnutrition and infection has long been recognized. For example, risk of death from infection is higher in severely malnourished infants. Of equal importance, infection often negatively affects nutritional status by increasing metabolic demands while decreasing nutrient intake and absorption. However, some infectious diseases (e.g., yellow fever and poliomyelitis) do not appear to be adversely influenced by malnutrition. Historically, because of the complexity of the relationship between infection and malnutrition and because single nutrient deficiencies are relatively rare, the influence of specific nutrients on immune function has been obscured. However, by using animal models, *in situ* techniques, and occasional clinical studies, researchers have begun to understand some of the immunologic implications of a variety of nutrients.[47]

A. PROTEIN-CALORIE MALNUTRITION

Protein-calorie malnutrition (PCM) produces defects in both cellular and humoral immunity. PCM reduces thymic size, delayed cutaneous hypersensitivity responses, NK cell activity, and the number of CD4$^+$ helper T cells.[47-49] Additionally, PCM alters migration of mucosal lymphocytes[50] and affects the complement system by decreasing complement C3 and factor B levels and complement hemolytic activity.[47] One clinical manifestation of altered immune function due to PCM is a decrease in nasopharyngeal secretory IgA levels in response to vaccination.[47,51] Specifically, the immune response to poliovirus vaccine does not produce adequate titers in these patients.[51]

B. VITAMIN A AND CAROTENOIDS

Vitamin A deficiency produces growth retardation and increases susceptibility to infection. Specifically, vitamin A deficiency reduces thymic weight, decreases *in vitro* lymphocyte proliferation, and enhances bacterial binding to respiratory epithelium.[52-54] Vitamin A deficiency, compounded by PCM, significantly alters migration of mesenteric lymphocytes to the intestinal lamina propria.[50] Supplementation with vitamin A or with carotenoids including beta-carotene, a vitamin A precursor, reverses the effects of vitamin A deficiency.[54-56] Recent evidence suggests an immunoregulatory role for carotenoids independent of vitamin A activity.[55,57,58]

C. VITAMIN B$_6$

Vitamin B$_6$ deficiency produces profound immune changes in animals including depression of *in vitro* proliferation of both B and T lymphocytes, impairment of delayed cutaneous hypersensitivity reactions, reduction of T lymphocyte cytotoxicity, delayed rejection of allografts, and inhibition of antibody response to immunization.[57,59-62] The elderly tend to be at greater risk for vitamin B$_6$ deficiency, and when such a deficiency is experimentally induced in previously healthy elderly subjects, changes in immune function include diminished IL-2 production.[60,61,63]

D. VITAMIN C

Controversy surrounds the role of vitamin C in immunity. The immune effects of its antioxidant properties are not yet completely understood. Deficiency of vitamin C impairs neutrophil and macrophage locomotion and bactericidal activity.[57,64,65]

E. VITAMIN D

Vitamin D deficiency impairs immunity in guinea pigs infected with *Mycobacterium tuberculosis*. Vitamin D-deficient mice and humans exhibit diminished macrophage function. Calcitriol, the active vitamin D metabolite, induces TNF production and antigen receptor expression in macrophages.[66]

F. VITAMIN E

Vitamin E deficiency impairs T cell function.[52,57,65,67,68] Supplementation of 2 to 10 times the recommended amount of vitamin E improves natural and specific immunity in animals and humans in a variety of studies.[63,67,69] Vitamin E supplementation particularly benefits the elderly who are at greater risk for nutrition-related immune dysfunction.[63,65] The use of vitamin E as an adjuvant to vaccination is currently being investigated in animals and has shown some promising results.[69] It should be noted that, while it is likely that optimal immune function is maintained at vitamin E doses significantly higher than currently recommended, extremely high levels of vitamin E produce immune dysfunction.[67,70]

G. SELENIUM

Lymphocyte proliferation decreases with selenium deficiency and reverses with correction of the deficiency. Selenium supplementation to above normal levels stimulates lymphocyte proliferation even further and improves lymphocyte tumor cell cytotoxicity. However, supplementation to extremely high concentrations inhibits cytotoxic function.[71–73] These immune effects are likely the result of modulation of the selenium-dependent enzymes, glutathione peroxidase and phospholipid hydroperoxide glutathione peroxidase.[74]

H. ZINC

Zinc deficiency increases susceptibility to a variety of infectious diseases. Specifically, zinc deficiency reduces thymulin activity, proliferation of lymphocytes, delayed cutaneous hypersensitivity, and neutrophil chemotaxis. Zinc deficiency produces atrophy of the cortical areas of the thymus and the thymus-dependent areas of the spleen and lymph nodes. Zinc supplementation in humans reverses the impaired NK cell cytotoxicity found in patients with sickle cell disease. However, oversupplementation with zinc reduces lymphocyte proliferation and decreases chemotactic and phagocytic activities.[52,63,75–79]

I. COPPER

Dietary copper deficiency also impairs immune function. In mice, low copper diets impair neutrophil and macrophage function, antibody production, and lymphocyte reaction to both T and B cell mitogens.[52,57,79–83] Copper deficiency also alters mouse cytokine production.[80]

J. IRON

The influence of iron on immunity has been controversial since early research suggested that iron was a necessary nutrient for growth of many microorganisms and that repletion to the point of overload was associated with increased incidence of infection.[52,53,57,79,84] However, we now know that prevention of iron deficiency in children reduces the incidence of infection. Iron deficiency is associated with reduced antibody and IL-1 production in response to antigenic challenge, diminished NK cell activity, and impaired lymphocyte blastogenesis. Because iron deficiency remains the most prevalent nutrient deficiency worldwide in children and women of reproductive age, the impact of immune dysfunction associated with iron deficiency is vast.[53,57,79,84,85]

IV. NUTRITIONAL IMMUNOMODULATION

Infection is the most frequent life-threatening complication in severe illness. Sepsis induces a hypermetabolic state which can worsen nutritional status. One goal of nutritional support is the maintenance of normal immune function in the critically ill, but simply preventing nutrient deficiency and meeting protein and energy needs may not achieve this goal. To maximize immune function, it may be necessary to supplement nutrient formulas with immune-enhancing components that meet the special metabolic needs of the critically ill patient. Current animal and clinical research focuses on nutrient formulas supplemented with specific triglycerides, amino acids, and nucleotides.

A. LIPIDS

Traditionally, nutritional supplements have contained triglycerides which are rich in long-chain (C14 to C24) omega-6 fatty acids including linoleic acid. Such supplementation prevents fatty acid deficiency, facilitates absorption of fat-soluble vitamins, provides concentrated calories, and minimizes hyperglycemia associated with nutritional support.[86,87] However, long-chain omega-6 triglycerides produce immunosuppressive effects when administered in quantities which significantly exceed the amount necessary to prevent fatty acid deficiency.[88] Omega-6 fatty acids are precursors for 2-series prostanoids (prostaglandins, prostacyclins, and thromboxanes) and 4-series leukotrienes. These molecules are potent inducers of vasoconstriction and platelet aggregation. Administration of long-chain omega-6 triglycerides inhibits cytotoxic T lymphocyte function,[89] cytokine secretion,[90,91] leukocyte migration,[92] and *in vitro* complement synthesis.[93] Intravenous infusion of long-chain triglyceride emulsions[94–98] impairs the function of the fixed mononuclear phagocyte cell system or reticuloendothelial system. In addition, long-chain omega-6 polyunsaturated fatty acids enhance transplant immunosuppression therapy resulting in improved graft survival in animals and humans.[99,100] The immunosuppressive effects of omega-6 long-chain fatty acids have stimulated a search for alternate lipid sources, such as omega-3 fatty acids, medium-chain triglycerides, structured lipids, and short-chain fatty acids.

Omega-3 fatty acids are found in high concentrations in the brain and retina. Provision of 0.5% to 0.6% of the total caloric intake in the form of alpha-linolenic acid (an 18 carbon omega-3 fatty acid) prevents deficiency and resultant visual and neurologic deficits.[87] Omega-3 fatty acids compete with omega-6 fatty acids for the enzymes cyclooxygenase and lipoxygenase and are the precursors of 3-series prostanoids and 5-series leukotrienes. These compounds are less inflammatory and immunosuppressive than eicosanoids derived from omega-6 fatty acids.[101] This is believed to be the mechanism by which dietary fish oils, rich in omega-3 fatty acids, enhance immune function in a variety of animal and human clinical trials. Omega-3 supplements improve the outcome and metabolic state of guinea pigs in endotoxin, burn, and experimental peritonitis models.[102–106] Fish oil supplements also suppress autoimmune disease in mouse lupus and nephritis models.[107–109] In clinical trials fish oil supplementation improves symptoms of atopic dermatitis, psoriasis, and rheumatoid arthritis.[110–113] Renal vascular resistance and mean arterial blood pressure is reduced in renal transplant patients receiving cyclosporine when randomized to fish oil rather than corn oil (rich in omega-6 fatty acids) supplementation. Pretherapy values also improved with fish oil treatment.[114] These findings suggest a potential role for fish oil in prevention and/or treatment regimens in a wide variety of conditions which alter immune function.

The addition of medium-chain triglycerides to parenteral and enteral nutrition has been investigated in an effort to prevent mononuclear phagocyte system dysfunction associated with long-chain triglyceride infusions. Because medium-chain triglycerides (C6 to C12) are easily absorbed without bile or pancreatic lipase, they have been used for many years to provide oral nutrition in patients with malabsorption and maldigestion syndromes. Medium-chain triglycerides derived from palm kernel or coconut oils provide no essential fatty acids and are quickly oxidized to ketone bodies. Unlike long-chain triglycerides, medium-chain triglycerides do not accumulate in the liver or adipose tissue. Infusions of mixtures of long- and medium-chain triglycerides result in lower bilirubin levels and better mononuclear phagocyte function in animal models and in humans requiring

TPN.[115-122] This improvement in mononuclear phagocyte function correlates with decreased pulmonary sequestration of bacteria in animal models.[115]

Structured lipids were designed in an attempt to provide essential fatty acids while minimizing the immunosuppressive effects of long-chain fatty acid infusion. Structured lipids are chemically synthesized by transesterification of medium- and long-chain triglycerides in a specified molar ratio which produces a rearranged triglyceride with a medium-chain fatty acid and essential long-chain fatty acids on the same glycerol molecule. Structured lipids appear to serve as a more efficient fuel than similar physical mixtures of unstructured triglycerides.[87,123,124] The effect of structured lipids on immune function remains to be seen.

Short-chain (C2 to C4) fatty acids are also being investigated as a possible energy supplement in enteral and parenteral formulas. Like medium-chain triglycerides, short-chain fatty acids provide a readily available energy source without immunosuppressive effects. In fact, short-chain fatty acids are the preferred energy source for colonic mucosa.[125] Intracolonic or i.v. infusion of short-chain fatty acids in rats promotes healing of colonic anastomoses and diminishes small intestine mucosal atrophy associated with lack of enteral nutrition.[126,127] In addition, short-chain fatty acid-supplemented TPN reduces mucosal atrophy following massive small bowel resection in rats.[128]

Thus, lipid supplementation prevents essential fatty acid deficiency in the patient who requires nutritional support. However, large amounts of omega-6 long-chain fatty acids increase immunosuppressive prostanoids and leukotrienes and diminish bacterial clearance by the mononuclear phagocyte system. A lipid formula derived from a combination of sources will likely provide optimal immune function, but it is unlikely that any one lipid formula will prove to be best for all clinical situations. Currently, much research is devoted to understanding the proper amount and type of lipid supplementation for a variety of disease states.

B. ARGININE

Traditionally, arginine has been considered a nonessential amino acid, although arginine depletion diminishes wound healing and Kupffer cell immune function.[129,130] Recently, investigators have shown that arginine supplementation enhances wound healing in traumatized rats.[130-134] Arginine also enhances immune function in animals and humans by increasing thymic size and cellularity, augmenting lymphocyte proliferation in response to mitogen and alloantigen, improving macrophage and NK cell function, and enhancing lymphocyte IL-2 production and receptor activity.[135-139] Arginine improves survival in some, but not all, animal models of sepsis.[132,140,141]

C. NUCLEOTIDES

Dietary nucleotides are also being investigated for their immunomodulatory effects. Deprivation of dietary nucleotides suppresses normal immunity in a mouse model.[142-144] Mice maintained on nucleotide-free diets have diminished macrophage phagocytic activity which is restored by supplementation with adenine, uracil, or RNA.[145] Replenishing nucleotides in nucleotide-deprived animals improves T-cell function and *in vitro* IL-2 expression.[144,146] It is interesting to note that *in vitro* IL-2 expression is maintained better by supplementation with RNA than by uracil or adenine. Nucleotide-free diets adversely affect survival in mouse models challenged with *Staphylococcus aureus* and *Candida albicans*.[145,147] RNA supplementation prior to starvation results in improved T-cell function when compared to non-supplemented and chow-fed controls. However, the chow-fed control and the RNA-supplemented groups consumed a similar amount of nucleotide. It is possible that the differences seen in the RNA-supplemented animals were due to the less complex dietary composition and decreased amount of animal fats in their feedings.[148]

In addition, spleen cells taken from mice fed a nucleotide-free diet showed decreased production of IL-3, thereby diminishing the ability to proliferate bone marrow stem cells. The same animals also showed diminished levels of adenosine deaminase and purine nucleotide phosphorylase in the popliteal lymph nodes. This correlated strongly with immunosuppression in response to antigen stimulation. The changes seen in the spleno-cytes and popliteal lymph nodes were reversed by RNA supplementation.[149] These data suggest a critical role for dietary nucleotides in maintenance of normal immune function. Clinical trials with dietary nucleotide supplementation are currently ongoing.

D. GLUTAMINE

Depressed glutamine levels *in vitro*[150] and *in vivo*[151,152] alter immune function. When glutamine levels are reduced in culture medium, human lymphocyte proliferation and mouse macrophage phagocytosis are inhibited in a dose-dependent manner.[150] Adminis-tration of standard glutamine-deficient parenteral feedings decreases the number of IgA-producing lymphocytes within the intestinal lamina propria as well as the amount of IgA within rodent biliary secretions. The addition of glutamine to these feedings prevents the immunologic changes.[151,152] Glutamine supplementation may enhance immune function in patient populations at risk for diminished plasma glutamine levels, i.e., patients with major burn injuries[150] or those receiving standard glutamine-deficient parenteral feedings.

V. CLINICAL STUDIES AND CONCLUSION

While it appears that malnutrition increases susceptibility to infection, it is clear that just the administration of nutrient formulas to hospitalized patients is not in itself sufficient to reduce septic complications. This was most convincingly demonstrated in the recently published VA Cooperative Study[153] where 395 malnourished patients were randomized to early operation vs. 7 to 10 d of aggressive preoperative i.v. nutrition. Not only was there no improvement in major non-infectious complications with perioperative nutrition at 85% of calculated nutrient goals, there was also a significant increase in major infec-tious complications in patients given TPN. When stratified by degree of malnutrition, major infectious complications were greater in TPN patients. Only in the presence of severe malnutrition was perioperative TPN beneficial in reducing major non-infectious complications.

Clinically, route of nutrient administration appears to be an important factor in im-proving host defense. Alexander et al.[154] first noted decreased septic morbidity and a higher survival rate in burned children randomized to a protein-enriched enteral diet com-pared to a standard enteral diet. They proposed that either the quality or the quantity of enteral protein positively influenced outcome following burn injury. Subsequently, Kudsk et al.[155,156] found a significantly lower mortality rate when uninjured malnourished or well-nourished rats were randomized to enteral rather than intravenous administration of a standard TPN solution and then subjected to a septic challenge. Applying these data to a select group of trauma victims at increased risk of septic complications, Moore et al.[157] noted a significantly lower intra-abdominal abscess rate in patients randomized to early enteral (via operatively placed feeding jejunostomy) vs. delayed feeding. Subsequently, the same group[158] confirmed a lower incidence of pneumonia in a select population of trauma patients randomized to early enteral vs. early parenteral feeding. In both of these trauma studies, patients with very severe injuries, excessive blood loss, or the need for reoperation were excluded.

Most recently, Kudsk et al.[159] defined the importance of route of nutrient administration and septic complications in severely injured trauma patients by including patients with very severe injuries, massive hemorrhage, and the need for reoperation in a randomized trial of early enteral vs. early parenteral feeding. Significantly fewer pneumonias, abscesses, and episodes of line sepsis occurred in patients randomized to early enteral feeding. Significant differences were present in the most severely injured patient population with injury severity scores greater than 20, and abdominal trauma indices greater than 24, or both. Patients fed enterally following blunt or penetrating trauma clearly experienced a lower incidence of septic morbidity with a majority of these significant changes occurring in the most severely injured patient population.

Administration of early enteral feeding following injury appears to be an important factor although the ideal timing of early enteral feeding which will provide maximum patient benefit remains undefined. Rapp[160] prospectively studied 38 patients randomized to early TPN or standard enteral nutrition via nasogastric tube. Because of the gastric atony which is usually associated with closed head injury, enterally fed patients received significantly less nutrition than the TPN patients, creating a study of early TPN vs. delayed enteral feeding. Although this initial study documented some improvement in neurologic outcome with early TPN, there was a high sepsis rate of approximately 30% in both groups. Subsequently, Grahm[161] randomized patients with severe closed head injury to either early enteral feeding via nasojejunal feeding tubes placed fluoroscopically within 36 h of injury or delayed enteral feeding after gastric atony resolved. Although there was no impact on neurologic outcome, the incidence of bacterial infection was significantly lower and the length of stay in the intensive care unit was significantly shorter with early enteral feeding.

The mechanisms for improved host defense and reduced septic morbidity with early enteral feeding are not clear. With the exception of glutamine supplementation in Moore's studies, the enteral products in the trauma studies mentioned above were not enriched with any of the "immune-enhancing" nutrients previously discussed. Investigators have found diminished secretory IgA in biliary secretions of animals fed i.v. TPN, while levels of secretory IgA were maintained in animals when identical nutrient solution was delivered enterally.[162] Animals fed i.v. TPN have also been shown to have an increased incidence of bacterial translocation to mesenteric lymph nodes.[163] Similarly, in an injury model, cellular defenses improved in animals randomized to enteral feeding but not in animals receiving i.v. solution.[164] Glutamine-supplemented i.v. solutions, however, appear to reverse both bacterial translocation and the depression in secretory IgA levels in animals,[151] although the benefit of i.v. glutamine on patient outcome has not been studied.

Clinical studies employing nutrient formulas enriched with glutamine, arginine, nucleic acids, and omega-3 fatty acids are just now being completed. Gottschlich et al.[165] employed a high-protein, low-fat, linoleic-restricted, modular tube feeding enriched with omega-3 fatty acids, arginine, cysteine, histidine, vitamin A, zinc, and ascorbic acid. When administered to burn patients, there was a significant reduction in wound infection and length of stay/percent body burn and a tendency toward decreased mortality in this patient population. Daly et al.[166] randomized patients undergoing operations for upper GI malignancies to a standard enteral diet or a diet supplemented with arginine, RNA, and omega-3 fatty acids. *In vitro* lymphocyte mitogenesis improved only in the supplemented group in association with significantly fewer infectious and wound complications and a shortened hospital stay. The mean nitrogen intake was significantly higher in the supplemented group, reflecting the higher total protein of the supplemented diet. Since infectious complications correlated best with the amount of nitrogen ingested, it remains to be seen whether the clinical improvement was secondary to protein loading or due to individual "immune enhancing nutrients". Bower et al.[167] recently concluded a multi-institutional study using an immune-enhancing enteral formula and demonstrated shorter hospital stay and fewer urinary tract infections in the supplemented group. The final analysis of these data is not yet complete.

Clearly, malnutrition correlates with increased infectious complications. Preventing PCM and specific nutrient deficiencies through aggressive nutritional support appears to help maintain immune function. However, nutritional support should not come at the expense of prompt appropriate therapy for a disease process except in the severely malnourished elective surgical patient. When possible, primary therapy and nutritional repletion should be accomplished simultaneously. Enteral nutrition support is preferable because it costs less and because enteral processing of nutrients appears to be an important factor in reducing septic morbidity through possible effects on the gut mucosal immune system. However, it remains to be seen whether immune-enhancing nutrients will positively affect patient outcome when used to supplement standard enteral or parenteral feedings.

REFERENCES

1. **Beisel, W. R.,** History of nutritional immunology: introduction and overview, *J Nutr,* 122, 591, 1992.
2. **Bower, R. H.,** Nutrition and immune function, *NCP,* 5, 189, 1990.
3. **Wan, J. M.-F., Haw, M. P., and Blackburn, G. L.,** Symposium on the interaction between nutrition and inflammation, *Proc Nutr Soc,* 48, 315, 1989.
4. **Abbas, A. K., Lichtman, A. H., and Pober, J. S.,** General properties of immune responses, in *Cellular and Molecular Immunology,* Abbas, A. K., Lichtman, A. H., and Pober, J. S., Eds., W. B. Saunders, Philadelphia, 1991, 3.
5. **Goodman, J. W.,** The immune response, in *Basic and Clinical Immunology,* 7th ed., Stites, D. P. and Terr, A. I., Eds., Appleton & Lange, Norwalk, 1991, 34.
6. **Abbas, A. K., Lichtman, A. H., and Pober, J. S.,** Cells and tissues of the immune system, in *Cellular and Molecular Immunology,* Abbas, A. K., Lichtman, A. H., and Pober, J. S., Eds., W. B. Saunders, Philadelphia, 1991, 13.
7. **Broide, D. H.,** Inflammatory cells: structure & function, in *Basic and Clinical Immunology,* 7th ed., Stites, D. P. and Terr, A. I., Eds., Appleton & Lange, Norwalk, 1991, 141.
8. **Abbas, A. K., Lichtman, A. H., and Pober, J. S.,** The complement system, in *Cellular and Molecular Immunology,* Abbas, A. K., Lichtman, A. H., and Pober, J. S., Eds., W. B. Saunders, Philadelphia, 1991, 259.
9. **Frank, M. M.,** Complement & kinin, in *Basic and Clinical Immunology,* 7th ed., Stites, D. P. and Terr, A. I., Eds., Appleton & Lange, Norwalk, 1991, 161.
10. **Kamani, N. R. and Douglas, S. D.,** Structure & development of the immune system, in *Basic and Clinical Immunology,* 7th ed., Stites, D. P. and Terr, A. I., Eds., Appleton & Lange, Norwalk, 1991, 9.
11. **Abbas, A. K., Lichtman, A. H., and Pober, J. S.,** Antibodies and antigens, in *Cellular and Molecular Immunology,* Abbas, A. K., Lichtman, A. H., and Pober, J. S., Eds., W. B. Saunders, Philadelphia, 1991, 37.
12. **Oppenheim, J. J., Ruscetti, F. W., and Faltynek, C.,** Cytokines, in *Basic and Clinical Immunology,* 7th ed., Stites, D. P., and Terr, A. I., Eds., Appleton & Lange, 1991, 161.
13. **Abbas, A. K., Lichtman, A. H., and Pober, J. S.,** Cytokines, in *Cellular and Molecular Immunology,* Abbas, A. K., Lichtman, A. H., and Pober, J. S., Eds., W. B. Saunders, Philadelphia, 1991, 225.
14. **Abbas, A. K., Lichtman, A. H., and Pober, J. S.,** Effector cells of cell-mediated immunity, in *Cellular and Molecular Immunology,* Abbas, A. K., Lichtman, A. H., and Pober, J. S., Eds., W. B. Saunders, Philadelphia, 1991, 244.
15. **Brandtzaeg, P., Nilssen, D. E., Rognum, T. O., and Thrane, P. S.,** Ontogeny of the mucosal immune system and IgA deficiency, *Gastroenterol Clin N Am,* 20, 397, 1991.
16. **Brandgtzaeg, P., Halstensen, T. S., Kett, K., Krajci, P., Kvale, D., Rognum, T. O., Scott, H., and Sollid, L. M.,** Immunobiology and immunopathology of human gut mucosa: humoral immunity and intraepithelial lymphocytes, *Gastroenterology,* 97, 1562, 1989.
17. **Langkamp-Henken, B., Glezer, J. A., and Kudsk, K. A.,** Immunologic structure and function of the gastrointestinal tract, *NCP,* 7, 100, 1992.
18. **Roux, M. E., McWilliams, M., Phillips-Quagliate, J. M., Weisz-Carrington, P., and Lamm, M. E.,** Origin of IgA-secreting plasma cells in the mammary gland, *J Exp Med,* 146, 1311, 1977.
19. **Weisz-Carrington, P., Roux, M. E., and Lamm, M. E.,** Plasma cells and epithelial immunoglobulins in the mouse mammary gland during pregnancy and lactation, *J Immunol,* 119, 1306, 1977.

20. **Hanson, L. A., Carlsson, B., Cruz, J. R., Garcia, B., Holmgren, J., Khan, S. R., Lindblad, B. S., Svennerholm, A.-M., Svennerholm, B., and Urrutia, J.,** Immune response in the mammary gland, in *Immunology of Breast Milk,* Ogra, P. L. and Dayton, D. H., Eds., Raven Press, New York, 145, 1979, 145.

21. **Jackson, D. E., Lally, E. T., Nakamura, M. D., and Montgomery, P. C.,** Migration of IgA-bearing lymphocytes into salivary glands, *Cell Immunol,* 63, 203, 1981.

22. **Lamm, M. E., Weisz-Carrington, P., Roux, M. E., McWilliams, M., and Phillips-Quagliata, J. M.,** Mode of induction of an IgA response in the breast and other secretory sites by oral antigen, in *Immunology of Breast Milk,* Ogra, P. L., and Dayton, D., Eds., Raven Press, New York, 1979, 105.

23. **Rudzik, R., Clancy, R. L., Perey, D. Y. E., Day, R. P., and Bienenstock, J.,** Repopulation with IgA-containing cells of bronchial and intestinal lamina propria after transfer of homologous Peyer's patch and bronchial lymphocytes, *J Immunol,* 114, 1599, 1975.

24. **McDermott, M. R. and Bienenstock, J.,** Evidence for a common mucosal immunologic system. I. Migration of B immunoblasts into intestinal respiratory and genital tissue, *J Immunol,* 122, 1892, 1979.

25. **Kagnoff, M. F.,** Immunology of the digestive system, in *Physiology of the Gastrointestinal Tract,* 2nd ed., Johnson, L. R., Ed., Raven Press, New York, 1987, 1699.

26. **Heatley, R. V. and Bienenstock, J.,** Luminal lymphoid cells in the rabbit intestine, *Gastroenterology,* 82, 268, 1982.

27. **Owen, R. L., and Nemanic, P.,** Antigen processing structures of the mammalian intestinal tract: an SEM study of lymphoepithelial organs, in *Scanning Electron Microscopy,* Becker, R. P. and Johari, O., Eds., SEM Inc., Chicago, 1978, 367.

28. **Sell, S., Raffel, C., and Scott, C. B.,** Tissue localization of T and B lymphocytes in lagomorphs: anatomical evidence for a major role of the gastrointestinal associated lymphoid tissue in generation of lymphocytes in the adult, *Dev Comp Immunol,* 4, 355, 1980.

29. **Strober, W. and James, S. P.,** The mucosal immune system, in *Basic and Clinical Immunology,* 7th ed., Stites, D. P. and Terr, A. I., Eds., Appleton & Lange, Norwalk, 1991, 175.

30. **Owen, R. L.,** Sequential uptake of horseradish peroxidase by lymphoid follicle epithelium of Peyer's patches in the normal unobstructed mouse intestine: an ultrastructural study. *Gastroenterology,* 72, 440, 1977.

31. **von Rosen, L., Podjaski, B., Bettmann, I., and Otto, H. F.,** Observations on the ultrastructure and function of the so-called "microfold" or "membraneous" cells (M cells) by means of peroxidase as a tracer, *Virchows Arch,* 390, 289, 1982.

32. **Marcial, M. A. and Madara, J. L.,** *Crytosporidium:* cellular localization structural analysis of absorptive cell-parasite membrane-membrane interactions in guinea pigs, and suggestion of protozoan transport by M cells, *Gastroenterology,* 90, 583, 1986.

33. **Wolf, J. L., Rubin, D. H., Finberg, R., Kauffman, R. S., Sharpe, A. H., Trier, J. S., and Fields, B. N.,** Intestinal M cells: a pathway for entry of reovirus into the host, *Science,* 212, 471, 1981.

34. **Sonoda, E., Hitoshi, Y., Yamaguchi, N., Ishii, T., Tominaga, A., Araki, S., and Takatsu, K.,** Differential regulation of IgA production by TGF-β and IL-5: TGF-β induces surface IgA-positive cells bearing IL-5 receptor, whereas IL-5 promotes their survival and maturation into IgA-secreting cells, *Cell Immunol,* 140, 158, 1992.

35. **Lebman, D. A., Nomura, D. Y., Coffman, R. L., and Lee, F. D.,** Molecular characterization of germ-line immunoglobulin A transcripts produced during transforming growth factor type β-induced isotype switching, *Proc Natl Acad Sci,* 87, 3962, 1990.

36. **Salmi, M. and Jalkanen, S.,** Regulation of lymphocyte traffic to mucosal associated lymphatic tissues, *Gastroenterol Clin N Am,* 20, 495, 1991.

37. **Strober, W. and Harriman, G. R.,** The regulation of IgA B-cell differentiation, *Gastroenterol Clin N Am,* 20, 495, 1991.

38. **Underdown, J. M.,** Immunoglobulin A: strategic defense initiative at the mucosal surface, *Ann Rev Immunol,* 4, 389, 1986.

39. **Brandtzaeg, P.,** Polymeric IgA is complexed with secretory component (SC) on the surface of human intestinal epithelial cells, *Scand J Immunol,* 8, 39, 1978.

40. **Crago, S. S., Kulhavy, R., Prince, S. J., and Mestecky, J.,** Secretory component on epithelial cells is a surface receptor for polymeric immunoglobulins, *J Exp Med,* 147, 1832, 1978.

41. **Brown, W. R., Newcomb, R. W., and Ishizaka, K.,** Proteolytic degradation of exocrine and serum immunoglobulins, *J Clin Invest,* 49, 1374, 1970.

42. **Mestecky, J., Lue, C., and Russell, M. W.,** Selective transport of IgA: cellular and molecular aspects, *Gastroenterol Clin N Am,* 20, 441, 1991.

43. **Freter, R.,** Mechanism of action of intestinal antibody in experimental cholera. II. Antibody-mediated antibacterial reaction at the mucosal surface, *Infect Immun,* 2, 556, 1970.

44. **Fubara, E. S. and Freter, R.,** Protection against enteric bacterial infection by secretory IgA antibodies, *J Immunol,* 111, 395, 1973.
45. **Walker, W. A. and Isselbacher, K. J.,** Uptake and transport of macromolecules by the intestine: possible role in clinical disorders, *Gastroenterology,* 67, 531, 1974.
46. **André, C., Lambert, R., Bazin, H., and Heremans, J. F.,** Interference of oral immunization with the intestinal absorption of heterologous albumin, *Eur J Immunol,* 4, 701, 1974.
47. **Chandra, R. K.,** Protein-energy malnutrition and immunological responses, *J Nutr,* 122, 597, 1992.
48. **Puri, S. and Chandra, R. K.,** Nutritional regulation of host resistance and predictive value of immunologic tests in assessment of outcome, *Pediatr Clin N Am,* 32, 499, 1985.
49. **Chandra, R. K.,** Numerical and functional deficiency in T helper cells in protein energy malnutrition, *Clin Exp Immunol,* 51, 126, 1983.
50. **McDermott, M. R., Mark, D. A., Befus, A. D., Baliga, B. S., Suskind, R. M., and Bienenstock, J.,** Impaired intestinal localization of mesenteric lymphoblasts associated with vitamin A deficiency and protein-calorie malnutrition, *Immunology,* 45, 1, 1982.
51. **Keusch, G. T.,** Nutritional effects on response of children in developing countries to respiratory tract pathogens: implications for vaccine development, *Rev Infect Dis,* 13, S486, 1991.
52. **Chandra, R. K.,** Micronutrients and immune function, *Ann N Y Acad Sci,* 587, 9, 1990.
53. **Keusch, G. T.,** Micronutrients and susceptibility to infection, *Ann N Y Acad Sci,* 587, 181, 1990.
54. **West, C. E., Rombout, J. H. W. M., Van Der Zijpp, A. J., and Sijtsma, S. R.,** Vitamin A and immune function, *Proc Nutr Soc,* 50, 251, 1991.
55. **Bendich, A.,** β-Carotene and the immune response, *Proc Nutr Soc,* 50, 263, 1991.
56. **Sommer, A.,** Vitamin A status, resistance to infection, and childhood mortality, *Ann N Y Acad Sci,* 587, 17, 1990.
57. **Chandra, R. K.,** 1990 McCollum award lecture. Nutrition and immunity: lessons from the past and new insights into the future, *Am J Clin Nutr,* 53, 1087, 1991.
58. **Schwartz, J. L., Flynn, E., and Shklar, G.,** The effect of carotenoids on the antitumor immune response *in vivo* and *in vitro* with hamster and mouse immune effectors, *Ann N Y Acad Sci,* 587, 92, 1990.
59. **Miller, L. T. and Kerkvliet, N. I.,** Effect of vitamin B_6 on immunocompetence in the elderly, *Ann N Y Acad Sci,* 587, 49, 1990.
60. **Meydani, S. N., Ribaya-Mercado, J. D., Russell, R. M., Sahyoun N., Morrow, F. D., and Gershoff, S. N.,** The effect of vitamin B_6 on the immune response of healthy elderly, *Ann N Y Acad Sci,* 587, 303, 1990.
61. **Meydani, S. N., Ribaya-Mercado, J. D., Russell, R. M., Sahyoun N., Morrow, F. D., and Gershoff, S. N.,** Vitamin B-6 deficiency impairs interleukin 2 production and lymphocyte proliferation in elderly adults, *J Clin Nutr,* 53, 1275, 1991.
62. **Bendich, A.,** Vitamins and immunity, *J Nutr,* 122, 601, 1992.
63. **Meydani, S. N.,** Micronutrients and immune function in the elderly, *Ann N Y Acad Sci,* 587, 196, 1990.
64. **Anderson, R., Smit, M. J., Joone, G. K., and Van Staden, A. M.,** Vitamin C and cellular immune functions, *Ann N Y Acad Sci,* 587, 34, 1990.
65. **Bendich, A.,** Antioxidant micronutrients and immune responses, *Ann N Y Acad Sci,* 587, 168, 1990.
66. **McMurray, D. N., Bartow, R. A., Mintzer, C. L., and Hernandez-Frontera, E. H.,** Micronutrient status and immune function in tuberculosis, *Ann N Y Acad Sci,* 587, 59, 1990.
67. **Kelleher, J.,** Vitamin E and the immune response, *Proc Nutr Soc,* 50, 245, 1991.
68. **Kowdley, K. V., Mason, J. B., Meydani, S. N., Cornwall, S., and Grand, R. J.,** Vitamin E deficiency and impaired cellular immunity related to intestinal fat malabsorption, *Gastroenterology,* 102, 2139, 1992.
69. **Tengerdy, R. P.,** The role of vitamin E in immune response and disease resistance, *Ann N Y Acad Sci,* 587, 24, 1990.
70. **Mino, M., Okano, T., and Tamai, H.,** Leukocyte function generating superoxide and vitamin E, *Ann N Y Acad Sci,* 587, 307, 1990.
71. **Turner, R. J.,** Selenium and the immune response, *Proc Nutr Soc,* 50, 275, 1991.
72. **Kiremidjian-Schumacher, L., Roy, M., Wishe, H. I., Cohen, M. W., and Stotzky, G.,** Selenium and immune cell functions. I. Effect on lymphocyte proliferation and production of interleukin 1 and interleukin 2, *Proc Soc Exp Biol Med,* 193, 136, 1990.
73. **Roy, M., Kiremidjian-Schumacher, L., Wishe, H. I., Cohen, M. W., and Stotzky, G.,** Selenium and immune cell functions. II. Effect on lymphocyte-mediated cytotoxicity, *Proc Soc Exp Biol Med,* 193, 143, 1990.
74. **Spallholz, J. E., Boylan, L. M., and Larsen, H. S.,** Advances in understanding selenium's role in the immune system, *Ann N Y Acad Sci,* 587, 123, 1990.
75. **Cunningham-Rundles, S., Bockman, R. S., Lin, A., Giardina, P. V., and Hilgartner, M. W.,** Physiological and pharmacological effects of zinc on immune response, *Ann N Y Acad Sci,* 587, 113, 1990.

76. **Keen, C. L.,** Zinc deficiency and immune function, *Ann Rev Nutr,* 10, 415, 1990.
77. **Ruz, M., Cavan, K. R., Bettger, W. J., Thompson, L., Berry, M., and Gibson, R. S.,** Development of a dietary model for the study of mild zinc deficiency in humans and evaluation of some biochemical and functional indices of zinc status, *Am J Clin Nutr,* 53, 1295, 1991.
78. **Schlesinger, L., Arevalo, M., Arredondo, S., Diaz, M., Lönnerdal, B., and Stekel, A.,** Effect of a zinc-fortified formula on immunocompetence and growth of malnourished infants, *Am J Clin Nutr,* 56, 491, 1992.
79. **Sherman, A. R.,** Zinc, copper, and iron nutriture and immunity, *J Nutr,* 122, 604, 1992.
80. **Lukasewyucz, O. A. and Prohaska, J. R.,** The immune response in copper deficiency, *Ann N Y Acad Sci,* 587, 147, 1990.
81. **Bala, S., Failla, M., and Lunney, J.,** Phenotypic and functional alterations in peripheral blood mononuclear cells of copper-deficient rats, *Ann N Y Acad Sci,* 587, 283, 1990.
82. **Babu, L. and Failla, M. L.,** Respiratory burst and candidacidal activity of peritoneal macrophages are impaired in copper-deficient rats, *J Nutr,* 120, 1692, 1990.
83. **Bala, S., Lunney, J. K., and Failla, M. L.,** Effects of copper deficiency on T-cell mitogenic responsiveness and phenotypic profile of blood mononuclear cells from swine, *Am J Vet Res,* 53, 1231, 1992.
84. **Sherman, A. R.,** Influence of iron on immunity and disease resistance, *Ann N Y Acad Sci,* 587, 140, 1990.
85. **Kuvibidila, S., Dardenne, M., Savino, W., and Lepault, F.,** Influence of iron-deficiency anemia on selected thymus functions in mice: thymulin biological activity, T-cell subsets, and thymocyte proliferation, *Am J Clin Nutr,* 51, 228, 1990.
86. **Barr, L. H., Dunn, G. D., and Brennan, M. F.,** Essential fatty acid deficiency during total parenteral nutrition, *Ann Surg,* 193, 304, 1981.
87. **Gottschlich, M. M.,** Selection of optimal lipid sources in enteral and parenteral nutrition, *Nutr Clin Pract,* 7, 152, 1992.
88. **Mochizuki, H., Trocki, O., Dominioni, L., Ray, M. B., and Alexander, J. W.,** Optimal lipid content for enteral diets following thermal injury, *JPEN,* 8, 638, 1984.
89. **Richieri, G. V. and Kleinfeld, A. M.,** Free fatty acids inhibit cytotoxic T lymphocyte-mediated lysis of allogeneic target cells, *J Immunol,* 145, 1074, 1990.
90. **Meydani, S. N.,** Modulation of cytokine production by dietary polyunsaturated fatty acids, *Proc Soc Exp Biol Med,* 200, 189, 1992.
91. **Blackburn, G. L.,** Nutrition and inflammatory events: highly unsaturated fatty acids (ω-3 vs. ω-6) in surgical injury, *Proc Soc Exp Biol Med,* 200, 183, 1992.
92. **Nordenström, J., Jarstrand, C., and Wiernik, A,** Decreased chemotactic and random migration of leukocytes during intralipid infusion, *Am J Clin Nutr,* 32, 2416, 1979.
93. **Strunk, R. C., Kunke, K., Nagle, R. B., Payne, C. M., and Harrison, H. R.,** Inhibition of *in vitro* synthesis of the second (C2) and fourth (C4) components of complement in guinea pig peritoneal macrophages by a soybean oil emulsion, *Pediatr Res,* 13, 188, 1978.
94. **Jensen, G. L., Mascioli, E. A., Seidner, D. L., Istfan, N. W., Domnitch, A. M., Selleck, K., Babayan, V. K., Blackburn, G. L., and Bistrian, B. R.,** Parenteral infusion of long- and medium-chain triglycerides and reticuloendothelial system function in man, *JPEN,* 14, 467, 1990.
95. **Seidner, D. L., Mascioli, E. A., Istfan, N. W., Porter, K. A., Selleck, K., Blackburn, G. L., and Bistrian, B. R.,** Effects of long-chain triglyceride emulsions on reticuloendothelial system function in humans, *JPEN,* 13, 614, 1989.
96. **Friedman, Z., Marks, K. H., Maisels, J., Thorson, R., and Naeye, R.,** Effect of parenteral fat emulsion on the pulmonary and reticuloendothelial systems in the newborn infant, *Pediatrics,* 61, 694, 1978.
97. **Meydani, S. N., Endres, S., Woods, M. M., Goldin, B. R., Soo, C., Morrill-Labrode, A., Dinarello, C. A., and Gorbach, S. L.,** Oral (n-3) fatty acid supplementation suppresses cytokine production and lymphocyte proliferation: comparison between young and older women, *J Nutr,* 121, 547, 1991.
98. **Hamawy, K. J., Moldawer, L. L., Georgieff, M., Valicenti, A. J., Babayan, V. K., Bistrian, B. R., and Blackburn, G. L.,** The effect of lipid emulsions on reticuloendothelial system function in the injured animal, *JPEN,* 9, 559, 1985.
99. **McHugh, M. I., Wilkinson, R., Elliott, R. W., Field, E. J., Dewar, P., Hall, R. R., Taylor, R. M. R., and Uldall, P. R.,** Immunosuppression with polyunsaturated fatty acids in renal transplantation, *Transplantation,* 24, 263, 1977.
100. **Perez, R. V., Munda, R., and Alexander, J. W.,** Augmentation of donor-specific transfusion and cyclosporine effects with dietary linoleic acid, *Transplantation,* 47, 937, 1989.
101. **Lee, T. H., Hoover, R. L., Williams, J. D., Sperling, R. I., Ravalese J., III, Spur, B. W., Robinson, D. R., Corey, E. J., Lewis, R. A., and Austen, K. F.,** Effect of dietary enrichment with eicosapentaenoic and docosahexaenoic acids on *in vitro* neutrophil and monocyte leukotriene generation and neutrophil function, *N Engl J Med,* 312, 1217, 1985.

102. **Peck, M. D., Ogle, C. K., and Alexander, J. W.,** Composition of fat in enteral diets can influence outcome in experimental peritonitis, *Ann Surg,* 214, 74, 1990.

103. **Pomposelli, J. J., Flores, E., Hirschberg, Y., Teo, T. C., Blackburn, G. L., Zeisel, S. H., and Bistrian, B. R.,** Short-term TPN containing n-3 fatty acids ameliorate lactic acidosis induced by endotoxin in guinea pigs, *Am J Clin Nutr,* 52, 548, 1990.

104. **Mascioli, E. A., Iwasa, Y., Trimbo, S., Leader, L., Bistrian, B. R., and Blackburn, G. L.,** Endotoxin challenge after menhaden oil diet: effects on survival of guinea pigs, *Am J Clin Nutr,* 49, 277, 1989.

105. **Mascioli, E., Leader, L., Flores, E., Trimbo, S., Bistrian, B., and Blackburn, G.,** Enhanced survival to endotoxin in guinea pigs fed iv fish oil emulsion, *Lipids,* 23, 623, 1988.

106. **Trocki, O., Heyd, T. J., Waymack, J. P., and Alexander, J. W.,** Effects of fish oil on postburn metabolism and immunity, *JPEN,* 11, 521, 1987.

107. **Kelley, V. E., Ferretti, A., Izui, S., and Strom, T. B.,** A fish oil diet rich in eicosapentaenoic acid reduces cyclooxygenase metabolites, and suppresses lupus in MRL-lpr mice, *J Immunol,* 134, 1914, 1985.

108. **Prickett, J. D., Robinson, D. R., and Steinberg, A. D.,** Effects of dietary enrichment with eicosapentaenoic acid upon autoimmune nephritis in female NZB × NZW/F$_1$ mice, *Arthritis Rheum,* 26, 133, 1983.

109. **Donadio, J. V., Jr.,** Omega-3 polyunsaturated fatty acids: a potential new treatment of immune renal disease, *Mayo Clin Proc,* 66, 1018, 1991.

110. **Bjorneboe, A., Soyland, E., Bjorneboe, G.-E. A., Rajka, G., and Drevon, C.A.,** Effect of dietary supplementation with eicosapentaenoic acid in the treatment of atopic dermatitis, *Br J Dermatol,* 117, 463, 1987.

111. **Ziboh, V. A., Cohen, K. A., Ellis, C. N., Miller, C., Hamilton, T. A., Kragballe, K., Hydrick, C. R., and Voorhees, J. J.,** Effects of dietary supplementation of fish oil on neutrophil and epidermal fatty acids, *Arch Dermatol,* 122, 1277, 1986.

112. **Bittiner, S. B., Cartwright, I., Tucker, W. F. G., and Bleehen, S. S.,** A double-blind, randomized, placebo-controlled trial of fish oil in psoriasis, *Lancet,* 378, 1988.

113. **Kremer, J. M., Jubiz, W., Michalek, A., Rynes, R. I., Bartholomew, L. E., Bigaquette, J., Timchalk, M., Beeler, D., and Lininger, L.,** Fish-oil fatty acid supplementation in active rheumatoid arthritis, *Ann Intern Med,* 106, 497, 1987.

114. **Van Der Heide, J. J. H., Bilo, H. J. G., Tegzess, A. M., and Donker, A. J. M.,** The effects of dietary supplementation with fish oil on renal function in cyclosporine-treated renal transplant recipients, *Transplantation,* 49, 523, 1990.

115. **Sobrado, J., Moldawer, L. L., Pomposelli, J. J., Mascioli, E. A., Babayan, V. K., Bistrian, B. R., and Blackburn, G. L.,** Lipid emulsions and reticuloendothelial system function in healthy and burned guinea pigs, *Am J Clin Nutr,* 42, 855, 1985.

116. **Dennison, A. R., Ball, M., Hands, L. J., Crowe, P. J., Watkins, R. M., and Kettlewell, M.,** Total parenteral nutrition using conventional and medium chain triglycerides: effect on liver function tests, complement, and nitrogen balance, *JPEN,* 12, 15, 1988.

117. **Mascioli, E. A., Bistrian, B. R., Babayan, V. K., and Blackburn, G. L.,** Medium chain triglycerides and structured lipids as unique nonglucose energy sources in hyperalimentation, *Lipids,* 22, 421, 1987.

118. **Mascioli, E. A., Babayan, V. K., Bistrian, B. R., and Blackburn, G. L.,** Novel triglycerides for special medical purposes, *JPEN,* 12, 127S, 1988.

119. **Hamawy, K. J., Moldawer, L. L., Georgieff, M., Valicenti, A. J., Babayan, V. K., Bistrian, B. R., and Blackburn, G. L.,** The effect of lipid emulsions on reticuloendothelial system function in the injured animal, *JPEN,* 9, 559, 1985.

120. **Sailer, D. and Muller, M.,** Medium chain triglycerides in parenteral nutrition, *JPEN,* 5, 115, 1981.

121. **Crowe, P. J., Dennison, A. R., and Royle, G. T.,** A new intravenous emulsion containing medium-chain triglyceride: studies of its metabolic effects in the perioperative period compared with a conventional long-chain triglyceride emulsion, *JPEN,* 9, 720, 1985.

122. **Mascioli, E. A., Lopes, S., Randall, S., Porter, K. A., Kater, G., Hirschberg, Y., Babayan, V. K., Bistrian, B. R., and Blackburn, G. L.,** Serum fatty acid profiles after intravenous medium chain triglyceride administration, *Lipids,* 24, 793, 1989.

123. **Teo, T. C., DeMichele, S. J., Selleck, K. M., Babayan, V. K., Blackburn, G. L., and Bistrian, B. R.,** Administration of structured lipid composed of MCT and fish oil reduces net protein catabolism in enterally fed burned rats, *Ann Surg,* 210, 100, 1988.

124. **Mok, K. T., Maiz, A., Yamazaki, K., Sobrado, J., Babayan, V. K., Moldawer, L. L., Bistrian, B. R., and Blackburn, G. L.,** Structured medium-chain and long-chain triglyceride emulsions are superior to physical mixtures in sparing body protein in the burned rat, *Metabolism,* 33, 910, 1984.

125. **Settle, R. G.,** Invited comment: short-chain fatty acids and their potential role in nutritional support, *JPEN,* 12, 104S, 1988.

126. **Koruda, M. J., Rolandelli, R. H., Bliss, D. Z., Hastings, J., Rombeau, J. L., and Settle, R. G.,** Parenteral nutrition supplemented with short-chain fatty acids: effect on the small-bowel mucosa in normal rats, *Am J Clin Nutr,* 51, 685, 1990.

127. **Rolandelli, R. H., Koruda, M. J., Settle, R. G., and Rombeau, J. L.,** Effects of intraluminal infusion of short-chain fatty acids on the healing of colonic anastomosis in the rat, *Surgery,* 100, 198, 1986.

128. **Koruda, M. J., Rolandelli, R. H., Settle, R. G., Zimmaro, D. M., and Rombeau, J. L.,** Effect of parenteral nutrition supplemented with short-chain fatty acids on adaptation to massive small bowel resection, *Gastroenterology,* 95, 715, 1988.

129. **Callery, M. P., Mangino, M. J., and Flye, M. W.,** Arginine-specific suppression of mixed lymphocyte culture reactivity by Kupffer cells—a basis of portal venous tolerance, *Transplantation,* 51, 1076, 1991.

130. **Seifter, E., Rettura, G., Barbul, A., and Levenson, S. M.,** Arginine: an essential amino acid for injured rats, *Surgery,* 84, 224, 1978.

131. **Barbul, A., Lazarou, S. A., Efron, D. T., Wasserkrug, H. L., and Efron, G.,** Arginine enhances wound healing and lymphocyte immune responses in humans, *Surgery,* 108, 331, 1990.

132. **Nirgiotis, J. G., Hennessey, P. J., and Andrassy, R. J.,** The effects of an arginine-free enteral diet on wound healing and immune function in the postsurgical rat, *J Pediatr Surg,* 26, 936, 1991.

133. **Barbul, A., Sisto, D. A., Wasserkrug, H. L., Yoshimura, N. N., and Efron, G.,** Metabolic and immune effects of arginine in postinjury hyperalimentation, *J Trauma,* 21, 970, 1981.

134. **Chyun, J.-H., and Griminger, P.,** Improvement of nitrogen retention by arginine and glycine supplementation and its relation to collagen synthesis in traumatized mature and aged rats, *J Nutr,* 114, 1697, 1984.

135. **Kirk, S. J., Regan, M. C., Wasserkrug, H. L., Sodeyama, M., and Barbul, A.,** Arginine enhances T-cell responses in athymic nude mice, *JPEN,* 16, 429, 1992.

136. **Reynolds, J. V., Daly, J. M., Zhang, S., Evantash, E., Shou, J., Sigal, R., and Ziegler, M. M.,** Immunomodulatory mechanisms of arginine, *Surgery,* 104, 142, 1988.

137. **Daly, J. M., Reynolds, J., Sigal, R., Shou, J., and Liberman, M. D.,** Effect of dietary protein and amino acids on immune function, *Crit Care Med,* 18, S86, 1990.

138. **Barbul, A., Wasserkrug, H. L., Yoshimura, N., Tao, R. T., and Efron, G.,** High arginine levels in intravenous hyperalimentation abrogate post-traumatic immune suppression, *J Surg Res,* 36, 620, 1984.

139. **Barbul, A., Sisto, D. A., Wasserkrug, H. L., and Efron, G.,** Arginine stimulates lymphocyte immune response in healthy human beings, *Surgery,* 90, 244, 1981.

140. **Madden, H. P., Breslin, R. J., Wasserkrug, H. L., Efron, G., and Barbul, A.,** Stimulation of T cell immunity by arginine enhances survival in peritonitis, *J Surg Res,* 44, 658, 1988.

141. **Gonce, S. J., Peck, M. D., Alexander, J. W., and Miskell, P. W.,** Arginine supplementation and its effect on established peritonitis in guinea pigs, *JPEN,* 14, 237, 1990.

142. **Van Buren, C. T., Kulkarni, A. D., and Rudolph, F.,** Synergistic effect of a nucleotide-free diet and cyclosporine on allograft survival, *Transplant Proc,* 15, 2967, 1983.

143. **Van Buren, C. T., Kulkarni, A. D., Schandle, V. B., and Rudolph, F. B.,** The influence of dietary nucleotides on cell-mediated immunity, *Transplantation,* 36, 350, 1983.

144. **Van Buren, C. T., Kulkarni, A. D., Fanslow, W. C., and Rudolph, F. B.,** Dietary nucleotides, a requirement for helper-inducer T lymphocytes, *Transplantation,* 40, 694, 1985.

145. **Kulkarni, A. D., Fanslow, W. C., Drath, D. B., Rudolph, F. B., and Van Buren, C. T.,** Influence of dietary nucleotide restriction on bacterial sepsis and phagocytic cell function in mice, *Arch Surg,* 121, 169, 1986.

146. **Kulkarni, A. D., Fanslow, W. C., Higley, H., Pizzini, R. P., Rudolph, F. B., and Van Buren, C. T.,** Expression of immune cell surface markers in vivo and immune competence in mice by dietary nucleotides, *Transplant Proc,* 21, 121, 1989.

147. **Fanslow, W. C., Kulkarni, A. D., Van Buren, C. T., and Rudolph, F. B.,** Effect of nucleotide restriction and supplementation on resistance to experimental murine candidiasis, *JPEN,* 12, 49, 1988.

148. **Pizzini, R. P., Kumar, S., Kulkarni, A. D., Rudolph, F. B., and Van Buren, C. T.,** Dietary nucleotides reverse malnutrition and starvation-induced immunosuppression, *Arch Surg,* 125, 86, 1990.

149. **Kulkarni, A. D., Fanslow, W. C., Rudolph, F. B., and Van Buren, C. T.,** Immunohemopoietic effects of dietary nucleotide restriction in mice, *Transplantation,* 53, 467, 1992.

150. **Parry-Billings, M., Evans, J., Calder, P. D., and Newsholme, E. A.,** Does glutamine contribute to immunosuppression after major burns?, *Lancet,* 336, 523, 1990.

151. **Burke, D. J., Alverdy, J. C., Aoys, E., and Moss, G. S.,** Glutamine-supplemented total parenteral nutrition improves gut immune function, *Arch Surg,* 124, 1396, 1989.

152. **Alverdy, J. C., Weisz-Carrington, P., Bushmann, R. J., Kelemen, P. R., Aoys, E., and Moss, G. S.,** Effect of parenteral nutrition on gut IgA plasma, *JPEN,* 14, 10S, 1990.

153. **The Veteran Affairs Total Parenteral Nutrition Cooperative Study Group,** Perioperative total parenteral nutrition in surgical patients, *N Engl J Med,* 325, 525, 1991.

154. **Alexander, J. W., Macmillan, B. G., Stinnett, J. D., Ogle, C. K., Bozion, R. C., Fischer, J. E., Oakes, J. B., Morris, M. S., and Krummel, R.,** Beneficial effects of aggressive protein feeding in severely burned children, *Ann Surg,* 192, 505, 1980.

155. **Kudsk, K. A., Carpenter, G., Petersen, S. R., and Sheldon, G. F.,** Effective enteral and parenteral feeding in malnourished rats with hemoglobin-*E. coli* adjuvant peritonitis, *J Surg Res,* 31, 105, 1981.

156. **Kudsk, K. A., Stone, J. M., Carpenter, G., and Sheldon, G. F.,** Enteral and parenteral feeding influences mortality after hemoglobin-*E. coli* peritonitis in normal rats. *J Trauma,* 23, 605, 1983.

157. **Moore, F. A., Moore, E. E., and Jones, T. N.,** Benefits of immediate jejunostomy feeding after major abdominal trauma—a prospective randomized study, *J Trauma,* 26, 874, 1986.

158. **Moore, F. A., Moore, E. E., Jones, T. N., McCroskey, B. L., and Peterson, V. M.,** TEN vs. TPN following major abdominal trauma — reduced septic morbidity, *J Trauma,* 29, 916, 1989.

159. **Kudsk, K. A., Croce, M. A., Fabian, T. C., Minard, G., Tolley, E. A., Poret, A., Kuhl, M. R., and Brown, R. O.,** Enteral vs. parenteral feeding: effects on septic morbidity following blunt and penetrating trauma, *Ann Surg,* 215, 503, 1992.

160. **Rapp, R. P., Young, B., Twyman, D., Bivins, B. A., Haack, D., Tibbs, P. A., and Bean, J. R.,** The favorable effect of early parenteral feeding on survival in head-injured patients, *J Neurosurg,* 58, 906, 1983.

161. **Grahm, T. W., Zadrozny, D. B., and Harrington, T.,** The benefits of early jejunal hyperalimentation in the head-injured patient, *Neurosurgery,* 25, 729, 1989.

162. **Alverdy, J. C., Chi, H. S., and Sheldon, G. F.,** The effect of parenteral nutrition on gastrointestinal immunity: the importance of enteral stimulation, *Ann Surg,* 202, 681, 1985.

163. **Alverdy, J. C., Aoy, S. E., and Moss, G. S.,** Total parenteral nutrition promotes bacterial translocation from the gut, *Surgery,* 104, 185, 1988.

164. **Birkhahn, R. H. and Rank, C. M.,** Immune response and leucine oxidation in oral- and intravenous-fed rats, *Am J Clin Nutr,* 39, 45, 1984.

165. **Gottschlich, M. M., Jenkins, M., Warden, G. D., Baumer, T., Havens, P., Snook, J. T., and Alexander, J. W.,** Differential affects of three enteral dietary regimens on selected outcome variables in burn patients, *JPEN,* 14, 225, 1990.

166. **Daly, J. M., Lieberman, M. D., Goldfine, J., Shou, J., Weintraub, F., Rosato, E. F., and Lavin, P.,** Enteral nutrition with supplemental arginine, RNA, and omega-3 fatty acids in patients after operation: immunologic, metabolic and clinical outcome, *Surgery,* 12, 56, 1992.

167. **Bower, R. H., Lavin, P. T., LiCari, J. J., Jensen, G. O., Hoyt, D. R., VanBuren, C. T., Cerra, F. B., Rothkopf, M. P., Daly, J. M., and Adelsberg, B. R.,** A modified enteral formula reduces hospital length of stay (LOS) in patients in intensive care units (ICU), presented at the 14th Congress of the European Society of Parenteral and Enteral Nutrition, Vienna, September 7–9, 1992.

Chapter 6

ENTERAL NUTRITION: THE CHALLENGE OF ACCESS

Donald F. Kirby and Mark H. DeLegge

TABLE OF CONTENTS

0-8493-7847-8/94/$0.00+$.50
© 1994 by CRC Press, Inc.

I. INTRODUCTION

Enteral nutrition refers to the delivery of nutrients and fluids to the GI tract for digestion and absorption. No benefit is realized unless absorption of these substrates is achieved. The GI tract has specialized areas that perform distinct functions with the ultimate goal of absorption of nutrients. While certain diseases or surgical removal may alter the integrity of the GI tract, there is great reserve in the system. We will not review the physiology of digestion and absorption in this chapter, but suggest a basic review by Cashman.[1]

While most people will consider the upper GI tract as the main route for enteral feeding, it is known that nutrient enemas, proctoclysis, were used in the time of the Egyptians. The Greeks also used nutrient enemas as a treatment of diarrhea and as part of a monthly ritual with enemas to purify the body.[2] Even in the early 20th century, proctoclysis was used up until World War II. While tube feeding into the stomach and small intestine was becoming more popular, rectal infusion of nutrients and fluids was still performed and could provide approximately 400 kcal/d. Rectal infusions were limited by irritation caused by the solutions, but the administration of saline or water was a common surgical practice in the early part of this century before i.v. infusions became commonplace.[3]

The approach to tube feeding has slowly advanced with improvements in technology. The first tube feeding is credited by His to Capivacceus in 1598.[4] He utilized a bladder with a hollow tube attached that delivered a feeding into the esophagus. In 1617, a monk named Aquapendente passed a silver tube through a nostril into the nasopharynx for feeding patients afflicted with tetanus. Later, leather catheters were fashioned by Van HelMont, and Boerhaave suggested that they place the tube in the stomach.[5,6] Hunter is known to have successfully fed patients in the stomach in the late 18th century.[7]

Current practice still utilizes the Levin tube for nasogastric feeding which was introduced in 1921.[8] In the 1950s polyethylene tubes were introduced to try to decrease the complications seen from other tubes that were too stiff. In 1954 polyvinyl plastic tubes were introduced. Shortly thereafter, silicone tubes that were weighted were reported by Keoshian and Nelsen.[9] Finally, polyurethane tubes began to replace the polyvinyl tubes.

Surgically placed gastrostomy tubes were placed in the late 19th century, but jejunostomy tubes did not appear until the early 20th century. Improvements in materials and surgical techniques have lead to many advances in accessing the GI tract for nutrition support. This chapter will focus on the current choices of enterally feeding patients and the risks and benefits of each.

II. OVERVIEW OF ENTERAL ACCESS

After it has been decided to enterally support a patient, it must be determined if it is safe to do so. Severe diarrhea, protracted vomiting, mechanical obstruction, or intestinal dysmotility can preclude the use of the GI tract. Until safe enteral use can be reasonably expected, parenteral nutrition either by peripheral vein or central vein may be more appropriate. Many patients have normal GI function, so that selecting an appropriate method of access to the GI tract is the key decision.

Figure 1 illustrates the potential sites for accessing the GI tract. When choosing a method of access, it should be considered whether the access will be needed short term (<3 weeks, usually) or long term, and the risk of potential complications should be assessed.

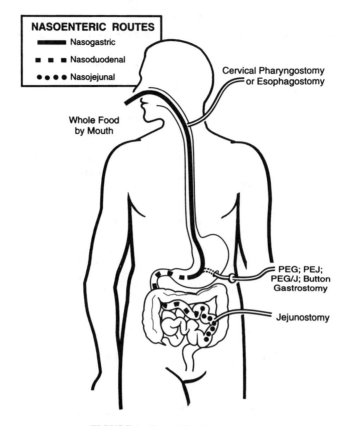

FIGURE 1. Enteral feeding options.

III. OPTIONS FOR ENTERAL ACCESS

A. CERVICAL PHARYNGOSTOMY

Cervical pharyngostomy was described in 1951 by Klopp as an open neck procedure for the placement of a feeding tube in a patient with a carcinoma of the cervical esophagus.[10] It has also been used for patients who have swallowing disorders secondary to maxillofacial trauma or neurological diseases. While it is unclear how frequently this procedure is presently being practiced compared to surgical gastrostomy, jejunostomy, or endoscopic methods, a percutaneous method was described in 1985 by Bucklin and Gilsdorf.[11] Using an over-the-wire technique through the lateral neck, they were able to provide access into the stomach or proximal duodenum in 17 patients. The procedure was well tolerated by all patients. Complications of this type of access include tube clogging due to the small caliber tube, tube migration with bolus delivery of feedings to the hypopharynx, aspiration, and local infection. By changing the tubes every 30 days, Bucklin and Gilsdorf were able to control local infections.

B. OROESOPHAGEAL OR OROGASTRIC TUBES

While orally placed tubes are not commonly used, they may occasionally be substituted for the nasal route in cases of severe facial trauma where it is not possible or safe to pass a tube nasally. It is unlikely that an alert patient would tolerate an orogastric tube as a

TABLE 1
Nasoenteric Tubes: Indications, Contraindications, and Complications

Indications	Contraindications
Feeding	Coagulopathy[a]
Gastric acid analysis	Combative patient[a]
Gastric decompression	Facial trauma with fractures[a]
? Luminal stenting after	Nasal obstruction
lye-induced	Severe esophageal obstruction[a]
esophageal injury	Patient refusal (competent patient)
Monitor gastric pH	
Monitor GI bleeding	
Medication delivery	

Complications[b]

Arrhythmia	Clogging	Duodenal perforation
Empyema	Epistaxsis	Esophageal perforation
Gastric rupture	GI bleeding	Knotted tubes
Myocardial infarction	Nasal mucosal ulceration	Nasal trauma
Otitis media	Pneumothorax	Pulmonary aspiration
Pulmonary intubation	Pyriform sinus perforation	Reflux esophagitis/ulceration/stricture
Rupture and leakage	Tracheobronchial trauma	Tracheoesophageal fistula
of mercury weight		
Tube feeding into	Tube dislodgement	Tube obstruction
pulmonary tree		

[a] Relative contraindication
[b] Does not include all problems related to tube feeding.

method of feeding for any significant length of time. However, short-term use is common for gastric lavage for GI hemorrhage prior to endoscopic evaluation, and intermittent placement of a tube for a gavage feeding has been practiced prior to the development of nasoenteric tubes.

C. NASOENTERIC TUBES

Initially, it was the goal to get a tube past the upper esophageal sphincter so that gross aspiration would not jeopardize the lungs. With time the development of tubes has progressed so that nasoenteric tubes may be placed in the esophagus, stomach, duodenum, and even jejunum. The main reasons for feeding more distal are to protect the lungs from aspiration of feedings and to eliminate dependence on gastric emptying, which may be altered in certain disease states. Nasoesophageal placement offers no significant advantage and is generally not practiced unless by error with a tube looping in the esophagus. In this setting aspiration is a high risk and underscores the importance of radiographic confirmation of tube placement. This potential access route will not be considered further.

1. Nasogastric Tubes

Nasogastric tubes (NGT) are a common form of access to the GI tract. However, they function in roles other than feeding. Table 1 shows indications, contraindications, and complications of nasoenteric tubes. As previously discussed, the first recorded NGT was made out of silver. Since that time rubber, polyethylene, polyvinyl, polyurethane, and silicone have been used in varying sizes.

For patients that are critically ill in an intensive care unit (ICU), nasogastric tubes are commonplace, especially if patients are receiving mechanical ventilation. These tubes then become a convenient method to decompress the stomach, to provide medications, to give feedings, to monitor gastric pH, and other functions.

The most feared complication is aspiration. This is a potentially serious risk for a nasogastric tube since the tube broaches two anatomical safeguards, the upper and lower esophageal sphincters. While it has always been taught that the risk of reflux—hence, aspiration—increases with the diameter of the nasogastric tube, it has recently been shown in several studies that patient position is also important.[12–14] Torres et al. showed that the supine position and length of time kept in this position were important variables in the number of episodes of tracheal aspiration in a series of ventilated patients with NGT. Patients were not fed during this study, and it was also shown that even a cuffed endotracheal tube was not protective in this group of patients.[13] In a similar study, Ibañez and colleagues showed that in a similar group of patients NGT feedings were associated with a higher incidence of aspiration in the supine position.[14] Also, 20 patients were studied after an isotope was delivered into the stomach and then the NGT was removed. There was a statistically significant reduction in aspiration by removing the NGT. They concluded that semirecumbency reduced the incidence of reflux compared to the supine position, but did not prevent reflux from occurring. It is our hospital's policy to discourage tube feeding by the nasogastric route except in the ICU or in highly selected patients when there is intensive patient monitoring.

Nasogastric tube sizes vary from 5 to 18 French (Fr). The smaller tubes are generally used for feeding in children and adults, but have a higher risk of clogging than the larger tubes. The smaller tubes also preclude the use of blenderized diets which generally require a 10 Fr tube for commercially prepared products and larger tubes for hospitalized or home blenderized diets. For the smallest tube sizes, elemental tube feedings may need to be used since they are the least viscous.

While NGT have been used for feeding for many years, they are prone to certain problems. Patient discomfort or agitation can lead to self-extubation. The risk of aspiration pneumonia is well known and can be a significant problem. Clogging and kinking of tubes can occur, and difficulties in placement can lead to problems.

The standard Levin tube or Salem sump tubes are stiff enough not to require a stylet, but the softer polyurethane and silicone elastomer tubes may require stiffening in ice water or more commonly are packaged with a stylet. Water-activated lubricated tubes help facilitate stylet removal without catheter dislodgement.

2. Nasoduodenal and Nasojejunal Tubes

There has been a proliferation of nasoduodenal (NDT) and nasojejunal tubes (NJT) in the marketplace. The assumption is that the more distally a feeding is placed, the smaller the risk of aspiration. Also, the tube itself being placed past another anatomic sphincter, the pyloric sphincter, may help to reduce aspiration. Unfortunately, controversial issues regarding aspiration have not been totally resolved. However, the fate of feeding tubes has been examined by Lipman and found to have a small chance of being functional over a 6-week observation period.[15]

There are many methods of placing NDT and NJT tubes. Traditionally, the tube is passed at the bedside, and motility is often required to pass the tube into the small intestine. Radiographs should be obtained to verify the position prior to instituting feeding. Metoclopramide (MET) and erythromycin have been used with variable success.[16–19] Whatley et al. using 8 Fr NDT found that MET works best if it is infused just prior to placement.[16] Kittinger and co-workers found that infusing MET after tube placement was ineffective except in diabetic patients; this study used 10 Fr tubes.[17] Seifert and colleagues used 12 Fr tubes and showed no significant benefit with MET infused 15 minutes prior to tube placement.[18] Kalafarentzos et al. used 8 Fr tubes and separated 30 patients into

3 equal groups: placebo, MET after placement, and MET prior to placement.[19] The latter group had a 90% passage rate after 4 h and was statistically different from the other 2 groups. Unfortunately, all of these studies suffer from a lack of adequate numbers and differ in the size of the nasoenteric tubes placed. We feel that the question of the utility of MET in facilitating NDT passage has not been adequately answered. Erythromycin has also been studied in a small group of patients and appears to be promising, but again, further studies are needed.[20]

Tubes that fail to pass spontaneously can be assisted endoscopically or fluoroscopically. Gutierrez and Balfe reported the results of a 1-year study in 448 patients referred for fluoroscopically guided nasoenteric feeding.[21] They were successful in placing the tube distal to the third portion of the duodenum in 86.6% of patients. They experienced 4 major complications (0.4%) either during or immediately after nasoenteric tube placement. Three patients with known cardiomyopathy had fatal arrhythmias, and one patient had a tube malpositioned in the tracheobronchial tree. One advantage to this technique is that after successful placement, tube feeding can begin immediately.[21] However, the cost is higher to place the tube fluoroscopically rather than by obtaining a radiograph after passing the tube. Rapid placement by whatever means and initiation of tube feeding may be the most cost-effective approach as well as providing intestinal fuels to protect against bacterial translocation. Local expertise and availability of ICU fluoroscopy will be limiting factors. Again, tube longevity is an important issue due to self-extubation, clogging, or migration. Some centers favor securing nasoenteric tubes by means of a bridle or as part of a modified nasal cannula if the patient also requires oxygen.[12,22]

Placement of any tube nasally in a patient with altered mental status can be particularly hazardous. Without a cough reflex, these tubes can be passed into the pulmonary tree even with a cuffed endotracheal tube in place. While intrapulmonary placement of feeding tubes occurs in only 0.3% of patients, serious complications such as pneumothorax, intrapulmonary feeding, empyema, and/or abscess have been reported.[21,23] Roubenoff and Ravich reported a two-stage placement technique in high-risk patients. The tube to be passed is measured from the tip of the earlobe to the xiphoid process. The tube is then passed to this predetermined distance and an anteroposterior radiograph obtained. This will determine if the tube is in the esophagus or the pulmonary tree. If esophageal placement is confirmed, then the tube is advanced further into the stomach or beyond and another radiograph obtained before tube feeding is initiated.[23]

Another technique for avoiding pulmonary intubation was reported by Raff and colleagues.[24] Here the nasoenteric tube is passed to 25 cm, which should bring the tube to the level of the carina. Then the tube is checked for sounds of air exchange and/or placed under water to look for air bubbles. If neither of these signs is present, then passage of the tube can continue; otherwise, removal and another trial at passage can be attempted. This technique is simple and is quicker than that reported by Roubenoff and Ravich, since an interim chest radiograph is not required.

Recently Ugo et al. have reported a bedside technique of postpyloric passage of weighted tubes.[25] Here they placed ICU patients in the right lateral decubitus position and used auscultation to track the tube and attempt placement into the duodenum and beyond. They had no adverse placements in the pulmonary tree and placed 85/103 of the tubes into the duodenum or jejunum. However, only 44/103 were in the preferred portions of the duodenum (third or fourth portion) or jejunum.

Baskin has helped to develop a new tube that provides NG suction with small intestinal feeding.[26] This can require either endoscopy alone or endoscopy and fluoroscopy to place this tube. However, this might be an acceptable option in those patients where early gut recovery is anticipated and an endoscopic PEG/J or surgically placed tube would be less appropriate.[27]

TABLE 2
Indications and Contraindications for Endoscopic or
Radiologic Tube Enterostomy Placement

Indications	Contraindications[a]
Decompression	Ascites
Feeding	Coagulopathy[a]
Long-term enteral route	Inability to transilluminate[a]
Medication delivery	Intestinal obstruction[a]
	Marked hepatomegaly[a]
	Morbid obesity[a]
	Peritoneal dialysis
	Peritoneal metastases
	Portal hypertension
	Previous gastrectomy[a]

[a] Relative contraindication.

D. TUBE ENTEROSTOMY

Tube enterostomy refers to the end product of a tube that enters the body through the skin into the stomach or intestine. There are multiple ways to perform a tube enterostomy: (1) percutaneous gastrostomy—placed either endoscopically (PEG) or radiologically; (2) percutaneous jejunostomy—either endoscopic (PEJ) or radiologic; (3) percutaneous endoscopic gastrojejunostomy (PEG/J); (4) surgical gastrostomy; and (5) surgical jejunostomy. While each technique has its own risks and benefits, local expertise will help dictate which technique is performed in a particular community.

1. Percutaneous Endoscopic Gastrostomy—Indications and Techniques

Gauderer and Ponsky first reported performing an endoscopic gastrostomy in 1980.[28] The first PEGs utilized a 14 French Pezzer catheter, but since that time multiple commercial kits and variations on the technique have been popularized. Table 2 lists the indications and contraindications for endoscopic or radiologic tube enterostomy placement. In general, it requires a functional GI tract and the need for prolonged (>3 weeks) or permanent enteral access. The endoscopic approach is generally contraindicated in patients with significant ascites, peritoneal dialysis, intestinal obstruction, or peritoneal metastases. While these are not absolute contraindications for a surgical gastrostomy, they can increase the morbidity and mortality. In addition, it should be carefully considered how long the patient will survive. Patients who are unlikely to survive the index hospitalization (<30 days) should carefully have the risks and benefits of this procedure reviewed before having this procedure done. A recent study by Taylor and co-workers identified several risk factors in their patients that were associated with a poor short-term survival. These included the following: diabetes mellitus, older age, male gender, and specific medical diagnoses.[29] While this study may not be applicable to all populations, it does point out that we must use our resources carefully and consider which patients will truly benefit from this type of technology.[30]

Marked esophageal obstruction is actually a relative contraindication to PEG placement. Success will be dependent on the ability to pass the esophageal obstruction, even temporarily. There are several techniques for placing PEGs endoscopically: Pull, Push, Introducer (Russell), and Versa methods.

The Pull technique is the method originally popularized by Ponsky (Appendix II, Part A).[28] The Push technique is a variation that places a guidewire into the stomach that is pulled out of the mouth, and a feeding tube is "pushed" over the guidewire and then pulled from the abdominal incision as the catheter appears (Appendix II, Part B). Hogan et al. performed a prospective, randomized study where they found no significant difference between the Pull and Push techniques.[31] Both techniques are capable of providing equivalent size tubes and are standard methods of PEG placement today. Because the catheters are pulled down the esophagus, there is a possibility that the internal bumper could become lodged in the esophagus if there is intrinsic pathology such as a stricture or carcinoma. In these higher risk patients, either a suture should be looped in such a way around the bumper so that it will be possible to retrieve the PEG tube or another method of PEG insertion should be considered.[32] In patients with a high-grade esophageal obstruction, it will need to be determined if a radiologic or surgical approach is more appropriate, but often this cannot be determined until it is seen if the endoscope can pass the lesion. If the endoscope passes into the stomach, it is almost assured that one of the methods discussed can provide PEG access.

The Introducer (Russell) method is a variation of the Seldinger technique where a J-wire is placed into the stomach under endoscopic control (Appendix II, Part C). A dilating catheter is then placed into the stomach and a feeding tube placed through a peel-away sheath.[33] This initially resulted in a small feeding tube (14 Fr) that had a higher than average dislodgement rate. However, larger tubes can now be placed. Kozarek and co-workers compared the Russell technique to the Push method and found both successful and associated with an acceptable complication rate.[34] However, these authors preferred the Push technique.

Recently, Ross Laboratories (Columbus, Ohio) has introduced a variation of this technique called the Flexiflo® Introducer Gastrostomy Kit. Here four Brown/Mueller T-fasteners™ are placed to affix the stomach to the anterior wall, and an introducer needle allows placement of a J-wire into the stomach that is snared to secure it. A dilating catheter is then placed over the wire and finally a replacement gastrostomy set is placed over an introducer/stylet. This allows an 18 Fr tube to be placed that does not require a second endoscopic look or endoscopy to remove to replace the tube.

Another recently available technique, the Versa PEG (Ross Laboratories, Columbus, Ohio), is an interesting variation and combination of techniques (Appendix II, Part D). The feeding tube site is secured by the placement of four Brown/Mueller T-fasteners™ prior to the placement of Seldinger catheter into the stomach through which a guidewire is placed. The guidewire is grasped with a forceps or snare via an endoscope and is removed from the mouth. A special ''stoma creator tube'' is passed over the guidewire and the mouth and then through the anterior abdominal wall. A 22 Fr balloon replacement PEG is placed through the ''stoma creator tube'' and pulled into the stomach and inflated. However, these T-fasteners are sometimes tricky to use and once dislodged cannot be retrieved, which can be a potential problem if they are not correctly positioned. This technique can have some potential advantages in patients where an endoscope can pass through certain esophageal lesions and the ''stoma creator tube'' will take no more space than the endoscope. The gastrostomy catheter will not have to be dragged through the esophagus so that the internal bumper of the tube will not cause trauma or become lodged in patients with esophageal disease. The authors have used this technique successfully in a patient with a bulky and irregular esophageal cancer and in a patient with achalasia with a sigmoid esophagus who was unsuitable for pneumatic dilatation or surgery.[35] One advantage is that because a balloon replacement catheter is used as a primary tube, a repeat endoscopy is not needed to replace the tube, thus making exchange or discontinuation very easy and cost effective. This may be quite appropriate in the patient with inoperable esophageal cancer where a surgical gastrostomy may be less appealing and repeat endoscopy will not be necessary, given the limited life expectancy of these patients. It affords these patients the opportunity to end their lives without an NGT in place. It also provides a route for giving fluids, nutrition, and pain medication and helps limit, but not eliminate, pulmonary aspiration from attempts at eating or drinking.

PEG tubes are available in many styles and sizes and are in prepackaged kits. It is generally standard to put larger bore catheters (>18 Fr) in adults, but smaller tubes are available. The larger tubes are less likely to clog with feedings and medications. Most tubes have an inner bumper that is firm or pliable or a crossbar shape. The firm internal bumper is preferred for the patient who may inadvertently pull out the PEG tube, because it provides a more rigid support. Some models have an inflatable internal bumper that passes esophageal lesion more readily compared to tubes with large attached internal bumpers. After insertion of all models, an outer retention system is placed to prevent slippage of the tube into the stomach. Care must be taken not to pull these bumpers too tightly, which can lead to pressure necrosis and migration of the tube from the stomach through tissue layers out to the skin.[36,37]

2. Radiologically Placed Gastrostomy Tubes

While surgical and endoscopic placement of tube enterostomies are most common, there are techniques for placing these tubes under radiologic control.[38–42] The main disadvantage of this technique is that it has generally yielded a small tube compared to those available by other methods. Again, local expertise is important in the method of choice.

Ho and co-workers published an interesting retrospective comparison of surgical and percutaneous nonendoscopic gastrostomy.[43] Here, a radiologic technique placed a tube through the stomach and placed the tip at the duodenojejunal flexure. This paper is actually misnamed since the nonendoscopic tube is actually in the small intestine and not in the stomach. There were significantly fewer complications with the radiologic approach, and there were no episodes of aspiration after this technique as compared to the surgical group. Despite the small size of the catheter, 9 Fr (90 patients) and 10 Fr (43 patients), no comment is made about clogged catheters. This technique may be underutilized and should be seriously considered when aspiration is an issue as well as the risk of surgery.

3. Removal of PEGs

Many PEG tubes are removed with a second endoscopy because PEG models often have a rigid inner bumper. After the internal bumper is snared, the external portion of the tube is cut, and the resultant small tube is pulled through the GE junction and out of the mouth. With the original Ponsky style PEGs utilizing the Pezzer catheter, many physicians would apply external pressure, causing the Pezzer catheter to come out and leave the small internal bumper to make its way through the GI tract. This was a very cost-effective maneuver, but until the bumper was seen to pass in the stool, there was the risk of intestinal obstruction. This potential complication was commented on by Craig, but apparently, this particular bumper passed fairly readily.[44] However, in a case report by Waxman et al., it is mentioned that Ponsky noted a case of bumper-related obstruction with the original homemade kit, but no details were given.[45] Waxman further reported a case where a silicone Ponsky-Gauderer PEG (Bard Interventional Products, Billerica, Massachusetts) was cut at the skin level and caused an intestinal obstruction requiring surgical removal. This internal bumper was much larger than the small crossbar in the original kits. Korula and Harma reported a series of 64 patients where they pulled the external portion of the tube tightly and cut it at the level of the abdomen.[46] A Foley catheter was then pushed into the fistula tract to push the internal bumper into the stomach, where it was expected to pass uneventfully into the stool. Only one patient failed to have the bumper pass. It lodged at the pylorus and was removed endoscopically. Recently, a case of bowel obstruction and death from this type of removal was reported in an elderly patient.[47] Certain tubes with large internal bumpers may not be appropriate for this method of removal. We have seen one patient whose PEG tube bumper eroded and fractured at the skin and passed to the level of the terminal ileum before causing obstructive symptoms. This patient had a laparotomy to "milk" the bumper into the large intestine. After it did not pass, she was referred to our hospital where colonoscopic removal was performed (personal experience). It is our practice to remove tubes with rigid inner bumpers endoscopically unless there is a contraindication to do so.

Tube dislodgement or inadvertent removal requires immediate attention to prevent closure of the fistula tract. If inadvertent removal occurs in the first few weeks after PEG placement, then the stomach may fall away from the parietal peritoneum. Some centers have considered this an indication for exploratory laparotomy. Galat et al. have reported that they have repeated the endoscopic procedure immediately and given antibiotics with excellent results, thereby eliminating laparotomy.[48] They have estimated this problem to occur in 1.8% of their PEG procedures. In a more mature PEG tract, a Foley catheter can be placed as a temporizing measure to insure the integrity of the tract prior to replacement with a more standard replacement tube. Kadakia et al. prospectively studied a group of 28 patients using silicone (18 or 20 Fr) Foley catheters as replacement catheters.[49] They found these to be an acceptable alternative to the replacement tubes which were many times more expensive. They suggested a randomized trial of available replacement tubes and Foley catheters.

Replacement PEG kits generally utilize an inflatable balloon that serves as the internal bumper; however, other nonballoon models are available. PEG buttons or low profile gastrostomy kits are also available as replacement devices. In these devices a semirigid dome or inflatable balloon serves as the internal bumper. These devices are particularly useful in children, where the skin level devices are cosmetically and functionally more acceptable, or in the confused, combative patient who is more prone to pull at an attached tube and dislodge it. However, we have found that buttons are not optimal in patients who have tracheostomies because when they cough and markedly increase their intraabdominal pressure, they can defeat most antireflux valves of these buttons. This allows tube feeding and stomach acid to spill onto the patient's skin which can cause a severe chemical burn if not dealt with urgently.[50] Recently, Olympus Corporation (Lake Success, NY) has introduced the One-Step PEG Button™ that can be used as a primary device and is available in 18 and 24 Fr sizes.

Even though most physicians assume that once a PEG has been removed there will be no further complications because most of the sites appear to close over in 24 h, this has recently been shown to be an incorrect assumption. Bender and Levison report two cases of complications after PEG removal.[51] One patient had a persistent gastrocutaneous fistula requiring operative closure, and a second patient developed pneumoperitoneum after an episode of severe vomiting 3 weeks after PEG removal. In the latter case, laparotomy showed separation of the stomach from the posterior abdominal wall and peritonitis. This underscores the need to inform these patients and/or families about potential problems after PEG removal as well as to increase physician awareness.

4. Percutaneous Endoscopic Jejunostomy and Gastrojejunostomy

The term percutaneous endoscopic jejunostomy (PEJ) is often a misnomer since the original description of this procedure by Ponsky et al. yielded a one-piece apparatus consisting of a gastrostomy tube and a smaller "jejunal" tube that was dragged into the duodenum.[52] This tube often clogged or fell back into the stomach. Many other variations of this technique have subsequently yielded similar tubes which have gone into the proximal duodenum. Technically, proper placement has been hampered by tubes falling back into the stomach as forceps and endoscope are withdrawn. The main impetus to develop the PEJ was to try to reduce the risk of aspiration. The previous devices have generally not fulfilled this function again because of suboptimal placement within the duodenum. Thus, articles on the success, or lack thereof, of the PEJ must be viewed in terms of the ability to place the catheter reliably into the third or fourth portion of the duodenum or past the ligament of Trietz.[53–55]

Our center has reported a modification of the PEJ technique in which an over-the-guidewire method has placed the intestinal feeding tube at or past the ligament of Trietz in the majority of patients (Appendix II, Part E).[56,57] This has been done with a tube that provides gastric suction (28 Fr PEG, Sandoz Nutrition, Minneapolis, MN) and small intesinal feeding (12 Fr tube); we call this a percutaneous endoscopic gastrojejunostomy (PEG/J). In our experience, this has provided a very stable tube that is less likely to clog, and there have been no episodes of tube feeding aspiration. However, the long-term applicability and optimal patient population have not been identified. We find this tube very useful in the head-injured patient where we can obtain enteral access usually within 72 h. As gastric emptying improves several weeks later, the ''J'' portion can be removed, and the tube converted into a PEG.

A true PEJ has been described by Shike et al. and an endoscopically guided jejunostomy by Adams.[58,59] Both reports are in patients who have had partial gastric resections. Shike and colleagues report on 10 patients where they placed a standard Pezzar catheter into the jejunum in 9 patients and duodenum in 1.[58] They removed the internal horizontal bar bumper in these patients. A standard external bumper was used. There were two patients where they were not able clearly to visualize the endoscopic light and placement was not attempted. There were two complications: leakage of intestinal fluid around the PEJ in a patient who was later found to have a partial small bowel obstruction distal to the PEJ, and a localized peristomal infection that responded to antibiotic therapy.

Adams describes a technique that uses a colonoscope to place the scope deep into the jejunum and choose an appropriate site in the left hypochondrium.[59] The surgeon then makes an incision, parts the tissue layer, and delivers 10 to 15 cm of jejunum into the operative field. The surgeon can then place a straight tube Witzel jejunostomy, needle catheter jejunostomy, Tenchkoff catheter jejunostomy, or a button jejunostomy. This procedure provides a more secure placement that better protects against dislodgement compared to the procedure previously described by Shike et al.

Rosenblum and co-workers described a radiologic method for placement of a direct percutaneous jejunostomy tube.[60] In their patient with a near-obstructing pancreatic cancer, they were able to place a 16 Fr tube into the jejunum for feeding and a 12 Fr gastrostomy tube in the stomach. Long-term follow-up of this patient was not done, and a large comparative series is not available on this procedure. However, this method does provide a guide for those interested.

5. PEG and PEJ Complications

Table 3 shows complications related to endoscopically or radiologically placed tubes, some of which may be unique to these procedures. Most of the problems with PEG placement are generally minor and can be handled fairly easily.[61] However, there are problems that do occur which require higher levels of care or even operative intervention. Also, most series report their short-term complications, but not long-term problems. A recent study by Taylor et al. provides a sobering look at short- and long-term PEG-related complications.[29] They noted complications in 70% of patients, with 88% being minor and most occurring in the first 3 months after placement. A similar study of long-term problems with surgical gastrostomies might be equally enlightening.

Colocutaneous fistulas have been described, but seem to be an infrequent occurrence considering how many tubes have been placed by these methods.[62–65] While verifying

TABLE 3
PEG and PEJ Complications

Aspiration	Bleeding	Bowel obstruction
Buried bumper syndrome	Candida cellulitis	Clogged tube
Colocutaneous fistula	Dehydration	Extrusion/migration[a]
Gastric outlet obstruction	Hematoma	Hypopharyngeal/esophageal tube impaction

Ileus
   Prolonged
   From migrated PEG
	Inability to transilluminate	Incisional pain

Intraperitoneal placement	Intraperitoneal displacement	Mallory-Weiss tear of esophagus
Misplaced T-fastener	MRSA skin infection[b]	Multiple punctures of stomach
Necrotizing fasciitis	Peritonitis	Placement/technical failure
Pneumoperitoneum	Pneumonia	Small bowel perforation
Stomal leakage	Suture/wire breakage	Subcutaneous emphysema
Tube deterioration	Tube displacement	Volvulus
Wound infection		

[a] May also be part of the buried bumper syndrome.
[b] MRSA = Methicillin-resistant *Staphylococcus aureus.*

transillumination in the proper region helps to limit this complication, there is no guarantee short of an open or laparoscopic approach.

Wound infection is a common occurrence, and preprocedure antibiotics are now the standard of care.[66,67] However, several other interesting reports have also emerged including the following: candida cellulitis,[68] methicilin-resistant staphylococcus aureus wound infection/colonization,[69] and necrotizing fasciitis.[70–74]

Bowel obstruction has been reported from PEG balloons obstructing the pylorus or duodenum.[75] Also, parts of tube that have purposely been cut or have eroded have occasionally caused problems necessitating endoscopic removal or surgery, as previously discussed.[45,46,76]

Pneumoperitoneum is generally a benign occurrence after PEG placement.[77–79] In a study by Gottfried et al., it occurred in 38% of their PEG patients.[78] It is generally of no consequence, but its presence can inappropriately alert those who are unaware of the relationship to think that there is a surgical abdomen that has developed. This is usually not the case, and one reason that our group has always resisted placing PEGs in patients who have significant gastric or duodenal ulceration where subsequent perforation could confuse the patient's care. However, Ghahremani and colleagues reported a case of PEG-related pneumoperitoneum leading to progressive volvulus.[80]

Subcutaneous emphysema is another uncommon post-PEG complication.[81] Its main importance is its need to be differentiated from a more serious problem, necrotizing fasciitis, which requires immediate, aggressive attention. Subcutaneous emphysema is a benign process that occurs 7 hours to 7 days after PEG placement. It is not associated with high fever, as is the presentation of necrotizing fasciitis. In necrotizing fasciitis, the tube site may also show signs of erythema, induration, purulent drainage, and crepitus, which can lead to sepsis, clinical deterioration, and potentially death.[70]

Tube migration or erosion of the tube from inside the stomach toward the skin has been reported, as previously mentioned. It appears that the major factor in the pathogenesis of this problem is traction, either from the outside by too tight apposition of the external fixation device or even internal from the pressure of jejunostomy tube against the inner bumper.[36,37] Chung and Schertzer reported a comparative series that showed that traction on the gastrostomy tube is not only unnecessary, but is also the etiology of many of the complications reported.[82]

6. Surgical Gastrostomy

The first planned surgical gastrostomy is credited to Sedillot in 1846.[83] Witzel and Janeway made modifications, but the Stamm gastrostomy is generally the standard procedure today.[84] This technique can be performed alone, with other intra-abdominal procedures while under general anesthesia, or under local anesthesia in an appropriate patient. Concentric pursestring sutures are placed around the gastrostomy site so that a serosa-lined invagination is formed.[84] The major complications of this procedure include the following: wound dehiscence or infection, separation of the gastric and abdominal walls, injury to the posterior gastric wall, and leakage from an enlarging stoma. In addition to the direct procedure-related complications, the gastrostomy tube has been reported to cause complications including the following: gastric outlet obstruction,[85,86] duodenal prolapse of the tube with and without obstruction,[87–89] gastric laceration,[86] perforation of the stomach,[86–88] intussusception of the small bowel,[88] gastric torsion,[86] small bowel volvulus,[90] entero-enteric fistula and intussusception,[91] esophageal perforation,[88] and obstructive jaundice.[92–93]

As previously mentioned, when a tube enterostomy is the primary procedure, then performing it endoscopically has a slight advantage. This is especially true if placement is not done in the operating room or under general anesthesia; then there should be a cost savings favoring the endoscopic approach.[61] Stiegmann and colleagues prospectively compared operative gastrostomy performed under local anesthesia to percutaneous placement with a Sacks-Vine PEG.[94,95] They found no statistical difference in the morbidity or mortality of the two procedures. However, there was a slight economic advantage to the endoscopic technique.

Laparoscopic gastrostomy has also been reported.[96–98] While it will likely have a significant niche in the placement of these tubes in the future, a large comparative series needs to be performed. This technique will be very useful when there is an obstructing esophageal lesion preventing an endoscopic approach. Since it generally requires an operating room setting, it will probably be more expensive than endoscopic placement. A laparoscopic version of a PEG kit is now available.

7. Surgical Jejunostomy

Surmay performed the first surgical jejunostomy in 1878.[99] While many modifications have been made, the techniques that are currently used are as follows: Witzel jejunostomy, needle catheter jejunostomy, Roux-En-Y jejunostomy, and percutaneous peritoneoscopic jejunostomy.[100–102] A Witzel jejunostomy secures a portion of jejunum approximately 8 cm distal to the ligament of Treitz and anchors a #16 Fr rubber catheter. In 1973 Delany et al. described a modification creating a needle catheter jejunostomy.[103] This utilizes a 16-gauge catheter generally used for subclavian vein access. The small size of the catheter limits the type of tube feeding that can be infused through it. Later variations of this technique created a serosal tunnel with fixation of a section of the jejunum to the parietal peritoneum. Yeung and co-workers found this technique not to be beneficial in routine colorectal surgeries, but suggested that patients be carefully selected for this procedure.[104] Cobb et al. found the serosal tunnel jejunostomy to be technically safe and very effective, especially in patients who were judged to require long-term nutritional support.[105]

Roux-en-Y jejunostomy creates a permanent jejunostomy (Figure 2). The free end of a Roux-en-Y limb is brought to the skin. This procedure has the advantage of not allowing the stoma to close when the feeding tube is removed for hours or even days. The Roux-en-Y limb allows feedings to be placed into the GI tract, but diverts digestive juices from refluxing onto the skin.[100]

Some physicians are concerned about the small size of the tube that most jejunostomy procedures produce. However, Walters and co-workers report a technique for replacing

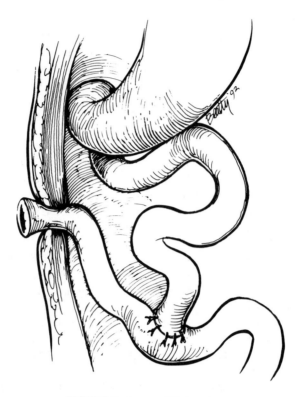

FIGURE 2. Roux-en-Y jejunostomy.

the 5 Fr tube that is standard in the needle jejunostomy kits with an 8 or 10 Fr tube after a simple dilating procedure in an established jejunostomy tract.[106] Another interesting modification of the jejunostomy operative technique is offered by Stellato and Gauderer, who have placed gastrostomy buttons in the jejunum as the primary tube.[107] This procedure allows for change of the button when needed, and generally a larger diameter tube can be used. This study reports their experience of 90 buttons in 50 children and 6 adults.

Some jejunostomy tubes are discontinued when it is believed that they are not required further; however, it may be discovered later that it is required again. Westfall et al. report a method for using an endoscope to go down to the site of an earlier surgical jejunostomy, and endoscopically to place a modified PEG catheter into the previously adhered area.[108] Transillumination and visible dimpling by an assistant's finger are key factors. The authors have utilized this technique in three patients; two patients had previous esophago-gastrectomy, and one patient had a vagotomy and pyloroplasty with Billroth II loop antecolic gastrojejunostomy.

Percutaneous peritoneoscopic jejunostomy provides a recent addition to the possible methods of placing a jejunostomy feeding tube.[101] The jejunum distal to the ligament of Treitz is identified in the left upper quadrant under laparoscopic control, and Endoclips® are used to clip the mesentery to the peritoneum. A needle introducer is placed into the jejunum subserosally and then into the gut lumen. The jejunum is additionally secured to the anterior abdominal wall to minimize tube dislodgement. Unfortunately, while this avoids a formal laparotomy, it yields a small feeding tube that is subject to the same problems as a standard needle catheter jejunostomy. Also, no large studies are available to provide any meaningful comparison of advantages or disadvantages of this procedure. Morris and colleagues offer a slightly different approach to the laparoscopic technique where they place a 12 Fr red rubber catheter as their final tube.[102] This procedure yields a good size tube with a minimally invasive procedure. This technique has promise for the future.

IV. CONCLUSION

The last decade has seen a rapid advancement in our knowledge and ability to provide enteral nutrition. New techniques that involve endoscopy, radiology, and surgery are being developed and refined at a frightening pace. Though we are seeing a technological explosion in our ability to provide enteral access, we must not lose sight of our duty to control and to choose wisely when we apply these principles and techniques to our patients. These techniques all have their risks and benefits, and we must be ever vigilant for complications as they develop. The next chapter will discuss the complications associated with enteral nutrition and a discussion of tube feeding choices.

REFERENCES

1. **Cashman, MD.** Principles of digestive physiology for clinical nutrition. *Nutr Clin Pract*, 1:241–9, 1986.
2. **Randall, HT.** The history of enteral nutrition. In *Enteral and Tube Feeding*, Rombeau, JL and Caldwell, MD, Eds., W. B. Saunders, Philadelphia, 1984, 1–9.
3. **Rhoads, JE.** Forward. In *Enteral and Tube Feeding*, Rombeau, JL and Caldwell, MD, Eds., W. B. Saunders, Philadelphia, 1984, ix–xi.
4. **His, W.** Zur geschichte der magenpumpe. *Med Klin*, 21:391–3, 1925.
5. **Pareira, MD, Conrad, EJ, Hicks, W, and Elman, R.** Therapeutic nutrition with tube feeding. *JAMA*, 156:810–6, 1954.
6. **Alcock, T.** On the immediate treatment of persons poisoned. *Lancet*, 1:372–7, 1823.
7. **Hunter, J.** A case of paralysis of the muscles of deglutition cured by an artificial mode of conveying food and medicines into the stomach. *Trans Soc Improve Med Chir Know*, 1:182–8, 1793.
8. **Levin, AL.** A new gastroduodenal catheter. *JAMA*, 76:1007, 1921.
9. **Keoshian, LA, and Nelsen, TS.** A new design for a feeding tube. *Plast Reconstr Surg*, 44:508–9, 1969.
10. **Klopp, CT.** Cervical esophagostomy. *J Cardiovasc Surg*, 21:490–1, 1951.
11. **Bucklin, DL, and Gilsdorf, RG.** Percutaneous needle pharyngostomy. *JPEN*, 9:68–70, 1985.
12. **Forlaw, L, and Chernoff, R.** Enteral delivery systems. In *Enteral and Tube Feeding*. Rombeau, JL and Caldwell, MD, Eds., W. B. Saunders, Philadelphia, 1984, 228–239.
13. **Torres, A, Serra-Battles, J, Ros, E, et al.** Pulmonary aspiration of gastric contents in patients receiving mechanical ventilation: the effect of body position. *Ann Intern Med*, 116:540–3, 1992.
14. **Ibañez, J, Penafiel, A, Raurich, JM, et al.** Gastroesophageal reflux in intubated patients receiving enteral nutrition: effect of supine and semirecumbent positions. *JPEN*, 16:419–22, 1992.
15. **Lipman, TO.** The fate of enteral feeding tubes. *Nutr Supp Serv*, 3:71, 1983.
16. **Whatley, K, Turner, WW, Jr, Dey, M, et al.** When does metoclopramide facilitate transpyloric intubation? *JPEN*, 8:679–81, 1984.
17. **Kittinger, JW, Sandler, RS, and Heizer, WD.** Efficacy of metoclopramide as an adjunct to duodenal placement of small-bore feeding tubes: a randomized, placebo-controlled, double-blind study. *JPEN*, 11:33–7, 1987.
18. **Seifert, CF, Cuddy, PG, Pemberton, B, et al.** A randomized trial of metoclopramide's effects on the transpyloric intubation of weighted feeding tubes. *Nutr Supp Serv*, 7:11–13, 1987.
19. **Kalafarentzos, F, Alivizatos, V, Panagopoulos, K, and Androulakis, J.** Nasoduodenal intubation with the use of metoclopramide. *Nutr Supp Serv*, 7:33–4, 1987.
20. **Wolf, DC, and Stern, MA.** Erythromycin elixir facilitates the transpyloric passage of enteral feeding tubes: preliminary results of a prospective randomized controlled trial. *Am J Gastroenterol*, 87:1278, 1992 (abstract).
21. **Gutierrez, ED and Balfe, DM.** Fluoroscopically guided nasoenteric feeding tube placement: results of a 1-year study. *Radiology*, 178:759–62, 1991.

22. **Armstrong, C, Luther, W, and Sykes, T.** A technique for preventing extubation of feeding tubes: "the bridle". *JPEN,* 4:603, 1980 (abstract).
23. **Roubenoff, R, and Ravich, WJ.** The technique of avoiding feeding tube misplacement. *J Crit Illness,* 4:75–9, 1989.
24. **Raff, MH, Cho, S, and Dale, R.** A technique for positioning nasoenteral feeding tubes. *JPEN,* 11:210–3, 1987.
25. **Ugo, PJ, Mohler, PA, and Wilson, GL.** Bedside postpyloric placement of weighted feeding tubes. *Nutr Clin Pract,* 7:284–7, 1992.
26. **Baskin, WN and Johanson, JF.** A novel approach to enteral nutrition in the ICU. *Gastrointest Endosc,* 38:272, 1992 (abstract).
27. **Baskin, WN.** Advances in enteral nutrition techniques. *Am J Gastroenterol,* 87:1547–53, 1992.
28. **Gauderer, MWL, Ponsky, JL, and Izant, RJ, Jr.** Gastrostomy without laparotomy: a percutaneous endoscopic technique. *J Pediatr Surg,* 15:872–5, 1980.
29. **Taylor, CA, Larson, DE, and Ballard, DJ, et al.** Predictors of outcome after percutaneous endoscopic gastrostomy: a community-based study. *Mayo Clin Proc,* 67: 1042–9, 1992.
30. **Kirby, DF.** To PEG or not to PEG—that is the costly question. *Mayo Clin Proc,* 67: 1115–7, 1992 (editorial).
31. **Hogan, RB, DeMarco, DC, and Hamilton, JK.** Percutaneous endoscopic gastrostomy—to push or pull: a prospective randomized trial. *Gastrointest Endosc,* 32:253–8, 1986.
32. **Patel, J and Wang, M.** Percutaneous endoscopic gastrostomy—secure the mushroom head. *Gastrointest Endosc,* 30:218–9, 1984 (letter).
33. **Russell, TR, Brotman, M, and Norris, F.** Percutaneous gastrostomy: a new simplified and cost-effective technique. *Am J Surg,* 148:132–7, 1984.
34. **Kozarek, RA, Ball, T, and Ryan, J.** Percutaneous endoscopic gastrostomy: when push comes to shove, a comparison of two insertion methods. *Am J Gastroenterol,* 81:642–6, 1986.
35. **Deal, SE and Kirby, DF.** Percutaneous Endoscopic Gastrostomy (PEG) placement using Ross Laboratories VERSA-PEG procedure: insertion and efficacy study. *Am J Gastroenterol,* 85:1232, 1990 (abstract).
36. **Klein, S, Heare, BR, and Soloway, RD.** The "Buried Bumper Syndrome": a complication of percutaneous endoscopic gastrostomy. *Am J Gastroenterol,* 85:448–51, 1990.
37. **Behrle, KM, Dekovich, AA, and Ammon, HV.** Spontaneous tube extrusion following percutaneous endoscopic gastrostomy. *Gastrointest Endosc,* 35:56–8, 1989.
38. **Preshaw, RM.** A percutaneous method for inserting a feeding gastrostomy tube. *Surg Gynecol Obstet,* 152:659–60, 1981.
39. **Willis, JS and Oglesby, JT.** Percutaneous gastrostomy. *Radiology,* 149:449–53, 1983.
40. **Tao, HH and Gillies, RR.** Percutaneous feeding gastrostomy. *AJR,* 141:793–4, 1983.
41. **vanSonnenberg, E, Cubberley, DA, Brown, LK, et al.** Percutaneous gastrostomy: use of intragastric balloon support. *Radiology,* 152:531–2, 1984.
42. **Brown, AS, Mueller, PR, and Ferrucci, JT, Jr.** Controlled percutaneous gastrostomy: nylon T-fastener for fixation of the anterior gastric wall. *Radiology,* 158:543–5, 1986.
43. **Ho, C-S, Yee, ACN, and McPherson, R.** Complications of surgical and percutaneous nonendoscopic gastrostomy: review of 233 patients. *Gastroenterology,* 95:1206–10, 1988.
44. **Craig, RM.** Removing percutaneously placed gastrostomy tubes. *Gastrointest Endosc,* 32:430, 1986 (letter).
45. **Waxman, I, Al-Kawas, FH, Bass, B, and Glouderman, M.** PEG ileus: a new cause of small bowel obstruction. *Dig Dis Sci,* 36:251–4, 1991.
46. **Korula, J and Harma, C.** A simple and inexpensive method of removal or replacement of gastrostomy tubes. *JAMA,* 265:1426–8, 1991.
47. **Garenani, CL, Setzen, G, Harvey, LP, and Bronzo, R.** PEG removal by traction technique: is it really safe? *Am J Gastroenterol,* 87:1355, 1992 (abstract).
48. **Galat, SA, Gerig, KD, Porter, JA, and Slezak, FA.** Management of premature removal of the percutaneous gastrostomy. *Am Surg,* 56:733–6, 1990.
49. **Kadakia, SC, Cassaday, M, and Shaffer, RT.** Prospective evaluation of Foley catheter as a replacement gastrostomy tube. *Am J Gastroenterol,* 87:1594–7, 1992.
50. **Sanyal, A, Jefferson, PA, and Kirby, DF.** Percutaneous endoscopic gastrostomy button malfunction with severe cough. *Gastrointest Endosc,* 35:118–9, 1989.
51. **Bender, JA, and Levison, MA.** Complications after percutaneous endoscopic gastrostomy removal. *Surg Laparosc Endosc,* 1:101–3, 1991.
52. **Ponsky, JL and Aszodi, A.** Percutaneous endoscopic jejunostomy. *Am J Gastroenterol,* 79:113–6, 1984.

53. **DiSario, JA, Foutch, PG, and Sanowski, RA.** Poor results with percutaneous endoscopic jejunostomy. *Gastrointest Endosc,* 36:257–60, 1990.
54. **Wolfsen, HC, Kozarek, RA, Ball, TJ, et al.** Tube dysfunction following percutaneous endoscopic gastrostomy and jejunostomy. *Gastrointest Endosc,* 36:261–3, 1990.
55. **Lewis, BS.** Perform PEJ, not PED. *Gastrointest Endosc,* 36:311–2, 1990 (editorial).
56. **Duckworth, PF, Jr, Kirby, DF, and McHenry L.** Percutaneous endoscopic gastrojejunostomy made easy: a simplified endoscopic technique. *Gastrointest Endosc,* 37:269, 1991 (abstract).
57. **DeLegge, MH, Duckworth, PF, Craig, RM, et al.** Percutaneous endoscopic gastrojejunostomy (PEG/J): simple and effective. *Am J Gastroenterol,* 87:1338, 1992 (abstract).
58. **Shike, M, Schroy, P, Ritchie, MA, et al.** Percutaneous endoscopic jejunostomy in cancer patients with previous gastric resection. *Gastrointest Endosc,* 33:372–4, 1987.
59. **Adams, DB.** Feeding jejunostomy with endoscopic guidance. *Surg Gynecol Obstet,* 172:239–41, 1991.
60. **Rosenblum, J, Taylor, FC, Lu, C-T, and Martich, V.** A new technique for direct percutaneous jejunostomy tube placement. *Am J Gastroenterol,* 85:1165–7, 1990.
61. **Kirby, DF, Craig, RM, Tsang, T-K, and Plotnick BH.** Percutaneous endoscopic gastrostomies: a prospective evaluation and review of the literature. *JPEN,* 10:155–9, 1986.
62. **Saltzberg, DM, Anand, K, Juvan, P, and Joffe, I.** Colocutaneous fistula: an unusual complication of percutaneous endoscopic gastrostomy. *JPEN,* 11:86–7, 1987.
63. **Berger, SA and Zarling, EJ.** Colocutaneous fistula following migration of PEG tube. *Gastrointest Endosc,* 36:86–88, 1991.
64. **Fernandes, ET, Hollabaugh, R, Hixon, SD, and Whitington, G.** Late presentation of gastrocolic fistula after percuatneous gastrostomy. *Gastrointest Endosc,* 34:368–9, 1988.
65. **van Gossum, A, DesMarez, B, and Cremer, M.** A colo-cutaneous-gastric fistula: a silent and unusual complication of percutaneous endoscopic gastrostomy. *Endoscopy,* 20:161, 1988 (letter).
66. **Jonas, SK, Neimark, S, and Panwalker, AP.** Effect of antibiotic prophylaxis in percutaneous endoscopic gastrostomy. *Am J Gastroenterol,* 80:438–41, 1985.
67. **Jain, NK, Larson, DE, Schroeder, KW, et al.** Antibiotic prophylaxis for percutaneous endoscopic gastrostomy: a prospective, randomized, double-blind clinical trial. *Ann Intern Med,* 107:824–8, 1987.
68. **Patel, AS, DeRidder, PH, Alexander, TJ, et al.** Candida cellulitis: a complication of percutaneous endoscopic gastrostomy. *Gastrointest Endosc,* 35:571–2, 1989.
69. **Nunley, D and Berk, SL.** Percutaneous endoscopic gastrostomy as an unrecognized source of methicillin-resistant Staphylococcus aureus colonization. *Am J Gastroenterol,* 87:58–61, 1992.
70. **Grief, JM, Ragland, JJ, Ochsner, MG, and Riding, R.** Fatal necrotizing fasciitis complicating percutaneous endoscopic gastrostomy. *Gastrointest Endosc,* 32:292–3, 1986.
71. **Cave, DR, Robinson, WR, and Brotschi, EA.** Necrotizing fasciitis following percutaneous endoscopic gastrostomy, *Gastrointest Endosc,* 32:294–6, 1986.
72. **Person, JL and Brower, RA.** Necrotizing fasciitis/myositis following percutaneous endoscopic gastrostomy. *Gastrointest Endosc,* 32:309, 1986 (letter).
73. **Korula, J, and Rice HE.** Necrotizing fasciitis and percutaneous endoscopic gastrostomy. *Gastrointest Endosc,* 33:335–6, 1987 (letter).
74. **Haas, DW, Dharmaraja, P, Morrison, JG, and Potts, JR.** III. Necrotizing fasciitis following percutaneous endoscopic gastrostomy. *Gastrointest Endosc,* 34:487–8, 1988 (letter).
75. **Fisher, LS, Bonell, JC, and Greenberg, E.** Gastrostomy tube migration and gastric outlet obstruction following percutaneous endoscopic gastrostomy. *Gastrointest Endosc,* 33:381–2, 1987.
76. **Wilson, WCM, Zenone, EA, and Spector, H.** Small intestinal perforation following replacement of a percutaneous endoscopic gastrostomy tube. *Gastrointest Endosc,* 36:62–3, 1990.
77. **Stassen, WN, McCullough, AJ, Marshall, JB, and Eckhauser, ML.** Percutaneous endoscopic gastrostomy: another cause of "benign" pneumoperitoneum. *Gastrointest Endosc,* 30:296–8, 1984.
78. **Gottfried, EB, Plumser, AB, and Clair, MR.** Pneumoperitoneum following percutaneous endoscopic gastrostomy: a prospective study. *Gastrointest Endosc,* 32:397–9, 1986.
79. **Schnall, HA, Falkenstein, DB, and Raicht, RF.** Persistent pneumoperitoneum after percutaneous endoscopic gastrostomy. *Gastrointest Endosc,* 33:248–50, 1987.
80. **Ghahremani, GG, Tsang, T-K, and Vakil, N.** Complications of endoscopic gastrostomy: pneumoperitoneum and volvulus of the colon. *Gastrointest Radiol,* 12:172–4, 1987.
81. **Stathopoulous, G, Rudberg, MA, and Harig, JM.** Subcutaneous emphysema following PEG. *Gastrointest Endosc,* 37:374–6, 1991.
82. **Chung, RS and Schertzer, M.** Pathogenesis of complications of percutaneous endoscopic gastrostomy: a lesson in surgical principles. *Am Surg,* 3:134–7, 1990.
83. **Cunha, F.** Gastrostomy: its inception and evolution. *Am J Surg,* 72:610–34, 1946.
84. **Stamm, M.** Gastrostomy by a new method. *Med News,* 65:324–6, 1894.

85. **Sherman, ML, Cosgrove, MJ, and Dennis, JM.** Gastrostomy tube migration. *Am Surg,* 39:122–3, 1973
86. **Vade, A, Jafri, SZH, Agha, FP, et al.** Radiologic evaluation of gastrostomy complications. *AJR,* 141:325–30, 1982.
87. **Wolf, EL, Frager, D, and Beneventano, TC.** Radiologic demonstration of important gastrostomy tube complications. *Gastrointest Radiol,* 11:20–6, 1986.
88. **Haws, EB, Sieber, WK, and Kiesewetter, WB.** Complications of tube gastrostomy in infants and children. *Ann Surg,* 164:284–90, 1966.
89. **Osborne, RO, and Toffler, RB.** Gastrostomy tube prolapse. *Am J Gastroenterol,* 60:602–6, 1973.
90. **Senac, MO, Jr and Lee, FA.** Small-bowel volvulus as a complication of gastrostomy. *Radiology,* 149:136, 1983
91. **Tom, W, Zachary, K, Fruchter, G, and Simko, V.** Case report: prolapse of gastrostomy tube resulting in entero-enteric fistula and intussusception. *Am Surg,* 54:245–7, 1988.
92. **Konda, J and Ruggle, P.** Prolapse of Foley catheter gastrostomy tube causing obstructive jaundice. *Am J Gastroenterol,* 76:353–5, 1981.
93. **Gustavsson, S, and Klingen, G.** Obstructive jaundice complication of Foley catheter gastrostomy. *Acta Chir Scand,* 144:325–7, 1978.
94. **Stiegmann, GV, Goff, J, VanWay, C, et al.** Operative versus endoscopic gastrostomy: preliminary results of a prospective randomized trial. *Am J Surg,* 155:88–91, 1988.
95. **Stiegmann, GV, Goff, JS, Silas, D, et al.** Endoscopic versus operative gastrostomy: final results of a prospective randomized trial. *Gastrointest Endosc,* 36:1–5, 1990.
96. **Edelman, DS and Unger, SW.** Laparoscopic gastrostomy. *Surg Gynecol Obstet,* 173:401, 1991.
97. **Edelman, DS, Unger, SW, and Russin, DR.** Laparoscopic gastrostomy. *Surg Laparosc Endosc,* 1:251–3, 1991.
98. **Reiner, DS, Leitman, IM, and Ward, RJ.** Laparoscopic Stamm gastrostomy with gastropexy. *Surg Laparosc Endosc,* 1:189–92, 1991.
99. **Surmay, M.** Observation d'enterosomie. *Bull Gen Ther,* 65:324–6, 1878.
100. **Rombeau, JL, Barot, LR, Low, DW, and Twomey, PL.** Feeding by tube enterostomy. In: *Enteral and Tube Feeding,* Rombeau, JL and Caldwell, MD, Eds., W. B. Saunders, Philadelphia, 1984, 275–91.
101. **Reed, DN.** Percutaneous peritoneoscopic jejunostomy. *Surg Gynecol Obstet,* 174:527–9, 1992.
102. **Morris, JB, Mullen, JL, Yu, JC, and Rosato, EF.** Laparoscopic-guided jejunostomy. *Surgery,* 112:96–9, 1992.
103. **Delany, HM, Carnevale, NJ, and Garvey, JW.** Jejunostomy by a needle catheter technique. *Surgery,* 73:786–90, 1973.
104. **Yeung, CK, Young, GA, Hackett, AF, and Hill, GL.** Fine needle catheter jejunostomy—an assessment of a new method of nutritional support after major gastrointestinal surgery. *Br J Surg,* 66:727–32, 1979.
105. **Cobb, LM, Cartmill, AM, and Gilsdorf, RB.** Early postoperative nutritional support using the serosal tunnel jejunostomy. *JPEN,* 5:397–401, 1981.
106. **Walters, AM, Bender, CE, and Sarr, MG.** Percutaneous conversion of needle catheter jejunostomy to large bore jejunostomy for long term use. *Surg Gynecol Obstet,* 173:397–8, 1991.
107. **Stellato, TA and Gauderer, MWL.** Jejunostomy button as a new method for long term jejunostomy feedings. *Surg Gynecol Obstet,* 168:553–4, 1989.
108. **Westfall, SH, Andrus, CH, and Naunheim, KS.** A reproducible, safe jejunostomy replacement technique by a percutaneous endoscopic method. *Am Surg,* 56:141–3, 1990.

APPENDIX II

DISCLAIMER

The illustrations on the following pages are intended for educational and instructional purposes only. Each manufacturer has a specific set of instructions for their products which should be adhered to when performing these procedures. The authors bear no responsibility for those attempting to use these illustrations as procedure-related instructions.

PART A

PULL TECHNIQUE OF PERCUTANEOUS ENDOSCOPIC GASTROSTOMY

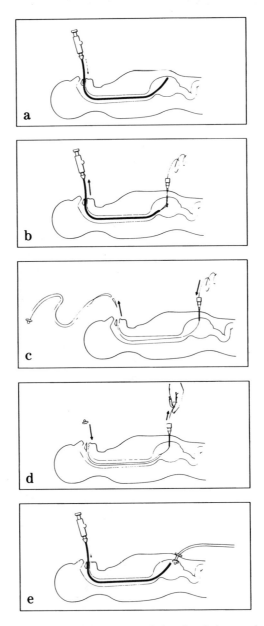

These drawings have been kindly provided and permission for their use given by Sandoz Nutrition, Minneapolis, MN.

PART A

PULL TECHNIQUE OF PERCUTANEOUS ENDOSCOPIC GASTROSTOMY (PEG) FIGURE EXPLANATION

a. The proper site for PEG insertion is identified.
b. After the overlying skin is cleansed and injected with local anesthetic, a skin incision is made. A needle cannula is placed into the stomach and a wire is placed through the cannula. The wire is grasped with either a snare or grasping forceps and removed with the endoscope from the patient.
c. The PEG assembly is attached to the wire and lubricated.
d. The PEG assembly is then pulled from the abdominal side until there is mild resistance from the inner stomach wall.
e. The endoscope is reinserted to verify the proper position of the internal bumper and to make sure that the proper amount of tension is placed on the outer bumper device used to help hold the PEG in the correct position.

PART B

PUSH TECHNIQUE OF PERCUTANEOUS
ENDOSCOPIC GASTROSTOMY

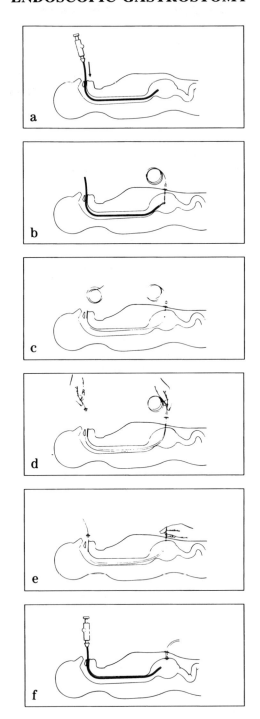

These drawings have been kindly provided and permission for their use given by Sandoz Nutrition, Minneapolis, MN.

PART B

PUSH TECHNIQUE OF PERCUTANEOUS ENDOSCOPIC GASTROSTYMY (PEG) FIGURE EXPLANATION

a. The proper site for PEG insertion is identified.

b. After the overlying skin is cleansed and injected with local anesthetic, a skin incision is made. A needle cannula is placed into the stomach and a wire is placed through the cannula. The wire is grasped with either a snare or grasping forceps and removed with the endoscope from the patient.

c. The wire is pulled through the mouth so that there is enough guidewire from the mouth to match the length of the tapered dilator/PEG tube assembly.

d. The wire is passed through the tapered end of the dilator so that the wire is visible from the PEG assembly. The dilator/PEG is then pushed down the wire while keeping tension on both pieces of the guidewire. Once in the stomach, the tapered tip of the dilator will meet the needle cannula and push out of the abdominal wall following the wire's path.

e. The dilator/PEG assembly is grasped and then pulled through the abdominal wall until there is mild resistance from the inner stomach wall.

f. The endoscope is reinserted to verify the proper position of the internal bumper and to make sure that the proper amount of tension is placed on the outer bumper device used to help hold the PEG in the correct position.

PART C

INTRODUCER (RUSSELL) TECHNIQUE OF PERCUTANEOUS ENDOSCOPIC GASTROSTOMY

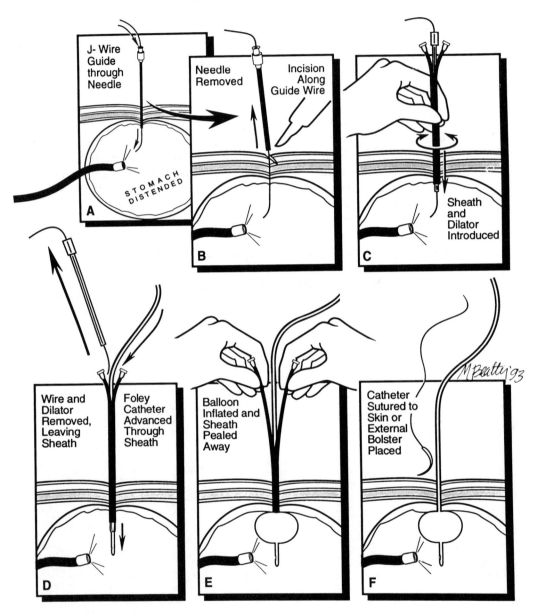

Illustrations by Mary Beatty and permission for use granted by the McGuire Veterans Affairs Medical Center, Richmond, VA.

PART C

INTRODUCER (RUSSELL) TECHNIQUE OF PERCUTANEOUS ENDOSCOPIC GASTROSTOMY (PEG) FIGURE EXPLANATION

a. The proper site for PEG insertion is identified. The site is cleansed and a Seldinger needle inserted into the stomach and verified by the endoscope. A J-wire is placed through the needle.

b. The needle is removed, but carefully maintaining the wire in the stomach. An incision is made along the guidewire.

c. A sheath and dilating catheter are threaded onto the guidewire and passed into the stomach.

d. The guidewire and inner dilator portion of the catheter are removed leaving the sheath in the stomach. A Foley catheter is advanced through the sheath.

e. The retention balloon of the catheter is inflated with water or saline, and the outer sheath is pealed away. The balloon is snugged up against the inner gastric wall.

f. The catheter is secured either by suturing it to the skin or placing an external bolster to help minimize movement or migration of the Foley catheter.

PART D

VERSA-PEG TECHNIQUE OF PERCUTANEOUS
ENDOSCOPIC GASTROSTOMY

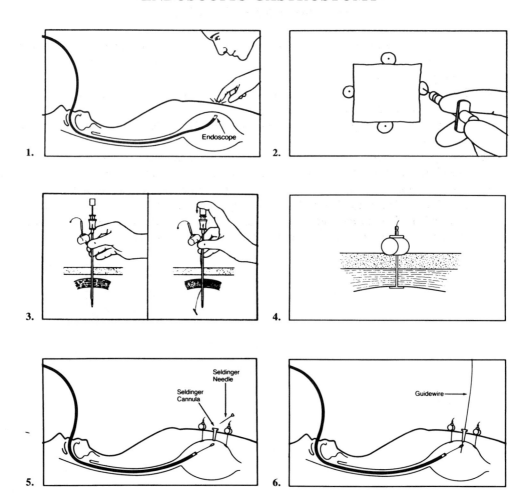

Reprinted with permission of Ross Laboratories, Columbus, OH.

PART D

VERSA-PEG TECHNIQUE OF PERCUTANEOUS ENDOSCOPIC GASTROSTOMY (PEG) FIGURE EXPLANATION

1. The proper site for PEG insertion is identified.
2. Place a 2 × 2 gauze over the insertion site as a guide for T-Fastener placement. Apply local anesthetic at midpoints of sides.
3. (A) insufflate stomach with air, and insert slotted needle (preloaded with T-Fastener). (B) Dislodge T-Fastener.
4. Withdraw the needle and stylet. Pull up "T" against gastric mucosa. Snug cotton pledget gently against skin surface. Slide nylon washer down and crimp aluminum crimps to hold T-Fastener in place. This procedure is repeated until all four T-Fasteners are in place.
5. Make incision. Insert Seldinger Needle. Remove inner stylet, leaving outer cannula in place. Loop endoscopic snare loosely over end of cannula.
6. Insert soft, floppy end of guidewire and grasp with snare. Remove endoscope to bring guidewire out through mouth.

PART D

VERSA-PEG TECHNIQUE OF PERCUTANEOUS ENDOSCOPIC GASTROSTOMY (Cont.)

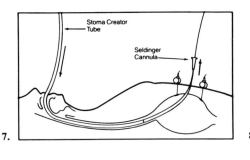

7.

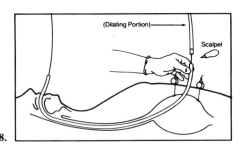

8.

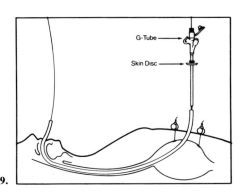

9.

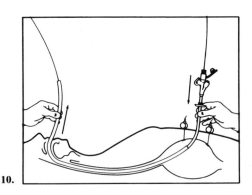

10.

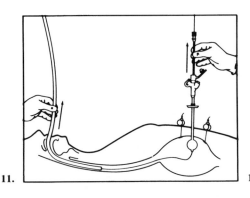

11.

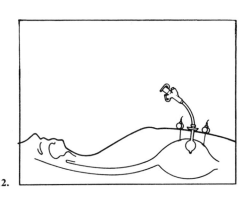

12.

Reprinted with permission of Ross Laboratories Columbus, OH.

PART D

VERSA-PEG TECHNIQUE OF PERCUTANEOUS ENDOSCOPIC GASTROSTOMY (PEG) FIGURE EXPLANATION (Continued)

7. Thread entire Stoma Creator Tube over guidewire, pass through oropharynx and into stomach, then out through abdominal wall, pushing cannula out.

8. Cut off dilating portion and remove from guidewire, leaving 2 to 3 inches of silicone tube protruding out from stoma.

9. Move skin disc up on Flexiflo Gastrostomy Tube and seat Introducer/Stylet firmly inside tube. Thread onto guidewire, lubricate tube nose, then insert G-Tube into protruding silicone tube up to lower end of balloon.

10. Simultaneously push G-Tube while pulling Stoma Creator Tube out of stomach, until the junction of the two tubes passes into stomach. Fill G-Tube with 10 to 20 ml of water or saline.

11. Pull Stoma Creator Tube out of stomach and remove from guidewire. Pull Introducer/Stylet out of G-Tube and remove from guidewire.

12. Slide skin disc down loosely against abdomen and verify there is some in-and-out play of G-Tube after the skin disc is positioned. This can be assessed by feel or, if desired, by direct visualization by reinserting the endoscope back into the stomach. Note: There should be no blanching of gastric mucosa.

PART E

PEG/J TECHNIQUE OF PERCUTANEOUS ENDOSCOPIC GASTROJEJUNOSTOMY

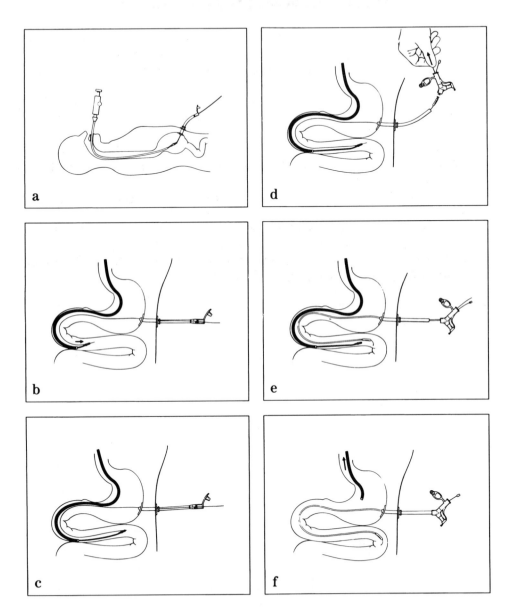

These drawings have been kindly provided and permission for their use given by Sandoz Nutrition, Minneapolis, MN.

PART E

PEG/J TECHNIQUE OF PERCUTANEOUS ENDOSCOPIC GASTROJEJUNOSTOMY FIGURE EXPLANATION

a. After an appropriate PEG assembly has been placed, the endoscope is reinserted into the stomach and a guidewire is grasped with a grasping forceps.

b. The endoscope with grasping forceps and guidewire are guided from the stomach through the pylorus and past the Ampulla of Vater and into the third portion of the duodenum.

c. Under direct vision of the endoscope the grasping forceps and guidewire are carefully advanced down the lumen of the intestine an additional 5 to 10 cm.

d. The jejunal feeding tube is then lubricated and passed over the guidewire until it is just about to enter the PEG tube. The guidewire is gently pulled from the outside until it feels tight.

e. The jejunal tube is guided over the guidewire while maintaining gentle tension on the wire. The feeding tube may be seen passing in front of the endoscope and may knock the forceps off the guidewire as it passes distally.

f. The endoscope is carefully removed from the small intestine and the tube position is verified by endoscope to ensure that there is not a large loop in the stomach. An abdominal radiograph is obtained to verify a distal placement of the small feeding tube.

Chapter 7

ENTERAL FEEDING: METHODS OF DELIVERY, FORMULA SELECTION, AND COMPLICATIONS

Mark H. DeLegge and Donald F. Kirby

TABLE OF CONTENTS

0-8493-7847-8/94/$0.00+$.50
© 1994 by CRC Press, Inc.

I. INTRODUCTION

The previous chapter has reviewed the state of the art regarding enteral access techniques. Once access has been established, then the focus must turn to providing safe and comprehensive enteral therapy. While being ever vigilant for potential complications, the method of delivery and choice of formula must be made. The purpose of this chapter will be to review the methods of delivery, to discuss enteral formula choices, and to review complications and strategies to limit them.

II. METHODS OF DELIVERY

Delivery methods for enteral feeding are either bolus, gravity, or mechanical pump systems. Each method has its own specific use and associated complications. Bolus feeding is the rapid delivery of formula, usually by syringe method, over 5 to 10 min every several hours. To meet a patient's caloric needs, 300 to 400 cc may need to be delivered at one sitting. This rate of delivery would usually not be tolerated if delivered to the small bowel, thus limiting its use to intragastric feedings. It is a reliable method of formula delivery that a family member or the patient can be easily taught. This method is especially useful for the alert, active patient as it frees him or her from any mechanical device. It is the preferred method for delivery of blenderized feedings, which might otherwise be too viscous for either gravity or mechanical pump delivery. It allows for an accurate delivery of feeding over a specified amount of time; however, bolus feedings are more likely to generate high residual volumes.[1]

Gravity feedings can be delivered via intermittent or continuous drip. The patient is dependent only on a bedside pole and not upon a power source. The rate of delivery can be inaccurate and predispose the patient to gastroesophageal reflux and aspiration. Intermittent feedings are generally the preferred modality for intragastric feedings. Gravity feeding is useful for the patient who requires intermittent feedings but cannot tolerate syringe bolus feedings. New closed enteral feeding systems allow the delivery of a specified amount of tube feeding measured out in a "drip" chamber, thus allowing the remainder of the feeding to be used later in the day. Alternatively, cans of tube feeding can be poured into a delivery system that is flushed and cleaned after each delivery. Continuous gravity feedings are important for intrajejunal feedings; close monitoring is required to assure a constant rate of delivery.

Pump feedings require a mechanical device and a source of power. Feedings can be delivered via a continuous or intermittent schedule. Formula delivery is more accurate, thereby reducing residual volume and the risk of aspiration. Continuous pump feedings are the preferred route for intrajejunal feedings. The mechanical device allows an even administration of formulation, helping to prevent clogging of smaller jejunal feeding tubes with viscous substances.[2] Too rapid a bolus of a hyperosmolar formulation into the jejunum results in abdominal distention, cramps, hyperperistalsis, and diarrhea. Continuous intragastric feedings can be performed in a monitored environment which would watch for signs of gastric retention and the possibility of subsequent aspiration.

There is literature supporting the use of continuous rather than intermittent tube feedings in the critically ill patient. In this population, continuous tube feedings have been associated with a positive nitrogen balance and weight gain as compared to intermittent tube feedings.[3] Continuous tube feeding requires less energy expenditure because of diet-induced thermogenesis and has been shown effective in the prevention of stress ulceration.[4,5]

Each institution generally has an established protocol for starting a patient on an enteral feeding regimen. These protocols vary with reference to flow rates, enteral formula dilution, and the use of intermittent or continuous feedings. Studies in healthy volunteers have demonstrated a tolerance of both elemental and complex tube feedings at starter flow rates of up to 150 cc/h and starter osmolalities of up to 690 mOsm/kg.[6] Obviously, it would be inappropriate to extrapolate this information to an ill population who may demonstrate problems with both gastrointestinal digestion and motility.

There is no clearly defined regimen for converting a patient from continuous to intermittent feedings. Many centers use a discontinuous method where continuous feedings are completely stopped and intermittent feedings are begun at slow rates and increased to the patient's tolerance. This often results in missing feedings or prolonged periods of hypocaloric feedings. An overlapping method of conversion was recently reported where continuous feeds were maintained at lower rates while intermittent feedings were introduced.[7] This resulted in improved nitrogen balance and early attainment of nutritional goals as well as fewer diarrheal episodes, aspiration events, and hospital days than the discontinuous method.

III. FORMULA SELECTION

Although most patient's needs can be met with one or two enteral formulations, there are a wide range of "disease specific" products now available which may provide advantages in selected patients. Enteral formulations are divided into seven classes: blenderized, lactose-containing, lactose-free, elemental, modular, specialized, and supplemental.

A. BLENDERIZED DIETS AND FORMULAS
Blenderized formulations are a combination of table foods with added vitamins and minerals. Although blenderized formulations are commercially available, patients can be instructed in home preparation. The commercial formulations contain about 1 kcal/cc and are approximately 85% water; 50% of the total calories are carbohydrates. They contain a large amount of fiber and must be delivered through a large bore nasoenteric tube (NET) or a percutaneous gastrostomy tube (PEG). The cost of the commercial products are a limiting factor.

B. LACTOSE-CONTAINING/LACTOSE-FREE FORMULAS
There are few lactose-containing products still in clinical use. Many patients referred for enteral feeding have lactase deficiency, thus precluding the use of lactose-based products because of diarrhea, abdominal pain, and abdominal distention.

Lactose-free mixtures are the basic feeding formulations and are designed for long-term use. They contain 85% free water. They generally provide 1 kcal/cc and derive 12 to 20% of its calories from protein, 45 to 60% from carbohydrates, and 30 to 40% from fat. They contain complex forms of carbohydrates, fats, and proteins and require some degree of digestion prior to absorption. Nutrient-dense formulations are available containing 1.5 to 2.0 kcal/cc. They are slightly hyperosmolar (400 to 700 mOsm/kg water) and are approximately 75% free water by content. These formulas may be beneficial in the fluid restricted patient.

C. HIGH NITROGEN FORMULAS
These formulations are designed to deliver a higher protein load to a patient without changing the overall caloric content. Standard formulations have a calorie to nitrogen

ratio of approximately 150:1. High nitrogen formulations reduce this ratio to approximately 120 to 130:1. These products are available as a 1 kcal/cc isosmolar or a 2 kcal/cc hyperosmolar formula. The more nutrient-dense formulations have a higher content of fat.

D. ELEMENTAL FORMULAS

Elemental or defined diets are designed for use by the patient with limited ability to digest nutrients. They are composed of free amino acids, dipeptides, and tripeptides and are absorbed via an active transport mechanism. They may be combined with easily absorbed fats (medium-chain triglycerides) or carbohydrates (maltodextrins). Elemental diets are fiber-free and highly osmotic secondary to small component particle size.

Intact proteins are broken down by the small intestinal brush border. There is significantly slower absorption of peptides with four to five amino acids as compared to two to three amino acids.[8] Elemental formulas have proven superior to intact protein diets in attaining nutritional goals in the intensive care unit where patients often experience poor small bowel nutrient absorption.[9] However, there is no advantage in using an elemental diet in a normal GI tract where absorption is not impaired.[10] Elemental diets are expensive compared to standard polymeric diets, and their taste generally precludes oral ingestion, necessitating a feeding tube. Newer flavor-pack additives are available and may help improve the overall taste.

E. SPECIALTY FORMULAS

Specialty formulations are available for patients with unique medical needs. These formulations are often disease specific and are designed to meet the nutritional needs of these disease states. These products are more expensive than standard enteral nutrition and may lead to complications if used inappropriately.

Glutamine is a nonessential amino acid which is stored in skeletal muscle. It is essential for rapidly dividing cells and as a fuel for the small intestinal mucosa.[11] The use of glutamine-free parenteral solutions has led to small bowel mucosal atrophy and loss of DNA content.[11,12] Nitrogen balance in physically stressed, ill patients may be improved with glutamine supplementation.[13] Large trials demonstrating the efficacy of glutamine in a fortified enteral formulation are still pending.

Arginine is a nonessential amino acid that promotes nitrogen retention, accelerates wound healing, and improves immune function. In animal studies, arginine supplements increased blood mononuclear response to stimulation with concanavalin A and phytohemagglutinin.[14] Arginine has been shown to significantly enhance lymphocyte blastogenesis and increase CD4 lymphocyte populations in a preoperative surgical population.[15] Postsurgical patients fed an enteral diet fortified with arginine, structured lipids, RNA, and mehhaden oil (rich in omega-3 fatty acids) had improved *in vitro* immune response and nitrogen balance as compared to controls fed a standard enteral diet.[16] A randomized prospective trial in patients with upper GI malignancy who received postoperative enteral nutrition noted fewer infections, complications, and a reduced hospital stay in the arginine-supplemented group as compared to the group receiving standard enteral nutrition.[17]

1. Pulmonary Formulas

Most enteral formulations provide a majority of their calories as carbohydrates. Glucose is metabolized to CO_2 and H_2O. New pulmonary formulations are available that provide a majority of the calories as fat (55%) and maintain a respiratory quotient below 1 such that less CO_2 is produced per unit of oxygen consumed.[18] This may be beneficial in the intubated patient with lung disease who may be difficult to wean off the ventilator. Ventilated patients fed a low carbohydrate, high fat enteral diet were shown to have a lower $PaCO_2$ and spent a reduced period of time on the ventilator as compared to patients fed a standard enteral diet.[19]

2. Renal Failure Formulas

Renal failure patients would benefit from a formulation that reduces blood urea nitrogen formation, slows the progression of renal disease, and meets nutritional goals. Current renal failure formulations are low in protein, phosphorous, magnesium, potassium, and sodium. The protein content of these formulations may vary. Protein consists of a combination of essential amino acids (EAA) and nonessential amino acids (NEAA). Formulations with a high EAA content are based on the premise that urea will be used to produce required nonessential amino acids, ultimately reducing the amount of nitrogenous wastes. Although there has been no evidence of improvement in survival with this formulation, there has been reported improvement in renal function with a decreased need for dialysis.[20] The use of BCAA as the only or majority source of protein in a group of patients on a low-protein diet improved their nitrogen balance and reduced the rise in blood urea nitrogen as compared to similar renal failure patients fed a standard enteral diet.[21] Nutrition and renal disease will be covered in more detail in Chapter 11.

3. Hepatic Failure Formulas

In patients with liver failure, serum branched-chain amino acid (BCAA) (leucine, isoleucine, and valine) levels are reduced and serum aromatic amino acid (AAA) (phenylalanine, tyrosine, and tryptophan) levels and methionine levels are elevated. The use of a high BCAA, low AAA designed formulation in this population may be helpful. This premise is founded in the belief that BCAA inhibit AAA from crossing the blood-brain barrier, thus preventing them from acting as false neurotransmitters and inducing encephalopathy. A review of multiple trials using BCAA in encephalopathic patients with chronic liver disease noted BCAA was no more effective than the use of lactulose or neomycin.[22] No improvement in nutritional parameters or the degree of encephalopathy was found among BCAA-supplemented patients with an episode of acute alcoholic hepatitis.[23] One study reported an improvement in inpatient mortality among malnourished patients with cirrhosis fed a BCAA-supplemented enteral diet as compared to a similar control group of patients fed a low-sodium diet.[24] However, there was no control for equivalent caloric or protein intake between the two groups.

4. Trauma Formulas

Critically ill patients exhibit significant proteolysis and hydrolysis of muscle BCAA for energy. It has been suggested that BCAA are necessary in the severely stressed or traumatized population. These patients may enter a period of negative nitrogen balance that may not be correctable by standard amino acid formulations.[25] While some clinical trials have shown an improvement in nitrogen balance with the use of BCAA-fortified nutritional support, other trials have shown no improvement.[26]

5. Postoperative Formulas

These formulas were designed for the postoperative patient who would normally be on a clear liquid diet. They have low caloric density (0.7 kcal/cc) and are approximately 95% water. They contain 50 to 60 g protein/1000cc and are low in fat content. These products are sometimes used in frozen (popsicle) form as a nutrient supplement, especially in patients with small bowel absorption dysfunction.

6. Glucose Intolerance Formulas

A low-carbohydrate, high-fat enteral formulation is available for glucose-intolerant patients. Thirty-three percent of total calories are available as glucose, whereas the other carbohydrate calories are provided as fructose, a sugar with low glycemic response. This formulation has been compared to standard enteral formulations in a type I diabetic population and produced a significantly lower glycemic response.[27] Side effects associated with fructose include incomplete GI absorption causing abdominal distention and cramping and its ability to elevate serum lipid levels.

7. Fiber-Containing Formulas

Standard enteral formulations were designed to contain low amounts of fiber. The major role for fiber in the diet is, by bacterial degradation, to form short-chain fatty acids, which are trophic for large bowel mucosa, and to impact on bowel function, possibly preventing diarrhea associated with the use of standard enteral formulations. Insoluble fiber such as wheat bran is the best suited for this role. However, this type of fiber has the propensity to clog small bore enteric tubes. The type of fiber most often added to enteral formulations is soy or oat. In a prospective trial no difference in stool weight or frequency was seen when fiber was added to fiber-free formulations in patients in a long-term care facility.[28] Another trial comparing a fiber-supplemented enteral formulation to a fiber-free enteral formulation in head trauma patients noted no difference in bowel function.[29] Fiber's potential role in the prevention of multiple disease states, including diverticulosis, colon cancer, and heart disease, may have a role in long-term care facilities or in patients on enteral feedings for a prolonged period of time.

8. Medium-Chain Triglyceride Formulas

Medium-chain triglyceride (MCT) supplemented formulations have been proposed as an alternative to long-chain fatty acids for patients with fat malabsorption. Long-chain fatty acids are hydrolyzed in the intestinal lumen to monoglycerides and free fatty acids by bile salts and pancreatic lipase prior to absorption. MCT are absorbed unchanged by the enterocyte from the intestinal lumen. MCT are also independent of carnitine transport into the mitochondria. MCT may be advantageous for the patient with malabsorption secondary to intestinal mucosal damage, biliary tract dysfunction, bile salt deficiency, or pancreatic exocrine insufficiency.

F. MODULAR DIETS

Modular feedings are individual nutrient components that are mixed to create an enteral formulation or to modify an existing one. They exist as separate nutrient units: fat, carbohydrate, or protein. This allows the formation of a custom enteral formulation or the nutrient-specific fortification of an existing commercial formula.

G. SUPPLEMENTS

Supplements are added to the diets of patients who cannot meet all their protein or caloric needs. They may be in the form of a liquid, a shake, or a pudding and may be taken with or between meals. There are a multitude of products available with conflicting information regarding their efficacy, thus making their role in aggressive nutritional support difficult to interpret.

IV. COMPLICATIONS

Most clinicians feel that enteral nutrition is much safer than parenteral nutrition. However, Powers et al. showed that there are many complications that occur during delivery

TABLE 1
Complications of Enteral Feeding

Mechanical (tube related)
    Difficulty with placement
    Nasal mucosal ulceration
    Otitis media
    Pharyngitis
    Pneumothorax
    Reflux esophagitis/ulceration/stricture
    Tube obstruction
    Tube migration
Gastrointestinal
    Aspiration
    Bloating and/or distention
    Constipation
    Diarrhea
    Nausea/vomiting
Metabolic
    Abnormal liver tests
    Dehydration
    Electrolyte disorders
    Hyperglycemia
    Vitamin and/or trace mineral
      deficiencies

of enteral nutrition, and that these can be reduced if a team-managed approach is used.[30] This study showed that complications with enteral therapy are, in fact, quite common.

We have already discussed the importance of enteral nutrition and its role in preventing bacterial translocation. Parenteral nutrition can be associated with a number of problems directly related to the i.v. catheters which do not occur with enteral nutrition. The major savings come from the low to moderate cost of the commercial or homemade tube feedings compared to the higher costs of parenteral nutrition. Depending on the medical condition of the patient, monitoring may need to be as rigorous as with parenteral nutrition or much less frequent in a stable patient.

Complications can be divided into three broad categories: mechanical, gastrointestinal, and metabolic. Table 1 shows a general list of complications.

A. MECHANICAL

For nasoenteric tubes (NET), problems related to passage through the nose and their effects on nasal structures can be significant. Generally, the smaller the tube, the better it is tolerated. Ten French (Fr) NETs provide a good balance between size and product selection. These tubes can be used to infuse the commercial blenderized formulas or homemade varieties that are composed of baby formulas. Tubes smaller than 8 Fr may require the least viscous formulas, the elemental formulas.

Complications to nasal structures can include nasal septal irritation, ulceration, or perforation, epistaxis, and sinusitis. The latter must be considered in febrile, unresponsive patients and treated aggresively so that more serious complications of sinusitis, such as cavernous sinus thrombosis, do not occur. Local care to the intubated nostril is indicated and attention to taping of the tube is important in preventing nasal necrosis.

Techniques for placement of nasoenteric tubes were discussed in the last chapter. However, pulmonary placement of NETs can have serious consequences. Pneumothorax, pulmonary feeding, and pleural effusions have been reported.[31-33] It is important to obtain and to review a radiograph to verify placement of smaller nasoenteric tubes where pulmonary placement may be less obvious compared to larger bore nasogastric tubes (NGT) that can be easily aspirated for gastric contents.

NET occlusion is related not only to size of the tube but also to the type of medications placed through the tube. When starting a patient on a tube feeding, medications should be reviewed and attempts to change medications to liquid equivalents, when available, should be made. Fiber-containing bulk laxatives and anion exchange resins are particularly notorious for causing occlusions. Also liquid phenytoin can coagulate with tube feedings. The basic principle of frequent flushing of the tube is key. While many articles have been published on using a variety of materials to help dislodge the obstruction, new declogging catheters are now available to carefully "brush" the interiors of the tubes. Care must be taken not to force these special catheters, and other guidewires are not recommended because perforation of the wall of the catheter can occur and lead to more dramatic consequences.

B. GASTROINTESTINAL
1. Aspiration

Aspiration is an important and controversial area. While the technology exists to place feeding tubes in multiple areas of the GI tract, the actual decision of which route of access to use is often not carefully evaluated. In the literature, the risk of aspiration pneumonia varies from 2 to 95%. Also, the criteria for aspiration in many articles are poorly defined.[34,35] What is most apparent is that aspiration is often multifactorial in nature and is an area that still requires active research. Important issues include the following: (1) differentiating between the risk of oropharyngeal and gastric aspiration, (2) evaluating the effect of tube size and presence across the gastroesophageal junction, (3) evaluating the effect of body position on gastric reflux/aspiration, (4) considering the effect of underlying disease (e.g., poor gastric emptying with head trauma or diabetes), (5) establishing access for short-term and long-term use, (6) evaluating the benefit between intermittent and continuous feeding regimens, and (7) documenting an advantage of jejunostomy feeding over nasogastric or gastrostomy feeding.[36]

Lazarus et al. attempted to critically analyze the literature from 1978 through 1989 regarding aspiration with long-term gastric or jejunal feeding in patients with severe neurogenic oropharyngeal dysphagia.[37] Due to poorly designed data collection methods, small sample sizes, marked differences in patient population, and inadequate definitions for aspiration, they were unable to conclude that one method of feeding was superior to another. In patients who are aspirating their oral secretions due to severe transfer dysphagia, it will be difficult to determine which feeding method will be best because a main source of pulmonary aspiration is not being dealt with. An interesting report used a radionuclide study as a salivagram, and it was effective in documenting oral aspiration in an infant.[38] We are unaware of a similar prospective evaluation in adult patients with oropharyngeal dysphagia and tube feeding. Huxley et al. have studied pharyngeal aspiration in man.[39] Using indium[111] chloride placed carefully into the pharynx in 20 normals and 10 patients with depressed consciousness while sleeping, they showed that 45% of normals and 70% of patients aspirate pharyngeal secretions. It would appear that pulmonary defense mechanisms efficiently prevent most people from developing pneumonia, but altered immunity or large volume aspiration may overwhelm these local defenses. Unfortunately, the only way to insure no pulmonary aspiration, especially from orpharyngeal secretions, is to surgically close the vocal cords and perform a tracheostomy. This is generally not a preferred option. There is also little agreement in the prevalence and mortality associated with aspiration. Cameron et al. found a 62% mortality rate when they reviewed 47 patients with documented aspiration.[40] In contrast, Mullan et al. prospectively evaluated the risk of aspiration in 276 patients and found a prevalence of 4.4% with an overall mortality of 17%; they concluded that there was little morbidity and no excess mortality associated with aspiration.[41] In this study, hospital location and advanced age were found to be major risk factors such that patients on medical and surgical wards were at higher risk for aspiration than in the intensive care units.

The presence and size of a nasoenteric tube as a risk factor has not been totally resolved. Mittal and associates have shown that a catheter in the pharynx may lead to more transient relaxations of the lower esophageal sphincter and have suggested that this may promote gastroesophageal reflux (GERD).[42] Catheter size was not evaluated in this study. Furthermore, Sloan and colleagues have nicely demonstrated that both a hiatal hernia and low LES pressure can interact with abrupt increases in intra-abdominal pressure which can increase the susceptibility to reflux.[43] The relationship between an increased susceptibility to reflux and the act of pulmonary aspiration has not been resolved in this area. In a small study of patients referred for PEG placement, Johnson et al. performed pre-PEG and post-PEG esophageal manometric studies and 24 pH monitoring.[44] There was a decrease in the reflux score and an increase in the LES pressure in nine patients. One patient was restudied 1 month later and did not appear to maintain the initial post-PEG improvement. Their conclusion was that PEG placement did not seem to increase the risk for reflux. Cole et al. documented gastroesophageal reflux and aspiration post-PEG in a patient who was known to have free GER on a pre-PEG barium study using technecium sulfur colloid tube feeding.[45] This technique may warrant further investigation.

The debate regarding the incidence of aspiration and large bore and narrow bore tubes and transpyloric tubes is also not settled.[46,47] These studies are too small to be truly meaningful, and while Strong et al. performed a randomized, prospective study, it is flawed by lack of documentation of where the ''postpyloric'' tubes really were or if the cases of aspiration were saliva or gastric secretions.[47] Gutske et al. showed that to reduce gastroduodenal reflux, catheter placement needed to be beyond the ligament of Treitz.[48] In a study with PEG/J catheters in the third portion of the duodenum and beyond, there was no gastric recovery of tube feeding colored with methylene blue.[49]

The effect of body position has been a concern to many investigators, especially with a large bore tube in place; two recent studies address the issue of position.[50,51] In a series of ventilated patients with NGT, Torres et al. showed that the supine position and the length of time kept in that position were important in the number of tracheal aspiration episodes recorded.[50] Also important in this study was that these patients were not being fed and that a cuffed endotracheal tube was not protective to aspiration episodes. Ibañez and co-workers showed that NGT feedings were associated with a higher incidence of aspiration in the supine position.[51] In addition, these authors delivered an isotope to the stomach in a small subset of patients and then removed the NGT. They noted a statistically significant reduction in aspiration after removing the NGT. They further concluded that the semirecumbent position decreased the incidence of reflux and aspiration, but did not prevent it.

Underlying disease pathophysiology must be considered when choosing a method of access. An example would include the high incidence of gastric emptying dysfunction due to elevations of intracranial pressure that are associated with head trauma.[52] A nasogastric feeding in a head trauma patient or diabetic gastroparesis may not be tolerated and can progress to gastric distention and aspiration.

Considerations of short-term vs. long-term requirements for feeding must also enter into the decision of a route of access. There may not be a significant difference between NGT feeding and gastrostomy feeding except in those patients with a higher risk for reflux before the index illness that may still have a higher risk of aspiration after PEG placement.

In a prospective study by Ciocon et al., 70 elderly patients in a skilled nursing facility were noted to have self-extubation and agitation as early and late problems in 39% and 67% of patients, respectively, when NGT were used.[53] Aspiration pneumonia was found early in 23% of patients and 44% late. This was compared to gastrostomy complications consisting of aspiration pneumonia 56% early, and 56% late; tube dysfunction 50% early, and 38% late; and agitation and self-extubation in 44% early, and 0% late. They concluded that tube feeding of the elderly can be continued for long periods, but was associated with multiple complications. They felt that agitation and self-extubation were best managed by gastrostomy, but aspiration was still a considerable problem. Cogen and Weinryb retrospectively reviewed 109 nursing home patients fed by gastrostomy.[54] They noted that 22.9% aspirated, and a previous history of pneumonia was the only risk factor that could be identified. They suggested considering jejunostomy placement in those patients.

Differences between long-term feeding by PEG and NET were retrospectively evaluated by Fay and co-workers.[55] Nonfatal aspiration pneumonia occurred within 14 days of tube placement in 6% and 24% of the PEG and NET patients, respectively. No differences were noted in follow-up of up to 559 days. They concluded that for those patients tolerating NET feeding, PEG placement was not needed.

Park and colleagues found PEG superior to NGT feeding in an interesting 28-day prospective comparison of the effectiveness of PEG vs. NGT feeding in patients with neurologic dysphagia. Tube dislodgement was responsible for most treatment failures in the NGT feeding group.[56] The NGT group received 55% of their prescribed feed, while the PEG group received 93%. Two PEG patients experienced minor aspiration. They concluded that PEGs were safe and useful for long-term enteral nutrition compared to NGT feeding.

Some authors suggest intermittent gastric feeding since it may be more physiologic, and the stomach can act as a reservoir.[57] However, continuous feeding is generally considered standard with jejunal feeding. In a study of 34 neurosurgical patients, Kocan and Hickisch could not show a significant difference between intermittent and continuous feeding looking at multiple parameters including aspiration.[58] Again, in the critical analysis of the literature by Lazarus et al., they concluded that there were not enough data to consider one method of feeding superior to the other.[37] Mullan et al. followed 276 tube-fed adults who received their feeding by continuous drip which they felt avoided the risk of gastric distention leading to aspiration.[41] Strong et al. also employed continuous feeding when comparing postpyloric and intragastric-placed small bore NET.[47] However, their higher rate of aspiration, 31.3% gastric and 40% postpyloric, is in contrast to the low prevalence rate (4.4%) found by Mullan et al.[41] The reasons for these different aspiration rates are not apparent.

Thus, the superiority of jejunal feeding has not been fully established even though it would seem to be a logical assumption. Few studies are actually available to evaluate this as a long-term option. This may be due in part to resistance of nursing homes which are not always able to provide the presumed level of care needed for jejunal feeding.[37,57,59] Weltz and co-workers followed 100 patients who underwent surgical jejunostomy placement.[60] They noted elimination of aspiration in 16/18 patients with preoperative aspiration and in all patients with known feeding-related preoperative aspiration. They concluded that jejunostomy feeding was very effective in patients with documented feeding aspiration. More comparative data are needed as well as true documentation of the source of aspiration as being oropharyngeal or tube feeding related.

2. Diarrhea

Diarrhea is the most common complication of enteral feeding ranging in incidence in as few as 2.3% and as high as 68% of patients.[61] The difficulty in reporting diarrheal complications is the variation in an author's interpretation of diarrhea. A specific diagnosis of diarrhea is often made on the number of stools per day or in other cases by the weight or volume of stools. There are many potential causes of diarrhea including diarrhea-inducing medications, formula composition, formula flow rate, bacterial flora, enteral formula contamination, hypoalbuminemia, and the disease state of the large and small intestine.

Multiple medications are often prescribed to hospitalized patients, and antibiotics often cause the growth of *Clostridium difficile* or other bacterial organisms.[62] Liquid medications used with an enteral feeding tube are often based in sorbitol, an obvious cathartic.

The composition of formula may affect the incidence of diarrhea. In the normal population, standard enteral formula osmolarities are tolerated at high flow rates. Normal volunteers were shown to tolerate full-strength small bowel feedings at rates up to 340cc/h without the development of diarrhea.[63] However, the critically ill patient who has an altered GI motility and absorptive capacity may demonstrate difficulties with the tolerance of any enteral formula. Generally, it is more appropriate to slow the rate of delivery of an enteral formula causing GI intolerance rather than attempt to dilute it.

Lactose-containing enteral formulations may lead to diarrhea secondary to the high incidence of lactase deficiency. High-fat concentration enteral products may precipitate diarrhea in the patient with disease states causing fat malabsorption, such as pancreatic or liver disease. The use of fiber-containing formulas to reduce the incidence of diarrhea is a matter of controversy. The fermentation of fiber leads to the generation of short-chain fatty acids. These short-chain fatty acids potentiate the absorption of sodium, chloride, and water.[64] One report noted an increase in diarrhea in a group of critically ill patients fed a fiber-free as compared to a fiber-supplemented formula, while another study found no significant differences in diarrheal episodes between critically ill patients receiving an isotonic tube feeding vs. a similar group receiving a fiber-supplemented formulation.[65,66]

Reduced gastric and small bowel motility or structural abnormalities of the small bowel may lead to bacterial overgrowth with a change in the intestinal microflora. Alterations in gastric pH, such as associated with the use of acid-suppressing agents, may precipitate bacterial overgrowth. Bacterial colonization of the GI tract begins when the gastric pH exceeds 4.[67] Bacterial overgrowth may cause diarrhea by direct damage to the small intestinal mucosa, impairment of brush-border enzyme activity, or deconjugation of bile acids.[68] Attempts at sterilization of the GI tract with an acidified enteral formulation have not impacted on diarrheal episodes.[69]

Contamination of an enteral formulation with a large number of microorganisms may precipitate diarrhea in an enterally fed patient. Residual enteral formulations cultured in feeding systems directly after feeding patients have been shown to contain 10^3 to 10^6 organisms, usually Gram negative bacilli. The relationship between bacterial contamination of enteral formula and diarrhea in gastric feeders is questioned because of the protective effect of gastric acid. However, contaminated enteral feedings have been cited as the cause of septicemia.[70]

Data suggested that hypoalbuminemia predisposed to diarrhea by causing edema in the intestinal mucosa and decreasing osmotic pressure. Critically ill patients who have serum albumins less than 2.6 g/dL may experience diarrhea with standard enteral nutrition.[71] This low level of albumin may have simply identified the sickest patients who may have been susceptible to diarrhea for many reasons. There has been reported good tolerance of both a peptide-based and free amino acid formulation in hypoalbuminemic, geriatric patients.[72]

The disease status of the small intestine and colon will have an obvious impact on the absorption of nutrients and water. The careful selection of a formula based on osmolarity, fat content, carbohydrate source, and protein content and careful attention to an acceptable delivery rate may have little effect on the development of diarrhea if the GI tract has significant disease precluding its ability to provide absorptive function.

3. Constipation

Constipation associated with tube feeding is generally related to a patient's hydration status. Previous enteral products with osmolarities >600 mOsm/kg were associated with marked dehydration, hyperglycemia, and hypernatremia.[73] Current formulations (300 to 600 mOsm) have reduced this complication. However, patients on fluid restriction in addition to enteral feeding may still be prone to dehydration. Geriatric patients, a population with reduced mobility, may be predisposed to the development of a high fecal impaction with liquid stool flowing around the impaction, thus presenting as diarrhea. A low residue diet has also been touted as the cause of constipation. However, there are conflicting reports on the importance of supplemental fiber to standard enteral formulas as related to stool weight or number of bowel movements.[74,75]

C. OTHER COMPLICATIONS

1. Medication Delivery

Medication delivery can be altered during tube feedings. Although phenytoin has not been shown to interact with various enteral formulas, it has been shown to bind to nasogastric tubing, thus reducing its availability.[76,77] The development of a precipitate mass has been reported with the use of a standard enteral feeding and over-the-counter cold preparations.[78] Resistance to warfarin has been reported secondary to the vitamin K found in enteral feedings.[79]

Hepatic and intestinal microsomes can also be influenced by diet. A decrease in the cytochrome P-450 content has been noted in rats fed a high-nitrogen, low-fat elemental formulation.[80] Human data suggest that a diet contain at least 10% fat calories to ensure proper drug metabolism.[81] The clinical significance of this fact remains unknown to date.

2. Metabolic

Metabolic complications of tube feeding include the following: electrolyte abnormalities, hyperglycemia, abnormal liver function tests, and vitamin and/or trace element deficiencies. Hyperglycemia may occur secondary to a high carbohydrate load of specific enteral formulas, especially in the ill or diabetic population. The use of a renal-specific enteral formulation may cause both potassium and phosphorous depletion if used in an ill, catabolic patient who may require high concentrations of these substances. The development of abnormal liver function tests has been reported with the use of an elemental formula.[82] Most enteral formulas are chromium deficient, which may be detrimental for some patients.[83] Appropriate use of specialized enteral formulas will often prevent these complications.

V. CONCLUSION

Enteral nutrition is a safe and effective modality for feeding most patients who require nutritional support, including patients with disease of the GI tract itself. Recent trends have seen a movement away from parenteral nutrition to enteral nutrition, often in patients who previously were thought not to be candidates for enteral support.

There are now many choices for standard enteral formulas, and the explosion of disease-specific enteral formulations in recent years has allowed us the opportunity for aggressive nutritional support in critically ill patients. This availability has also opened the door for the potential development of enteral formula-related complications. Although a multitude of complications are possible, the judicious use of enteral access devices and formula diets will minimize morbidity. Continuing developments will focus enteral nutrition support as a vital modality in the overall treatment of the critically ill.

REFERENCES

1. **Newark, SR, Koelzer, C, and McCowan, MH.** Current concepts in nutrition: enteral tube feeding. *JOSMA,* 80:163–165, 1987.
2. **Ciocon, JO, Galindo-Ciocon, DJ, Tiessen, C, et al.** Continuous compared with intermittent tube feeding in the elderly. *JPEN,* 16:525–528, 1992.
3. **Parker, P, Stroop, S, and Greene, H.** A controlled comparison of continuous vs intermittent feeding in the treatment of infants with intestinal disease. *J Pediatr,* 99:360–364, 1981.
4. **Hemyfield, S, Casper, K, and Grossman, G.** Bioenergetic and metabolic response to continuous vs intermittent nasoenteric feeding. *Metabolism,* 36:570–575, 1987.
5. **Solem, LD, Strate, RG, and Fischer, RP.** Antacid therapy and nutritional supplementation in the prevention of Curling's ulcers. *Surg Gynecol Obstet,* 148:367–370, 1979.
6. **Zarling, EJ, Parmar, JR, Mobarhan, S, et al.** Effect of enteral formula infusion rate, osmolality and chemical composition upon clinical tolerance and carbohydrate absorption in normal subjects. *JPEN,* 10:588–590, 1986.
7. **Powers, T, Cowan, GSM, Deckard, M, et al.** Prospective randomized evaluation of two regimens for converting from continuous to intermittent feedings in patients with gastrostomies. *JPEN,* 15:405–407, 1991.
8. **Grimble, RG, Rees, PA, Keohane, T, et al.** Effect of peptide chain length on absorption of egg protein hydrolysates in normal human jejunum. *Gastroenterology,* 92:135–142, 1987.
9. **Peterson, VM, Moore, EE, Jones, TN, et al.** Total enteral nutrition versus total parenteral nutrition after major torso injury: attenuation of hepatic protein repriorization. *Surgery,* 104:199–207, 1988.
10. **Jones, BJM, Andrews, J, Frost, P, et al.** Comparison of an elemental and polymeric diet in patients with normal gastrointestinal function. *Gut,* 24:78–84, 1983.
11. **O'Dwyer, ST, Smith, RS, and Wilmore, DW.** Maintenance of small bowel mucosa with glutamine enriched parenteral nutrition. *JPEN,* 13:579–585, 1990.
12. **Hwang, TI, O'Dwyer, ST, Smith, RJ, et al.** Preservation of small bowel mucosa utilizing glutamine-enriched parenteral nutrition. *Surg Forum,* 36:56–58, 1986.
13. **Dechelotte, P, Darmaun, D, Rongier, M, et al.** Absorption and metabolic effects of enterally administered glutamine in humans. *J Physiology,* 260:G677–682, 1991.
14. **Barbul, A, Rettura, G, Levenson, SM, et al.** Arginine: thymotropic and wound healing promoting agent. *Surg Forum,* 28:101–103, 1977.
15. **Nirgiotis, JG, Hennessey, PJ, and Andrassay, RJ.** The effects of an arginine-free enteral diet on wound healing and immune function in the postsurgical rat. *J Pediatr Surg,* 26:936–941, 1991.
16. **Daly, JM, Lieberman, MD, Goldfine, J, et al.** Enteral nutrition with supplemental arginine, RNA and omega-3 fatty acids in patients after operation: immunologic, metabolic and clinical outcome. *Surgery,* 112:56–67, 1992.
17. **Benya, R, and Mobrahan, S.** Enteral alimentation: administration and complications. *J Am Coll Nutr,* 10:209–212, 1991.
18. **Angelillo, VA, Bedi, S, Durfee, D, et al.** Effects of a low and high carbohydrate feedings in ambulatory patients with chronic obstructive pulmonary disease and chronic hypercapnia. *Ann Intern Med,* 103:883–885, 1985.
19. **Al-Saady, N, Blackmore, C, and Bennett ED.** High fat, low carbohydrate enteral feeding reduces $PaCO_2$ and the period of ventilation in ventilated patients. *Chest,* 94(Suppl.):94S, 1989.
20. **Abel, RM, Beck, CH, Jr, Abbott, WM, et al.** Improved survival from acute renal failure after treatment with intravenous essential L-amino acids and glucose: results of a prospective, double-blind study. *N Engl J Med,* 288:695–699, 1973.
21. **Sofio, CA, Nicora, RW, and Osborn, TM, et al.** Oral essential amino acids in the management of acute and chronic renal failure. *JPEN,* 3:506, 1979.
22. **Eriksson, LS, and Conn, HO.** Branched chain amino acids in the treatment of encephalopathy: an analysis of variants. *Hepatology,* 10:228–246, 1989.
23. **Marchesini, G, Dioguardi, FS, and Bianchi, GP, et al.** Long-term oral branched-chain amino acid treatment in chronic hepatic encephalopathy: a randomized double-blind casein-controlled trial. *J Hepatol,* 11:92–101, 1990.
24. **Calvey, H, Davis, M, and Williams, R.** Controlled trial of nutritional supplementation with and without branched-chain amino acid enrichment in treatment of alcoholic hepatitis. *J Hepatol,* 1:141–151, 1985.
25. **Cerra, FB, Mazuski, JE, Chute, E, et al.** Branched chain metabolic support: a prospective, randomized, double-blind trial in surgical stress. *Ann Surg,* 199:286–291, 1984.
26. **Numer, N, Cerra, FB, Shronts, EP, et al.** Does modified amino acid parenteral nutrition alter immune-response in high level surgical stress. *JPEN,* 7:521–524, 1983.

27. **Peters, AL, Davidson, MB, and Isaac, RM.** Lack of glucose elevation after stimulated tube-feeding with a low-carbohydrate, high-fat enteral formulation in patients with type I diabetes. *Am J Med,* 87:178–182, 1989.

28. **Fisher, M, Adkins, W, Hall, L, et al.** The effect of dietary fiber in a liquid diet on bowel function of mentally retarded individuals. *J Ment Defic Res,* 29:373–381, 1985.

29. **Frankenfield, DC, and Beyer, PL.** Soy-polysaccharide effect on diarrhea in tube-fed head-injured patients. *Heart Lung,* 20:404–408, 1991.

30. **Powers, DA, Brown, RO, Cowan, GSM, et al.** Nutritional support vs nonteam management of enteral nutritional support in a Veterans Administration medical center teaching hospital. *JPEN,* 10:635–638, 1986.

31. **Miller, KS, Tomlinson, JR, and Sahn, SA.** Pleuropulmonary complications of enteral tube feedings: two reports, review of the literature, and recommendations. *Chest,* 88:230–233, 1988.

32. **Ghahremani, GG, and Gould, RJ.** Nasoenteric feeding tubes: radiographic detection of complications. *Dig Dis Sci,* 31:574–585, 1986.

33. **McWey, RE, Curry, NS, Schabel, SI, and Reines, HD.** Complications of nasoenteric feeding tubes. *Am J Surg,* 155:253–257, 1988.

34. **Cataldi-Betcher, EL, Seltzer, MH, Slocum, BA, and Jones, KW.** Complications occurring during enteral nutrition support: a prospective study. *JPEN,* 7:546–552, 1983.

35. **Winterbauer, RH, Durning, RB, Barron, E, and McFadden, MC.** Aspirated nasogastric feeding solution detected by glucose strips. *Ann Intern Med,* 95;647–668, 1986.

36. **Kirby, DF, DeLegge, MH, and Fleming, CR.** AGA Technical guidelines on tube feeding. *Gastroenterology,* in press.

37. **Lazarus, BA, Murphy, JB, and Culpepper, L.** Aspiration associated with long-term gastric versus jejunal feeding: a critical analysis of the literature. *Arch Phys Med Rehabil,* 71:46–53, 1990.

38. **Heyman, S.** The radionuclide salivagram for detecting the pulmonary aspiration in an infant. *Pediatr Radiol,* 19:208–209, 1989.

39. **Huxley, EJ, Viroslav, J, Gray, WR, and Pierce, AK.** Pharyngeal aspiration in normal adults and patients with depressed consciousness. *Am J Med,* 64:564–568, 1978.

40. **Cameron, JL, Mitchell, WH, and Zuidema, GD.** Aspiration pneumonia: clinical outcome following documented aspiration. *Arch Surg,* 106:49–52, 1973.

41. **Mullan, H, Roubenoff, RA, and Roubenoff, R.** Risk of pulmonary aspiration among patients receiving enteral nutrition support. *JPEN,* 16:160–164, 1992.

42. **Mittal, RK, Stewart, WR, and Schirmer, BD.** Effect of a catheter in the pharynx on the frequency of transient lower esophageal sphincter relaxations. *Gastroenterology,* 103:1236–1240, 1992.

43. **Sloan, S, Rademaker, AW, and Kahrilas, PJ.** Determinants of gastroesophageal junction incompetence: hiatal hernia, lower esophageal sphincter, or both? *Ann Intern Med,* 117:977–982, 1992.

44. **Johnson, DA, Hacker, JF, III, Benjamin, SB, et al.** Percutaneous endoscopic gastrostomy effects on gastroesophageal reflux and the lower esophageal sphincter, *Am J Gastroenterol,* 82:622–624, 1987.

45. **Cole, MJ, Smith, JT, Molnar, C, and Shaffer, EA.** Aspiration after percutaneous gastrostomy: assessment by Tc-99m labeling of the enteral feed. *J Clin Gastroenterol,* 9:90–95, 1987.

46. **Sands, JA.** Incidence of pulmonary aspiration in intubated patients receiving enteral nutrition through wide- and narrow-bore nasogastric feeding tubes. *Heart Lung,* 20:75–80, 1991.

47. **Strong, RM, Condon, SC, and Solinger, MR, et al.** Equal aspiration rates from postpylorus and intragastric-placed small-bore nasoenteric feeding tubes: a randomized, prospective study. *JPEN,* 16:59–63, 1992.

48. **Gutske, RF, Varma, RR, and Soergel, KH.** Gastric reflux during perfusion of the proximal small bowel. *Gastroenterology,* 59:890–895, 1970.

49. **DeLegge, MH, Duckworth, PF, and Craig, RM, et al.** Percutaneous endoscopic gastrojejunostomy (PEG/J): simple and effective. *Am J Gastroenterol,* 87:1338, 1992.

50. **Torres, A, Serra-Battles, J, Ros, E, et al.** Pulmonary aspiration of gastric contents in patients receiving mechanical ventilation: the effect of body position. *Ann Intern Med,* 116:540–543, 1992.

51. **Ibañez, J, Penafiel, A, Raurich, JM, et al.** Gastroesophageal reflux in intubated patients receiving enteral nutrition: effect of supine and semirecumbent positions. *JPEN,* 16:419–422, 1992.

52. **Norton, JA, Ott, LG, McClain, C, et al.** Intolerance to enteral feeding in the brain-injured patient. *J Neurosurg,* 68:62–66, 1988.

53. **Ciocon, JO, Silverstone, FA, Graver, M, and Foley, CJ.** Tube feedings in elderly patients: indications, benefits, and complications. *Arch Intern Med,* 148:429–433, 1988.

54. **Cogen, R, and Weinryb, J.** Aspiration pneumonia in nursing home patients fed via gastrostomy tubes. *Am J Gastroenterol,* 84:1509–1512, 1989.

55. **Fay, DE, Popausky, M, Gruber, M, and Lance, P.** Long-term enteral feeding: a retrospective comparison of delivery via percutaneous endoscopic gastrostomy and nasoenteric tubes. *Am J Gastroenterol,* 86:1604–1609, 1991.

56. **Park, RHR, Allison, MC, Lang, J, et al.** Randomized comparison of percutaneous endoscopic gastrostomy and nasogastric tube feeding in patients with persisting neurolgical dysphagia. *BMJ,* 304:1406–1409, 1992.

57. **Rombeau, JL, and Jacobs, DO.** Nasoenteric tube feeding. In: *Enteral and Tube Feeding.* Rombeau, JL, and Caldwell, MD, Eds., W. B. Saunders, Philadelphia, 1984, 228–239.

58. **Kocan, MJ, and Hickisch, SM.** A comparison of continuous and intermittent enteral nutrition in NICU patients. *J Neurosci Nurs,* 18:333–337, 1986.

59. **Grant, JP.** Comparison or percutaneous endoscopic gastrostomy with Stamm gastrostomy. *Ann Surg,* 207:598–603, 1988.

60. **Weltz, CR, Morris, JB, and Mullen, JL.** Surgical jejunostomy in aspiration risk patients. *Ann Surg,* 215:140–145, 1992.

61. **Kelly, TWJ, Patrick, MR, and Hillman, KM.** Study of diarrhea in critically ill patients. *Crit Care Med,* 11:7–9, 1983.

62. **Broom, J, and Jones, K.** Causes and prevention of diarrhea in patients receiving enteral support. *J Hum Nutr,* 35:123–127, 1981.

63. **Kandil, HE, Opper, FH, Switzer, BR, et al.** marked resistance to tube-feeding-induced diarrhea: the role of magnesium. *Am J Clin Nutr,* 57:73–80, 1993.

64. **Binder, HJ, and Mehta, P.** Short chain fatty acids stimulate active sodium and chloride absorption in vitro in the rat distal colon. *Gastroenterology,* 96:989–996, 1989.

65. **Guenter, PA, Seth, R, Perlmutter, SS, et al.** Tube feeding-related diarrhea in acutely ill patients. *JPEN,* 15:277–280, 1991.

66. **Hart, GK, and Dobb, GJ.** Effect of a fecal bulking agent on diarrhea during enteral feeding in the critically ill. *JPEN,* 12:465–468, 1988.

67. **Hillman, KM, Riordan, R, O'Farrell, SM, et al.** Colonization of gastric contents in critically ill patients. *Crit Care Med,* 10:444–447, 1982.

68. **Isaacs, PET, and Kim, YS.** Blind loop syndrome and small bowel bacterial contamination. *Clin Gastroenterol,* 12:395–401, 1983.

69. **Heyland, D, Bradley, C, and Mandell, LA.** Effect of acidified enteral feedings on gastric colonization of the critically ill patient. *Crit Care Med,* 10:444–447, 1982.

70. **Caswell, MW, Cooper, JE, and Webster, M.** Enteral foods contaminated with *Enterobacter cloacae* as a cause of septicemia. *Br Med J,* 289:973–979, 1981.

71. **Brinson, RR, and Kolts, BE.** Hypoalbuminemia as an indicator of diarrheal disease in the critically ill patient. *Crit Care Med,* 15:506–509, 1987.

72. **Borlase, BC, Bell, SJ, Lewis, EJ, et al.** Tolerance to enteral tube feeding diet in the hypoalbuminemic, critically ill, geriatric patients. *Surg Gynecol Obstet,* 174:181–188, 1992.

73. **Edes, TE, Walk, BE, and Austin, JL.** Diarrhea in tube-fed patients: feeding formula not necessarily the cause. *Am J Med,* 88:91–93, 1990.

74. **Kapadia, SA, Raimundo, A, and Silk, DBA.** Intestinal function in normal volunteers consuming normal diet and polymeric enteral diet with and without added soy polysaccharide. *Clin Nutr,* 10(Suppl. 2):38, 1991.

75. **Scheppach, W, Burghardt, W, and Bartram, P, et al.** Addition of dietary fiber to liquid formula diets: the pros and cons. *JPEN,* 14:204–209, 1990.

76. **Fleisher, D, Sheth, N, and Kou, J.** Phenytoin interaction with enteral feeding administrated with nasogastric tubes. *JPEN,* 14:513–516, 1989.

77. **Marvel, M, and Bertino, J.** Comparative effects of elemental and a complex enteral feeding formulation on the absorption of phenytoin suspension. *JPEN,* 15:316–318, 1991.

78. **Strom, JG, and Miller, JW.** Stability of drugs with enteral nutrient formulas. *DICP,* 24:130–134, 1990.

79. **Howard, PA, and Hannaman, KN.** Warfarin resistance linked to enteral nutrition products. *J Am Diet Assoc,* 85:713–715, 1985.

80. **Laitinen, M, Hienaren, E, and Vainio, H.** Dietary fats and properties of endoplasmic reticulum: dietary lipid induced changes of the microsomal membranes in the liver and gastroduodenal tissue of rats. *Lipids,* 10:461–466, 1975.

81. **Knodell, RG.** Effect of formula composition on hepatic and intestinal drug metabolism during enteral nutrition, *JPEN,* 14:34–38, 1988.

82. **Zachary, JM, Lipman, TO, and Finkelstein, JD.** Elevated transaminases associated with an elemental diet. *Ann Intern Med,* 89:221–222, 1978.

83. **Bunker, VW, and Clayton, BE.** Trace element content of commercial enteral feeds. *Lancet,* 2:426–428, 1983.

Chapter 8

TOTAL PARENTERAL NUTRITION

Stanley J. Dudrick and Rifat Latifi

TABLE OF CONTENTS

0-8493-7847-8/94/$0.00+$.50
© 1994 by CRC Press, Inc.

I. INTRODUCTION

Among physicians, surgeons have demonstrated the greatest interest and have made the most concerted effort in developing innovative, comprehensive, and effective methods for providing adequate nutritional support to patients in the widest range of conditions and clinical situations. Several factors account for the consistent and continual stimulation of thoughtful surgeons and physicians to maintain or improve the nutritional status of their patients. The primary impetus is the observation and acknowledgment throughout the years that operative results, in terms of morbidity and survival, were usually best when patients were in good nutritional condition and worst when patients were in poor nutritional condition. Additionally, surgical patients often present with conditions that have either impaired their ability to maintain their nutrition prior to operation or have made it impossible or unlikely for them to obtain optimal nourishment by conventional means after operation. Moreover, the primary pathophysiologic condition necessitating surgery, such as a major burn, multiple trauma, or extensive neoplasm, often increases the metabolic expenditure of the body stores of calories, protein, and other substrates for energy and repair. The nutrient requirement for metabolic homeostasis, recovery, and rehabilitation are also substantially above normal. The problem is compounded if the surgical patient is an infant or child, because of the accentuated requirements for growth and development beyond those needed for maintenance of metabolic equilibrium. Furthermore, surgical procedures themselves not only induce or intensify catabolism, but often temporarily, and sometimes permanently, interfere significantly with the digestive, absorptive, and assimilative functions of the body at a time when nutritional requirements are increased. Finally, complications of operative procedures, general anesthesia, or trauma, such as wound infection, peritonitis, pneumonia, ileus, bowel obstruction, enterocutaneous fistula, anastomotic disruption, sepsis, shock, or multiple systems organ failure, can adversely affect the nutritional status of the patient.

II. HISTORICAL BACKGROUND OF PARENTERAL NUTRITION

The concept of feeding patients parenterally by injecting nutrient substances or fluids subcutaneously or even directly intravenously was advocated and attempted long before its successful achievement. The realization of this seemingly fanciful dream required centuries of fundamental investigation and discovery coupled with technological developments and judicious applications. The prerequisites to rational clinical studies included knowledge of the anatomy and physiology of the circulation; knowledge of the basic biochemical nature of nutrient substrates; their interrelationships with microbiology, immunology, asepsis, and antisepsis; and some knowledge of the complex interactions of food substances, metabolism, pharmacologic agents, and pathophysiologic processes.

The history of the development of safe and efficacious parenteral nutrition had its beginning with the discovery and demonstration by Harvey of the circulation of the blood, thus establishing the physiologic basis for introducing various fluids and foods by vein directly into the bloodstream where they could be carried to the various tissues of the body (Table 1). Although this landmark discovery occurred in 1616, Harvey did not publish his findings and results until 1628.[1] The credit for first injecting fluids intravenously belongs to Wren, who in 1656, infused ale, wine, and opium into the veins of dogs using a goose quill attached to a pig's bladder as his ingenious administration apparatus.[2] He subsequently made the observation that alcohol injected intravenously had the same effect as alcohol given orally.[3]

TABLE 1
Historical Highlights in the Development of Total Parenteral Nutrition

Year	Published accomplishment	Author
1628	Discovery of the circulation of the blood	Harvey[1]
1656	First intravenous injection (ale, wine, opium) in animals	Wren[2,3]
1831	Intravenous injection of saline solution in man	Latta[7]
1859	Intravenous injection of sugars, egg white, milk, etc., in animals	Bernard[8]
1870	Aseptic and antiseptic techniques in man	Lister[11]
1873	Intravenous infusion of milk in man	Hodder[9]
1877	Discovery of microbes and microbial relationship to infection	Pasteur[12]
1891	Intravenous infusion of saline solution in treatment of shock in man	Matas[14,15]
1895	Discovery of colloidal osmotic function of plasma proteins	Starling[16]
1896	Intravenous infusion of glucose in man	Biedl and Kraus[17]
1905	Development of methods for analysis of urea, creatinine, and other nitrogenous fractions	Folin[18,19]
1911	Intravenous infusion of glucose for nutritional purposes after operations in man	Kausch[20]
1912	Discovery of vitamins as an etiology of nutritional deficiencies	Funk[22]
1913	Demonstration of nutritional utilization of intravenously infused hydrolyzed protein in animals	Henriques and Andersen[21]
1915	Demonstration of nutritional utilization of intravenously infused fat in animals	Murlin and Riche[23]
1915	Demonstration of the rate of nutritional utilization of intravenously infused glucose in man	Woodyatt, Sansum, and Wilder[24]
1920	Intravenous infusion of emulsified fat in man	Yamakawa[25]
1923	Discovery of the cause of pyrogenic substances in sterile distilled water	Seibert[26]
1932	Description of increased nitrogen losses in urine resulting from catabolic response to trauma	Cuthbertson[27,28]
1935	First cottonseed oil emulsions infused in man	Holt[32]
1938	Identification of the essential amino acids and their requirements in man	Rose[30,31]
1939	Demonstration of nutritional utilization of the amino acids of hydrolyzed casein infused intravenously in man	Elman and Weiner[34]
1940	Demonstration of nutritional utilization of a complete mixture of pure crystalline amino acids infused intravenously in man	Shohl and Blackfan[35]
1944	Infusion of hypertonic dextrose, insulin, and plasma protein by peripheral vein in man	Dennis[36,37]
1945	Infusion of improved fat emulsion, dextrose, and protein hydrolysate by peripheral vein	McKibbin, Hegsted, and Stare[38]
1945	Description of indwelling peripheral venous catheter for intravenous feeding	Zimmerman[39]
1949	Development of first continous delivery technique for long-term intravenous infusion of nutrients in dogs	Rhode, Parkins, and Vars[42]
1952	Description of subclavian venipuncture to achieve rapid transfusion	Aubaniac[43]
1959	Demonstration of optimal nonprotein calorie:nitrogen ratio as 150:1	Moore[47]
1961	Development of first safe, standardized, and stable fat emulsion	Schuberth and Wretlind[49]
1962	Achievement of positive nitrogen balance by infusing high-volume nutrient solutions and diuretics by peripheral vein	Rhoads[51,52]
1967	Demonstration of normal growth and development in puppies nourished entirely by central venous infusion	Dudrick, Vars, and Rhoads[55,56]
1968	Demonstration of normal growth and development in an infant nourished entirely by central venous infusion; first use of in-line filter	Dudrick and Wilmore[57,59]
1968	First comprehensive technique for long-term TPN in man	Dudrick, Wilmore, Vars, and Rhoads[44]

By 1665, techniques of i.v. entry and infusion were described and illustrated in a book entitled *Clysmatica Nova,* published in Amsterdam.[4] In 1678, Courten recorded his results of injecting olive oil, vinegar, salt solutions, purgatives, and urine intravenously into animals and was followed by many others who injected a variety of other substances with variable consequences.[4-6] Considering the relative ignorance at that time of the fundamentals of biochemistry, microbiology, and immunology, the magnitude of the problems encountered with i.v. infusion is not surprising, and very little progress was made in this area for more than a century.

During a severe cholera epidemic in England in 1831, a major milestone in the history of i.v. infusion was achieved by Latta, who was the first to conceive of the idea of replacing the lost water and salts intravenously in order to replace the great losses of fluids resulting from severe vomiting and diarrhea.[7] Unable to replace the fluid by mouth or rectum he successfully used the i.v. route as the only alternative available to him. He was the first to inject salt solutions intravenously for the relief of severe dehydration and circulatory collapse. In a series of physiology experiments initiated in 1843, Bernard infused various sugar solutions into animals, and over the next two decades, injected egg whites, milk, and other nutrients into animals with some degree of success.[8] In 1859 he first reported these results, together with the important observation that cane sugar injected intravenously was promptly excreted in the urine, but if it had previously been converted to glucose by gastric juice, it was apparently utilized in the body and did not appear in the urine.[8]

In 1873, Hodder infused fresh cow's milk strained through gauze and administered by syringe intravenously in a desperate attempt to correct fluid and nutrient losses in three patients with cholera.[9] Although he considered his results generally good, he was forced to resign from the hospital staff and barred from the practice of medicine by his colleagues as a result of this experimental venture.[10]

Obviously, the field of i.v. nutrition could not progress meaningfully until additional basic scientific knowledge was acquired. It was not until the late 19th century, following Lister's investigations into aseptic and antiseptic procedures and Pasteur's discovery of microbes and their relationship to infection and sepsis, that i.v. infusions could be performed with a reasonable potential for success.[11,12]

In 1887, Landerer reported the beneficial results of treating a patient with severe postoperative hemorrhage with i.v. sugar solutions. He appreciated that intravenously infused glucose could possibly be used as food and might thereby serve as the basis for "artificial nutrition."[13] In 1891, Matas reported 20 surgical patients in whom he injected saline solution intravenously in the treatment of hemorrhagic shock.[14,15] Four years later, Starling published his classic paper on the colloidal function of the plasma proteins in maintaining blood volume, but blood transfusions could not be used safely for at least another decade until the blood groups were discovered.[16] The following year, Biedl and Kraus were the first to infuse glucose solutions intravenously in humans.[17] Using a 10% glucose solution, they observed no glycosuria or polyuria; however, severe fever resulted following infusions of either glucose or salt solutions in these early studies. The terms "glucose fever" and "salt fever" were used as explanations of these adverse reactions which were thought to be secondary to the unphysiological i.v. infusion of these ordinary substances.

Much of the methodology used in nutritional studies was developed in the early 1900s by Folin, who realized that urine constituents reflect the metabolic state of the body.[18,19] His goal was to determine accurately the quantities of the main solutes of the urine, which he assumed to be an index and measure of the chemical reactions within the body that produces them. He developed analytic methods for measuring urea, uric acid, ammonia, creatinine, nitrogen, and a number of other by-products in the urine. From his large numbers of analyses, he concluded that the amount of urea excreted in the urine fluctuated with the protein intake, whereas the creatinine and uric acid did not. He referred to the protein metabolism, which tended to be constant, as tissue or endogenous metabolism, and to the protein metabolism, which tended to be variable, as exogenous or intermediate metabolism. He later developed methods for analyzing nitrogen fractions in blood and showed the prompt disappearance of amino acids from the bloodstream as they were metabolized, hypothesizing correctly that their metabolism occurred to a large extent in the liver. By providing several novel analytic tools, he did much to advance the studies of nitrogen and carbohydrate metabolism to its current level of sophistication.

At the turn of the 20th century, Kausch was the first to give i.v. injections of glucose for nutritional purposes after operations, insisting that postoperative patients unable to take food by mouth or rectum urgently needed nourishment and must be fed "artificially".[20] By this time it was known that dietary proteins were hydrolyzed in the intestinal tract to peptides and amino acids which were rapidly absorbed. Therefore, it appeared logical to investigate the effects of i.v. infusion of amino acids and protein hydrolysates. Henriques and Andersen conducted the first successful studies in this area in 1913 when they maintained goats in nitrogen equilibrium for 16 days by infusing a protein hydrolysate, which was prepared by digesting goat muscle with pancreatic extract, combined in solution with glucose, sodium, and potassium.[21]

It was also early in the 20th century that most of the major discoveries of vitamins were made. Funk advanced the theory that beriberi was due to a nutritional deficiency rather than an infection or toxicity and called the deficiency substances "vital amines or vitamines".[22] Eventually the final "e" was dropped resulting in the word vitamin, which permitted it to represent a neutral substance of undefined composition.[4]

In 1915, Murlin and Riche infused emulsified fat intravenously into two dogs, monitored their respiratory quotients, and found changes comparable to those observed in dogs receiving fat by mouth.[23] That same year Woodyatt and his co-workers demonstrated for the first time that glucose could be injected intravenously indefinitely into human beings at a maximum rate of 0.85 g/kg body weight/hour without glycosuria.[24]

Using lecithin as the emulsifying agent, Yamakawa was the first to infuse emulsified fat in man in 1920.[25] Although he and his co-workers conducted many experiments during the next decade, very little progress was made toward developing a safe and practical fat emulsion for clinical use. The serious problem of pyrogenic reactions, which had plagued investigators interested in i.v. infusions for three centuries, was solved by Seibert in 1923, when she found that a specific bacterium that grew in distilled water produced a filterable, stable substance capable of inducing fever and chills when it entered the bloodstream even in minute amounts.[26] The discovery of this pyrogen eventually led to the production of safer i.v. solutions, and to the development of the commercial i.v. solution industry, but pyrogen-free water was not available generally for another decade.[10]

The 1930s and 1940s were characterized by a great number of investigations related to defining the specific nutritional needs of human beings during physiologic and various pathophysiologic conditions. In 1932, Cuthbertson reported observations on the catabolic response to major limb injuries and quantitated the surprisingly high nitrogen losses in the urine after major skeletal trauma.[27-29] In 1934, Rose first suggested the i.v. use of amino acids for nutritional purposes.[30] Three years later he defined the amino acid requirements for man and developed a formula for providing man's essential amino acid needs.[31] Working with fat emulsions produced from cottonseed oil, Holt and his co-workers reported some clinical successes in 1935, but noted that the emulsions were relatively unstable.[32]

In 1937, Elman infused a casein hydrolysate intravenously into dogs, and two years later, he and his co-worker, Weiner, reported the first i.v. infusions with nutritional utilization of protein hydrolysates in humans.[33,34] The following year, Shohl and Blackfan reported the first i.v. administration in man of a crystalline amino acid mixture, which was based on the amino acid formula recommended for rats.[35] The mixture promoted positive nitrogen balance in infants comparable to that obtained with commercially available protein hydrolysates, but because it was much more expensive to manufacture, it did not gain wide acceptance. In the mid-1940s, Dennis reported that surgical patients could be sustained for extended periods of time by peripheral i.v. infusions of 20% dextrose, in combination with insulin to improve utilization efficiency and human plasma as a source of protein.[36,37]

In 1945, an improved version of the original cottonseed oil emulsions used by Holt 15 years previously was successfully infused by McKibben and co-workers, together with dextrose and protein hydrolysates for i.v. alimentation.[38] Eventually, their emulsion was commercially available for a limited period of time. That same year, Zimmerman reported the use of a flexible, small diameter, plastic tubing inserted percutaneously through a needle, advanced 5 to 6 cm into the peripheral vein and, after removing the needle, left in place for as long as 12 days for "total intravenous feeding".[39] His nutrient mixture consisted of 10% dextrose, amino acids, and vitamins. Similarly, in 1948, Dennis and co-workers reported the use of a polyethylene catheter advanced into the superior vena cava for infusing hypertonic dextrose, thus taking advantage of the rapid dilution by the high blood flow in this large vein to avoid the complications of phlebitis and secondary thrombosis.[40] The following year, Dennis reported having maintained such catheters in place for as long as 3 weeks and again suggested the simultaneous use of i.v. insulin to minimize urinary glucose losses and subsequent osmotic diuresis and dehydration.[41] In 1949, Rhode and his co-workers reported the development of the first continuous delivery apparatus for long-term i.v. feedings of protein hydrolysates, 50% dextrose, and other nutrients in adult dogs.[42]

In 1952, Aubaniac first described the technique of percutaneous subclavian vein puncture as a means to achieve access for rapid transfusion in battle casualties in Vietnam.[43] This technique was subsequently modified and popularized by Dudrick and co-workers for safe and reliable access to the superior vena cava for long-term continuous central venous infusion of hypertonic nutrient solutions.[44-46] Although a great number of clinical investigations were carried out in the 1950s with fat emulsions, protein hydrolysates, and hypertonic dextrose, the results were largely equivocal or fell short of expectations primarily because of technological shortcomings and great reluctance on the part of clinicians to use central venous catheters for infusion.[10]

In 1959, Moore established the fact that the optimal non-protein calorie-to-nitrogen ratio was 150 kcal:1 g nitrogen in order to achieve anabolism.[47] The following year, Geyer published a comprehensive review of the world's literature on parenteral nutrition.[49] Until this time, the only route regularly used for i.v. infusion was by peripheral vein, and the only means of providing adequate energy intravenously was by infusing fat emulsions. In 1961, Shuberth and Wretlind reported the development and successful clinical application of the first safe, stable, and reliable fat emulsion which was derived from soybean oil and stabilized by egg phosphatides.[49] Conversely, because of the high incidence of side effects and the relative instability of the cottonseed oil emulsions, they were withdrawn from the commercial market in 1964.[50]

In 1962, Rhoads first reported on the use of diuretics as an adjuvant to excreting the extra water used as a vehicle in infusing 5 to 7 l/d of solutions containing 10% dextrose and protein hydrolysate by a technique called "parenteral hyperalimentation".[51] Subsequently in 1965, Rhoads and his co-workers reported a series of surgical patients with prolonged disability of the gastrointestinal tract nourished sufficiently by this technique to achieve positive nitrogen balance.[52] Eventually, problems related to fluid overload and electrolyte imbalance secondary to the unpredictability of the diuretic response led to the abandonment of this feeding technique. However, since this was the first i.v. feeding technique by which positive nitrogen balance had been reliably achieved, its success was the stimulus for a fresh attack on the problem, which culminated in the development of total parenteral nutrition.

III. GENESIS OF TOTAL PARENTERAL NUTRITION

The prevailing attitude among clinicians in the early 1960s regarding the potential of adequately feeding a patient entirely by vein was that it was probably impossible; that even if it were possible, it would probably be impractical; and even if it were practical, it would probably be unaffordable. Moreover, the catabolic response to injury was thought to benefit the patient by mobilizing tissue protein moieties for transport by the circulation to serve as substrates for repair and healing. Indeed, it was thought and taught that it was likely unnecessary and perhaps disadvantageous to attempt to overcome the catabolic response by increasing nutrient intake. It was commonly believed that a more natural approach would be to allow the post-traumatic or post-operative negative nitrogen balance to run its course and attempt to compensate for it later by increased food intake during the later phases of convalescence and rehabilitation.[47] However, in a significant number of patients who were malnourished prior to a major injury or operation and who could not be fed adequately for prolonged periods afterward for a variety of reasons, adherence to this philosophy resulted in unacceptable morbidity and mortality rates. Accordingly, it was absolutely essential to direct efforts and resources toward the development of a safe and efficacious i.v. feeding technique which could provide all required nutrients for patients who could not eat, should not eat, would not eat, or could not eat enough.

If the quality and quantity of nutrient solutions which could be infused by vein were to be improved, several obstacles had to be considered and overcome. An obvious limitation was the volume of fluid which could be tolerated safely per day by the average adult patient (2500 to 3500 ml). Another limitation was the requirement that solutions infused by peripheral veins be isosmotic with the body fluids (290 to 310 mOsm/l) in order to minimize physical and chemical trauma to the intima of the veins and the formed elements of the blood. Additional limitations were the immutable inherent caloric values of the individual nutrients (3.5 to 4.0 kcal/g carbohydrate, 4.0 to 4.25 kcal/g protein, 9.0 to 9.1 kcal/g fat and 7.0 kcal/g ethanol) and the maximum effective metabolic rate of utilization of these and other required nutrients (electrolytes, trace elements, and vitamins), together with the potentially toxic or other untoward effects of administering the necessarily multiple biochemical substrates simultaneously. Finally, the commercial availability of nutrient substrates for i.v. administration had to be determined, and the cost of formulating the solutions, infusing them, and monitoring their safety and effectiveness had to be reasonable. Moreover, at that time, several of the i.v. nutrient components now taken for granted, such as crystalline amino acids, trace elements, and fat-soluble vitamins, were not available for infusion in human beings.

Regarding the delivery system, the physicochemical characteristics of the existing metal needles and cannulas and the available plastic and rubber catheters had to be established in order to minimize thrombosis, phlebitis, and other inflammatory or toxic reactions in the circulatory system. Indeed, the safety of the entire administration system, i.e., the bottle, infusion tubing, syringes, pumps, etc., had to be guaranteed. The requirements for total parenteral nutrition had to be determined or estimated from known oral nutritional requirements because precise parenteral recommendations for nutrients were not available. Then the required nutrients had to be formulated, using individual molecular components whose solubility and compatibility could be assured. Finally, the risk of infection had to be eliminated or minimized to an acceptable level. Therefore, aseptic and antiseptic principles and practices had to be established for the preparation and administration of the nutrient solutions. In view of the fact that a foreign body, such as a cannula or catheter, had to be inserted through the skin into the bloodstream, it was likely that the incidence of infection would eventually approach 100% during prolonged periods of catheterization. Therefore, meticulous and conscientious aseptic and antiseptic techniques were mandatory to maximize safety and success.

Procedures and laboratory tests had to be established to monitor the efficacy and safety of total parenteral nutrition. In order to insure the administration of maximal doses of each of the nutrients daily, continuous infusion of the solution at a constant rate throughout each 24-h period had to be maintained. This was contrary to the customary infusion practices at that time. Financial, physical, and personnel resources had to be appraised to determine the feasibility of an undertaking of this magnitude. Finally, it was essential to overcome decades of written or verbal expressions by prominent physicians and scientists that total parenteral nutrition was either impossible or, at best, improbable and impractical. Convincing evidence had to be generated if these prejudices and teachings were to be neutralized or overcome and if widespread clinical acceptance of total i.v. feeding technique was to be gained. It was obvious that investigative efforts had to be directed toward designing an experiment in the laboratory to verify the theory, efficacy, and safety of total parenteral nutrition, with the ultimate goal of applying the basic knowledge of techniques generated in animals to human beings.

One approach to increasing the total caloric ration, which could be delivered by vein, was to add the experimental cottonseed oil emulsion to the nutrient regimen. As many as 3000 total calories daily had been provided by some investigators to a limited number of patients by infusing high doses of this fat emulsion intravenously.[53] However, the multiple and unpredictable adverse effects of the cottonseed oil emulsion severely restricted its usefulness. Fever, abdominal pain, anaphylactic reactions, coagulation defects, impaired hematopoiesis, and liver dysfunction were among the more serious sequelae to its infusion, and very few patients could tolerate more than 10 days of treatment with this emulsion. For these reasons, the cottonseed oil emulsion was withdrawn from clinical i.v. use.[50]

The next approach was to formulate solutions from available i.v. nutrients known to be safe and effective and to increase the total quantities infused to maximum levels of tolerance and utilization. Although ethyl alcohol could be infused intravenously as a source of calories, the total adult dose per day was limited to 700 to 1000 calories in order to avoid inebriation. Moreover, its known toxicity to the central nervous system, liver, kidneys, and other tissues, together with its associated mental obtundity, depressed reflexes, and aggravation of GI tract inflammation, even when infused by vein, limited its widespread acceptance as a caloric source. Fructose, or invert sugar, offered no particular advantage over dextrose, nor did the sugar-alcohols, sorbitol and xylitol, which were much more expensive than dextrose. Therefore, the only practical way to deliver adequate calories intravenously sufficient to promote maximum incorporation of administered nitrogen moieties into tissue synthesis was to increase the ration of the infused dextrose. Crystalline amino acids for i.v. use were not yet available, and the only nitrogen-containing nutrient substrates accessible for parenteral infusion were fibrin and casein hydrolysates.

The fundamental investigative plan to determine the feasibility of long-term total parenteral nutrition consisted of concentrating the nutrients known to be required for growth and development of beagle puppies into the quantity of water the animals could tolerate per day, and to infuse the resultant 30% hypertonic solution (1800 to 2400 mOsm/l) into a large diameter, high-flow central vein where it could be rapidly diluted to isotonicity. Continuous infusion for the entire 24-h day at the maximum rates of utilization and tolerance was required in order to avoid exceeding renal threshold for the individual nutrients. Starting with a continuous infusion apparatus designed for adult dogs by Rhode and co-workers,[42] an effective, practical, counterbalanced apparatus incorporating a specially designed swivel in order to permit maximum mobility of the animal in the cage evolved over a period of several months for continuous infusion into active, unrestrained puppies.[46,54] The induction of weight gain in a fully grown adult dog would be modest at best and likely to be interpreted as undesirable accumulation of extracellular water rather than as the synthesis of new tissue. Experimental methods were available for measuring total body water and some other water compartments, but they were rather tedious, complicated, and fraught with error, leading to skepticism of the validity of the data. However, if puppies were to be used as experimental subjects, the weight gain, growth, and development would likely be so dramatic as to avert any criticism that changes in body weight were secondary to excess water retention. Accordingly, over the next several months, an i.v. dietary regimen was formulated which most closely approximated that of the known oral dietary requirements for growth and development in beagle puppies. Although the initial goal was to grow puppies from birth for a few months, the technical, biochemical, and immunological difficulties encountered in this ambitious endeavor were so overwhelming that this idealistic goal was temporarily abandoned. Therefore, the next logical hallmark of growth and development at which to initiate the total parenteral feeding experiments was at 8 to 10 weeks of age, when puppies are normally weaned from the breast.

Although the recommended daily allowance of protein for a beagle puppy is 8 g/kg body weight/day, only 4 g protein equivalent/kg body weight/day, in the form of fibrin hydrolysate, could be infused without inducing toxic reactions in the puppies. Accepting this limitation as inevitable, it was decided to give the daily recommended carbohydrate dose, plus an additional 4 g/kg body weight as dextrose in order to spare the administered nitrogen substrates maximally and to maintain the recommended daily total caloric ration. Because cottonseed oil emulsion was still available at that time, it was possible to give the exact recommended ration of fat in this form. Over a period of approximately 2 to 4 h/d, 2.6 g fat/kg body weight were infused into the puppies during the initial experiments. However, when cottonseed oil emulsion was withdrawn abruptly from the market, the i.v. diet was modified in the second group of animals, so that the daily dose of fat was calculated to provide only the minimal requirements for linoleic acid (0.6 g emulsion/kg body weight/day). In the third set of animals, fat was, of necessity, eliminated completely. As the fat in the i.v. diet was decreased, carbohydrate calories in the form of dextrose were increased equivalently in order to maintain an isocaloric ration of 130 kcal/kg body weight/day.[44]

In order to provide all electrolyte requirements in one solution, it was necessary to bind the calcium and phosphate ions as separate organic compounds to prevent their precipitation in the solution as calcium phosphate. Calcium was added in the form of calcium gluconate and/calcium heptonate, and phosphate was supplied as sodium or potassium glycerophosphate. Several months of tedious trial-and-error experimentation were required in order to formulate a trace element solution in which all of the components were mutually soluble and compatible. When finally a combination of salts was found which initially would go into solution, precipitation would occur to varying degrees when the final nutrient mixture was autoclaved. Moreover, color changes occurred which indicated the probable formation of unknown chemical complexes. Therefore, it was necessary to add the individually sterile components together as aseptically as possible immediately prior to infusion without further sterilization procedures. During the course of the experiments, a trace element solution evolved which contained cobalt, copper, iodine, manganese, molybdenum, and zinc. The rest of the elements in the solution had to be added individually.

Providing the recommended vitamins for growth in beagle puppies presented a problem. First of all, no available vitamin preparation contained all of the vitamins required for growth in beagle puppies in parenteral form. Moreover, vitamin C, essential for man, is not required by dogs; biotin and choline, which were of questionable essentiality for man, were required for dogs; and PABA is a vitamin in dogs, but not in man. Biotin, choline, and PABA were obtained in crystalline form, dissolved in water, and added to the solution individually. Commercial mixtures of the B-complex vitamins, vitamin A, vitamin D, and vitamin K were added separately. Vitamin B_{12}, folic acid, and vitamin K had to be added individually to the solution immediately prior to infusion because of relative instability. Although some of the vitamins could have been given intramuscularly with less risk of decomposition or interaction in the solution, one of the goals of the investigation was to provide all nutrients entirely by vein if at all possible.

In order for the experiment to be successful, the following major problems had to be overcome: sepsis, either as a result of contamination of the solution during manufacture or administration, or as a result of indwelling catheter-associated infection; mechanical problems related to the continuous infusion of nutrients intravenously into an unrestrained, active, young animal; clotting, hemolysis, or other untoward effects on the intima of the circulatory system; and choosing the appropriate nutrients in the proper dosage in order to promote normal growth and development with minimal or no adverse metabolic effects on the various tissues and organs of the body.

The superior vena cava was chosen as the best venous channel for delivery of the hypertonic nutrient mixture. To confirm that adequate mixing of the continuously infused solution occurred within a reasonable distance of the tip of the catheter, two catheters were inserted into the superior vena cava, one via a jugular vein and one via an iliac vein, so that the tips of the catheters were virtually touching each other. As the solution was infused at the appropriate rate, the lower catheter was withdrawn 1 cm at a time sequentially, and blood samples were obtained at each level for determination of osmolarity and glucose concentration. In this way, it was shown repeatedly that the blood in the superior vena cava had normal osmolarity and normal glucose concentration within 1.5 to 2.5 cm from the tip of the infusion catheter because of the high volume blood flow.

All commercially available infusion catheters known to exist were tested for tissue reactivity, initially by implanting them subcutaneously in adult dogs, and observing the relative tissue reactivity to the various plastic products. Subsequently, under meticulously aseptic and antiseptic conditions, the least reactive catheters were inserted into the external jugular veins of dogs, threaded into the superior vena cava distally until the tips were just above the right atrium of the heart, secured with sutures, and threaded proximally subcutaneously from the base of the neck to emerge through the skin at a point midway between the scapulae. A custom-made soft canvas harness was attached to an aluminum or stainless steel support apparatus which secured the catheter to the animal at its exit site while providing a point of attachment to the infusion apparatus. Polyethylene was found to be most thrombogenic, least durable, and associated with the highest incidence of kinking, spontaneous rupture, and other mechanical difficulties. Teflon® was rather rigid and was, therefore, associated frequently with perforation of the venous system. Silicone rubber was the least reactive catheter material, but was the most difficult to insert and advance into the proper position, the most difficult to maintain secured in place, and the most likely to rupture spontaneously. Polyvinyl chloride had the best overall characteristics and was, therefore, chosen for use in the puppy study. The polyvinyl tubing used was not medical grade, but was designed for use as insulation for electrical wire. One such catheter remained *in situ* and useful for 170 days before it polymerized and fractured. It was successfully replaced by another catheter which survived for the 12 subsequent weeks in that experiment.

To minimize the introduction of microorganisms around the catheter exit site, a 2-in square area of skin was kept shaved and was prepared with 2% tincture of iodine followed by the application of 1 cc of antibiotic ointment daily.

Although the solutions were formulated in a relatively clean area of the laboratory with the usual aseptic and antiseptic precautions taken during addition of the components to the reservoir bottle, about 18 individual manipulations were required to complete the preparation of the solution. The high risk of contamination during preparation was obvious. To assess the degree to which inadvertent contamination was occurring, hundreds of bottles of solution were prepared and refrigerated, and samples were taken daily for a week thereafter for bacterial and fungal cultures. About 25% of the solutions prepared in this manner grew organisms. To reduce solution contamination to a more acceptable level, formulation was eventually carried out in a laminar-flow, filtered-air environment. This reduced solution contamination to 1 to 3%. To reduce further the risk of delivery of microorganisms to the puppies' circulations, a 1-in diameter filter having an average pore size of 0.22 μm, was incorporated into the delivery system in order to prevent the inadvertent infusion of any microorganismal contaminants which might have been introduced into the solution during preparation. The reduction in the incidence of sepsis in animals following this innovation was dramatic and significant.

The two longest-term animals were fed for 235 and 255 days while they more than tripled their body weights and developed comparably to their control littermates. In both groups the deciduous teeth were shed and replaced with permanent teeth at the same time. The intravenously fed animals were just as energetic as the controls, and there were no obvious abnormalities of their skin, coats, or bony development. Having demonstrated beyond a doubt that it was possible and practical to feed animals entirely by vein for prolonged periods of time without excessive risks or compromise of growth and development potential,[55] the research team then directed efforts to applying what was learned and developed in the laboratory to the treatment of patients.[44,56]

Although several critically ill adults were studied first, the puppy experience was soon applied directly to a human infant. In 1967, a serendipitous opportunity arose to feed entirely by vein a newborn female infant with near-total small bowel atresia.[57] Following massive intestinal resection, her duodenum had been anastomosed to the terminal 3 cm of ileum; her weight had declined to 4 lb at 19 days of age; she appeared hypometabolic and moribund; and it was obvious that she was dying of starvation. After extensive consideration of the moral and ethical aspects of her problems, all were in accord that the risks of attempting to provide total parenteral nutrition by means of a central venous catheter in this infant were justifiable.

A polyvinyl chloride catheter was inserted via cut-down into the right external jugular vein and threaded into the superior vena cava; the other end of the catheter was passed subcutaneously behind the ear to emerge through the parietal scalp. It was hoped that the skin tunnel would reduce the chances of microorganisms reaching the circulatory system. Initially, the infant was infused cautiously with a basic nutrient mixture containing hypertonic dextrose, fibrin hydrolysate, electrolytes, and vitamins. Each day or so, something new was added to the mixture so that if the infant experienced an adverse reaction, there would have been some indication as to its cause. The infusion was delivered continuously by a peristaltic pump through a closed system containing an in-line 0.22 μm membrane filter.[58] Fear of infection was foremost because the anticipated infection rate associated with an indwelling central venous foreign body inserted percutaneously was 100% if left in place indefinitely. The initial decision was to leave the catheter *in situ* until clinical evidence of infection was manifested. If no other logical explanation for an infection was apparent, the blood was cultured, the catheter was removed and cultured, and antimicrobial treatment was instituted. If the baby survived the septic episode, another catheter was inserted, and the feeding was continued. According to this plan, catheters could be maintained sepsis-free clinically for 35 to 40 days by following meticulous aseptic and antiseptic techniques in insertion and maintenance.

The baby weighed 5.1 lb at birth and 4 lb when the catheter was inserted. After 45 days, she had gained 3.5 lb in weight and had increased 5.5 cm in length. Her head circumference increased by 6.5 cm, her chest circumference increased by 8.5 cm, and she manifested normal activity and development.[57] She was fed for 22 months primarily by vein and achieved a maximum weight of 18.5 lb.[59] She had undergone central venous catheterization via her jugular veins six times, a saphenous vein once, a cephalic vein once, and the subclavian veins eight times. Although she eventually died, an unprecedented and invaluable metabolic and technological experience was gained during her management, and her legacy to total parenteral nutrition (TPN) is unparalleled.[60]

In the first few adult patients to whom the technique of central venous feeding was applied via the superior vena cava, the catheters were inserted through an external jugular vein by cut-down or percutaneously. However, because of problems either in advancing the catheter or maintaining it free of infection, a more proximal and less mobile site of insertion was desirable. Thus, percutaneous subclavian vein catheterization, which had been used infrequently clinically since its inception in 1948[43] for monitoring central venous pressure,[61,62] was explored as an access route for continuous hypertonic central venous feeding and has become commonplace.[63] The principles and techniques of asepsis and antisepsis which subsequently developed during the initial clinical trials have minimized the risks of infection and have allowed long-term feeding catheters to remain in place for months or even years.[64] The components of total parenteral nutrition solutions have improved over the years and will continue to undergo further modification as more knowledge and experience are gained in this vital area of clinical biochemistry and nutritional support.[65]

IV. GENERAL INDICATIONS FOR TOTAL PARENTERAL NUTRITION

For the well-nourished patient who has a normally functioning GI tract, provision of adequate nutritional support is usually not a great problem in the majority of hospitalized patients. However, in patients who exhibit signs and symptoms, or have a history, of malnutrition prior to hospitalization, or who are likely to develop them during hospitalization as a result of stressful periods of diagnosis and therapy, a significantly higher morbidity and mortality may result if adequate efforts have not been directed toward their nutritional maintenance or restitution.

The primary general indication for the use of TPN is to provide adequate nutrition to support and maintain normal metabolism when use of the GI tract is impractical, inadequate, ill-advised, or impossible. The decision to initiate TPN should be based upon the achievement of a specific, definable, and realistic goal for each patient, in order to prolong meaningful life and not merely to prolong an active process of inevitable death. A fundamental goal of nutritional support is to provide nutrients adequate in quality and quantity to meet the normal or increased metabolic requirements for the following:

1. Growth and development
2. "Regrowth" of a depleted adult to ideal weight
3. Restoration of optimal bodily function
4. Achievement of homeostasis
5. Positive nitrogen balance
6. Improved protein status
7. Repair of tissues
8. Improved response to all forms of therapy

9. Increased physical activity
10. Recovery from stress
11. Restoration of immunocompetence
12. Reduced morbidity
13. Reduced mortality
14. Accelerated convalescence and rehabilitation

A second general indication for TPN is the reduction of mechanical and secretory activity of the alimentary tract to basal levels in order to achieve a state of "bowel rest". The combination of bowel rest and adequate nutrition by vein has been of paramount value in the management of many GI diseases including granulomatous enterocolitis, ulcerative colitis, tuberculous enteritis, and infectious or parasitic enterocolitis; severely malnourished patients requiring prolonged periods of bowel preparation during diagnostic studies and prior to major surgical procedures; patients with malignant diseases receiving chemotherapy, radiotherapy, immunotherapy, or multimodal therapy; and paraplegics, quadriplegics, or debilitated patients with indolent decubitus ulcers in the pelvic or perineal area. Detailed and specific indications for use of TPN have been extensively described elsewhere.[66,67]

A third general indication for TPN is to provide specially tailored diets and to improve nutritional status in patients with renal or hepatic decompensation, without significantly elevating the blood urea nitrogen or blood ammonia levels. A fourth general indication is to reduce the urgency for surgical intervention in patients who might eventually require operation, but in whom prolonged, progressive malnutrition is likely to increase greatly the risk of operation and postoperative complications. A fifth general indication for TPN is to avoid, reduce, or correct protein deficiencies and the complications of hypoproteinemia and to achieve a steady, definable metabolic or nutritional state. The overall goal is to provide the protein moieties that are required both for repair and for restoration of injured tissues. The specific goals for protein repletion are outlined in Table 2.

V. NUTRITIONAL ASSESSMENT

A number of indices have been developed for clinical evaluation and have proved valuable in assessing the nutritional status of a broad spectrum of patients. A comprehensive discussion of nutritional assessment is presented in Chapter 1 of this volume. However, this aspect of nutritional support is sufficiently important in this era of managed care to merit additional emphasis of some practical clinical considerations. Among these, a history of an unintentional or unexplained weight loss of 10 lb or 10% of body weight during the previous 2 months, a serum albumin concentration of less than 3.4 g/dl, an impaired immunocompetence as determined by a standard battery of immunologic tests, and an abnormally low total lymphocyte count ($<1200/mm^3$) are the most important. If any one of these indices is manifested, the patient is malnourished to a mild degree; if any two of these indices are present, the patient is malnourished to a moderate degree; if any three of these indices are apparent, the patient is malnourished to a moderately severe degree; and if all four indices are documented, the patient is severely malnourished.

These fundamental clinical criteria are especially important in establishing the nutritional status of a patient who is a candidate for an elective or semi-elective major operative procedure because of the well-known correlation between the degree of preoperative malnutrition and the incidence of postoperative complications and death. In general, a rule of thumb derived from a vast collective experience is that the incidence of lethal and potentially lethal complications associated with a major GI tract operation is increased

TABLE 2
Indications for Protein Repletion

1. Increase resistance to blood loss.
2. Decrease susceptibility to shock.
3. Restore plasma and tissue proteins.
4. Increase plasma and blood volume.
5. Reduce edema locally at the wound and generally.
6. Accelerate wound healing.
7. Restore immunocompetence.
8. Improve gastrointestinal motility.
9. Restore digestive enzymes to normal.
10. Reverse the protein deficiency of malabsorption.
11. Improve metabolic rate.
12. Improve cardiovascular function.
13. Decrease weakness and lassitude.
14. Reverse mental depression.
15. Reduce morbidity.
16. Reduce mortality.
17. Reduce time and expense of convalescence.
18. Reduce time and expense of rehabilitation.

by about 10% in patients with mild malnutrition, about 25% in patients with moderate malnutrition, about 40% in patients with moderately severe malnutrition, and about 90% in patients with severe malnutrition.[68]

Evidence of malnutrition may not be easily detected during a casual clinical examination. However, a reasonably accurate evaluation of the nutritional status of most patients can be obtained readily from a carefully directed history, physical examination, and combination of clinical and laboratory studies.[69] A clinical impression or determination can often be made whether the patient's malnourished state consists primarily of marasmus (pan-starvation), kwashiorkor (protein-calorie deficiencies), or a mixture of both. Although all three of these forms of malnutrition can result in common adverse clinical consequences, each individual form exhibits characteristic clinical and biochemical manifestations which must be recognized and taken into consideration when planning specific nutritional rehabilitation regimens.

An accurate determination of the dietary intake of the patient is of paramount importance in evaluating nutritional status, especially as it relates to the degree and time course of weight loss. The presence of anorexia, dysphagia, nausea, vomiting, diarrhea, weakness, lethargy, loss of vitality, and a decreased sense of well-being may be consistent with malnutrition and may further compound the effects of weight loss. A focused systemic review and past medical history may elicit other signs, symptoms, or causes of malnutrition. A comprehensive family history may establish genetic, metabolic, endocrine, neoplastic, or other etiologies for primary or secondary nutritional problems. The social and economic status of the patient is essential in determining the quality and quantity of food usually ingested. The age and reliability of the patient are also important in evaluating the dietary history, especially in the geriatric population.

Weight loss is the most common measurement considered in assessing nutritional status, as there is a definite correlation between significant weight loss and morbidity. However, the overall limitation of weight loss as a nutritional assessment index is that it does not identify the specific body compartments that contribute to the weight loss. A patient may be in a state of negative nitrogen balance and relative malnutrition as a result of a recent or current catabolic pathological process although appearing physically to be adequately nourished. Careful examination may reveal that tissues which appear normal on visual inspection are actually edematous as a result of hypoproteinemia. On the other hand, a severe case of malnutrition can be obvious and easily recognized. Diagnosis of specific vitamin or mineral deficiencies can often be made by recognition of characteristic signs on physical examination. In the hospitalized patient, however, nutritional depletion often develops subtly and becomes clinically significant before overt deficiencies are manifested. In such cases, clinical anthropometric measurements such as serial triceps skinfold thickness, midarm circumference, midarm muscle circumference, and creatinine-height index may be helpful in improving accuracy and reproductibility of the clinical assessment of nutritional status.

Biochemical and hematologic studies are usually helpful in estimating the nutritional status of a patient. Determinations of the hemoglobin concentration and hematocrit in correlation with deviations in hydration and body weight may be very useful, although both measurements can be misleading and inaccurate, especially following recent blood loss or blood transfusions. Routine urinalysis may show significant protein, sugar, or electrolyte losses. A fasting blood sugar or 2-h postprandial determination may indicate previously unsuspected diabetes mellitus. The blood urea nitrogen or nonprotein nitrogen levels may reflect a catabolic state or GI bleeding. Measurement of serum total protein, albumin, and globulin levels should be obtained, although these determinations may also be misleading during periods of metabolic instability. The serum total protein level alone is of questionable value because a high serum globulin may mask a significant decrease in the serum albumin level, which is the best available indicator of visceral protein status. The critical levels of serum proteins, below which obligatory edema forms, have been defined as 5.5 g/dl for total protein and 3.0 g/dl for albumin, the latter fraction being responsible for most of the colloid osmotic pressure of plasma. There is poor correlation between serum protein levels and deviations in body weight; the serum protein levels usually are maintained for a considerable period of time after initial weight loss, and then suddenly decrease in the latter stages of protein depletion.

An important and rapidly responding index of protein nutrition can be obtained by measuring serial fasting plasma amino acid levels. However, this is still an expensive procedure and is generally reserved for only the most complex nutritional problems.

Other indices that have gained increasing importance and application in the serial evaluation of protein nutritional status include the serum transferrin, prealbumin, complement, and retinol-binding protein concentrations. These proteins have respectively shorter half-lives and accordingly respond more rapidly to protein depletion or repletion, thus providing indicators for the short-term effectiveness of nutritional therapy. In the presence of known or suspected hepatic disease, liver function studies should be performed, because the patient with liver insufficiency is particularly unable to compensate well for metabolic imbalances. In selected patients, it can be helpful to determine the serum lipid profile, specific individual serum vitamin levels, and serum levels of most of the biologically active electrolytes in addition to assessment of acid-base balance.

VI. FORMULATION AND COMPOSITION OF TOTAL PARENTERAL NUTRITION SOLUTION

The basic parenteral nutrient mixture is a hypertonic solution about six times more concentrated (1800 to 2400 mOsm/l) than blood and consists of approximately 20 to 35% dextrose and 4 to 5% crystalline amino acids. This provides about 6.5 to 8.0 g nitrogen, equivalent to about 40 to 50 g protein, and approximately 1000 cal/l (Table 3).[70] Although the base solution may contain various quantities of some of the essential minerals and electrolytes, other micronutrients, such as vitamins, iron, and trace elements; must be

TABLE 3
Total Parenteral Nutrition Solution Formulation

Base solution	
40–70% dextrose in water	500–1500 ml
8.5–15% crystalline amino acids	500–1500 ml
Additives to each liter	
Sodium chloride, acetate, or lactate	40–50 mEq
Potassium chloride or acetate	20–30 mEq
Potassium or sodium acid phosphate (10–20 mM phosphorus)	15–30 mEq
Magnesium sulfate	15–18 mEq
Calcium gluconate or chloride	4.6–9.2 mEq
Additives to total daily regimen	
Zinc sulfate	5–10 mg
Copper sulfate	1–2 mg
Selenium (sodium selenate)	60 μg
Chromium chloride	10–20 μg
Manganese chloride	0.5 mg
Iron-dextran[a]	5 mg
Multivitamin infusion	10 ml
A	3300 IU
D	200 IU
E	10 IU
Ascorbic acid	100 mg
Folic acid	400 μg
Niacin	40 mg
Riboflavin	3.6 mg
Thiamine	3.0 mg
B$_6$ (pyridoxine)	4.0 mg
B$_{12}$ (cyanocobalamin)	5.0 μg
Pantothenic acid	15 mg
Biotin	60 μg
Additive to any one liter twice weekly	
Vitamin K (phytonadione)	10 mg
IV fat emulsion 10% or 20%	
200–500 ml 2 to 7 times weekly	20–100 g
Average daily TPN ration provides	
Carbohydrate energy	850 kcal/l
Protein energy	150 kcal/l
Fat energy	1000–2000 kcal/l
Nitrogen	6.5–8.0 g/l
Amino acids	40–50 g/l

[a] Sensitivity test prior to infusion

added immediately prior to infusion in order to satisfy specific nutrient and metabolic requirements of individual patients.[67]

Appropriate modifications of the standard adult formula, or administration of specially formulated solutions, are required for treatment of patients with congestive heart failure, lung failure, renal insufficiency, acute pancreatitis, liver disease associated with encephalopathy, massive nutritional edema, and in the geriatric population. Modifications of the solution are often necessary following the initiation of TPN, depending upon the patient's metabolic response to the disease, trauma, operation, infection, or other intercurrent conditions. It is essential to recognize that no single i.v. nutrient solution can be ideal for all conditions in all patients at all times, or for the same patient during all of the various phases of a pathological process.

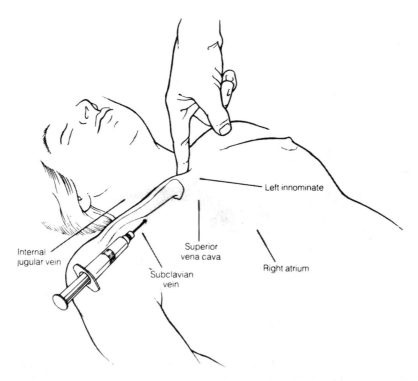

FIGURE 1. The needle is advanced beneath the clavicle in a horizontal plane with its tip aimed at the posterior aspect of the sternal notch.

VII. TECHNIQUES OF ADMINISTRATION OF TOTAL PARENTERAL NUTRITION

The method of choice for the infusion of hypertonic TPN solutions is via a subclavian vein catheter with its tip in the superior vena cava.[71,72] The percutaneous catheterization can be accomplished safely and effectively in most patients if the established principles for this procedure are conscientiously applied (Figures 1 and 2).

1. The patient is placed in the supine position with the head 15° lower than the feet to promote filling and dilatation of the subclavian vein by gravity.
2. The shoulders are extended backward over a rolled sheet placed under the thoracic vertebrae, and the head is turned to the opposite side, allowing the ipsilateral subclavian vein to become more easily accessible for percutaneous puncture.
3. The skin of the lower neck, shoulder, and upper chest is shaved, cleansed with acetone or adhesive remover, and prepared with povidone-iodine solution in a manner identical to skin preparation prior to a major operation.
4. With strict aseptic technique, including sterile gloves and surgical instruments, the prepared area of skin is draped into a sterile field.
5. Local anesthetic solution is infiltrated into the skin and subcutaneous tissue at the inferior aspect of the midpoint of the clavicle.
6. A needle 5 cm long and 0.5 mm in diameter, attached to a 5 ml syringe, is inserted beneath the clavicle in a horizontal plane, with its tip aimed at the posterior aspect of the sternal notch. Gentle negative pressure is applied to the syringe barrel as the

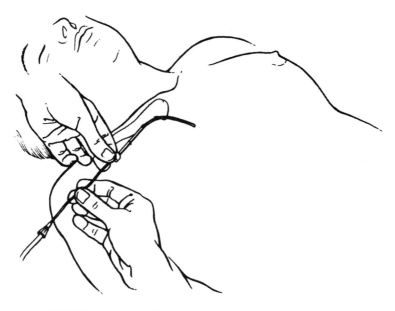

FIGURE 2. Correct position of the catheter in the superior vena cava.

syringe and needle are advanced, and a prompt flashback of venous blood indicates accurate puncture of the targeted vein.

7. The syringe is then disconnected from the needle, the bevel of which has been directed caudally, and a flexible guidewire (J wire) is advanced through the needle into the vein while monitoring heart rate and rhythm.

8. The needle is removed, and a dilator is passed over the wire to create a suitable tract for the catheter.

9. The dilator is removed, and the catheter is advanced over the wire through the subclavian vein into the superior vena cava.

10. The wire is withdrawn leaving approximately 15 cm of catheter in place, which should allow the tip to rest in the middle or distal portion of the superior vena cava.

11. A syringe is attached to the catheter and aspirated to confirm unimpeded backflow of venous blood.

12. The catheter is then flushed with heparin solution and locked.

13. The catheter is secured firmly to the skin with a monofilament suture, and povidone-iodine ointment is applied around the catheter exit site.

14. A sterile gauze pad is then applied and fixed in place with a transparent occlusive adhesive dressing.

15. After a chest roentgenogram has been obtained to confirm that the catheter is correctly positioned, infusion of the concentrated nutrient solution can begin.

However, if a catheter is malpositioned in a vein other than the superior vena cava, it should be redirected by withdrawing it 4 to 6 cm, inserting a J wire through the catheter aseptically into the superior vena cava, and then advancing the catheter again over the wire. Malfunctioning central venous feeding catheters can also be replaced by inserting the J wire into the catheter, removing the defective catheter, and then advancing a new catheter over the wire. Fluoroscopic guidance can be helpful in achieving and confirming optimal catheter placement, especially in difficult cases.

In patients who require prolonged or permanent home TPN, a silicone rubber catheter having a velour cuff is inserted into the central vein and implanted in a subcutaneous tunnel.[72,73] Catheter implantation is accomplished preferably in an operating room with the patient under local or light general anesthesia and using C-arm fluoroscopic guidance. The catheter is tunneled subcutaneously from the anterior upper abdominal wall inferior and lateral to the xiphoid to a second incision in close proximity to the vein to be cannulated. The cuff, into which fibrous tissue is expected to grow, is positioned about 6 cm proximal to the skin exit site. The risk of infection and the likelihood of inadvertent removal of the central venous feeding catheter have been shown to be less with an implanted catheter than with a percutaneous temporary catheter.

Other accessible veins that may be catheterized include the pectoral, cephalic, subclavian, thyroid, facial, internal jugular, external jugular, or femoral veins. Although fluoroscopic confirmation precludes the possibility of unrecognized catheter misplacement into the right atrium, an intercostal vein, azygous or hemiazygous vein, or elsewhere in the venous system, chest X-rays to confirm correct catheter position must be obtained before beginning infusion of TPN solution.[74]

VIII. ADMINISTRATION AND MONITORING OF TOTAL PARENTERAL NUTRITION

The average daily ration of TPN solution contains about 25 to 30% solute and should be infused continuously over 24 h at a constant rate, into a large-diameter, high-flow blood vessel, preferably the superior vena cava.[67] Starting at generally safe levels of water metabolism (1500 to 2500 ml/d in adults) and dextrose utilization (0.4 to 1.2 g/kg body weight/hour), the daily i.v. nutrient ration is gradually increased as indicated and tolerated (up to 3000 to 4000 ml/d in adults).[75]

Initial basic guidelines for safe TPN include accurate determinations of body weight daily; water balance every 4 to 8 h; fractional urine sugar concentration every 6 to 24 h; serum electrolytes, blood sugar, and blood urea nitrogen daily until stable, then every 2 to 3 days thereafter; and complete blood count, serum proteins, calcium, phosphorus, and magnesium weekly. Renal and hepatic function tests, prothrombin time, and accelerated partial thromboplastin time should be evaluated initially and every 1 to 3 weeks during TPN therapy. Intermittent measurements of serum osmolality; zinc, copper, and vitamin levels; and urine specific gravity, osmolality, and electrolytes are helpful in monitoring certain patients. Periodic determinations of arterial and central venous pressures, blood gases, and pH may also be indicated in the management of critically ill patients with significant cardiovascular, respiratory, or metabolic derangements.

Adjustments of water volume, sugar ration and concentration, amino acid composition and concentration, or colloid supplementation may be necessary during the treatment of a critically ill patient, or in the presence of shock, sepsis, or multiple systems organ failure. To avoid excessive glycosuria, which may result in significant water and electrolyte imbalances or in hyperosmolar, hyperglycemic, nonketotic coma, the infusion is maintained at a rate that will not allow quantitative urinary glucose to exceed 1 g/dl (3+ nitroprusside reaction). Ideally, the patient will not excrete any sugar in the urine. However, trace amounts of glucose in the urine do not represent significant losses of the total quantity of sugar administered, and such small amounts of glycosuria will induce a mild diuresis that may actually be helpful in excreting any excess infused water and in indicating that the limit of the patient's capacity to metabolize glucose has been reached.

In all patients with diabetes mellitus, regular human insulin is administered and evenly distributed in the i.v. nutrient solution. At times in non-diabetic patients with relative glucose intolerance, insulin is added to the nutrient solution in amounts of 5 to 60 units/1000 kcal.

Albumin and packed erythrocytes are sometimes infused early in the course of TPN to restore normal colloid osmotic pressure and red blood cell mass in patients with marked hypoproteinemia, hypoalbuminemia, and/or severe anemia. In patients with borderline serum protein concentrations and in the presence of only mild to moderate stress, administration of the nutrient solution alone is usually sufficient to correct these deficiencies, but may require weeks of TPN infusion to do so.

Special formulations of amino acids are available for infusion in selected patients whose primary gastrointestinal disorder or malnourished state is complicated by renal, hepatic, or multiple systems organ failure.[76-78] However, in patients with severe renal failure requiring hemodialysis, standard TPN amino acid solutions are infused, but adjustments are made in the total nitrogen ration relative to the effectiveness of dialysis while attempting to meet requirements for protein synthesis.

Fat has a high caloric density of 9 kcal/g, and it can be an efficient energy substrate for i.v. feeding. The 10 and 20% fat emulsions contribute little to osmotic pressure and yield 1100 and 2000 kcal/l, respectively. Their use can also meet essential fatty acid requirements, allowing parenteral nutrition regimens to be truly complete. On the other hand, fat emulsions should be avoided or limited in patients with hyperlipidemias, symptomatic atherosclerosis, or acute pancreatitis, and administered cautiously in the presence of pulmonary insufficiency and renal or hepatic failure. It is our practice to add fat emulsions to the parenteral nutrition regimen in quantities sufficient (2 to 5% of total calories) at least to provide essential fatty acid requirements (250 ml 10% emulsion three times a week) or at most to provide no more than 30% of total calories per day as fat. Periodic determination of the serum triene:tetraene ratio (normal >0.4) can be helpful in monitoring the efficacy of the fat emulsion in preventing or correcting essential fatty acid deficiency (EFAD).

Recent clinical investigations have indicated that long-chain triglycerides (LCT), such as those in soybean and safflower oil emulsions, may not be utilized optimally by septic patients.[76] Medium-chain triglycerides (MCT), on the other hand, are metabolized as rapidly as glucose in septic patients and appear to have a beneficial effect on immune function.[79]

IX. POTENTIAL COMPLICATIONS OF TOTAL PARENTERAL NUTRITION

Prevention of infection or sepsis is of paramount importance to the successful application of TPN. The occurrence of infection is rare if the aseptic and antiseptic principles previously discussed are conscientiously observed in the insertion and maintenance of the central venous feeding catheters. Because hypertonic nutrient solutions are excellent culture media for many species of bacteria and fungi, meticulous asepsis must also be maintained during solution preparation, additive injection, and long-term administration if infection is to be avoided or minimized (Table 4).[75] However, if fever does occur in a patient receiving TPN, the physician must immediately attempt to define its source in the ears, nose, throat, chest, urinary tract, GI tract, wound, or other possible foci. Should the fever persist or even intensify, the infusion must be terminated, the indwelling central venous catheter must be removed, and the distal tip of the catheter must be cultured for bacteria and fungi together with determination of microbiological sensitivities. Another central venous feeding catheter may be inserted into the opposite subclavian vein or may be inserted over a J-wire through the existing catheter tract. Administration of isotonic dextrose solution may be started via a peripheral vein at a rate to insure against postinfusion rebound hypoglycemia until central venous access and infusion can be safely reinstituted. Empiric systemic broad-spectrum antibiotic therapy or antifungal therapy is not always required. However, if the patient exhibits persistent signs of sepsis, an antimicrobial regimen may be instituted at this time and modified appropriately when specific sensitivity testing has been completed.

TABLE 4
Potential Catheter-Related Complications

Infectious	Technical
Insertion-site contamination	Pneumothorax
Contamination during insertion	Tension pneumothorax
Contamination during routine care	Hemothorax, hydrothorax
Catheter contamination	Hydromediastinum
Improper technique of catheter insertion	Tracheal injury
Administration of blood via feeding catheter	Esophageal injury
Use of catheter to measure central venous pressure	Cardiac tamponade
Use of catheter to obtain blood samples	Brachial plexus injury
Use of catheter to administer medications	Horner's syndrome
Contaminated solution during preparation of additives	Phrenic nerve paralysis
Contaminated tubing via connections	Carotid artery injury
Three-way stopcocks in system	Subclavian artery injury
Secondary contamination	False aneurysm
Septicemia, bacterial or fungal	Thrombosis of subclavian vein or
Septic emboli	superior vena cava
Osteomyelitis of clavicle	Catheter misplacement, knotting
Septic arthritis	Cardiac arrhythmia
Endocarditis	Cardiac perforation
Intercurrent infectious disorder	Endocarditis
Invasive dental procedures	Thoracic duct laceration
Concurrent invasive vascular access	Chylothorax
Hemodialysis	Innominate or subclavian vein laceration
Swan–Ganz catheter	Air embolism
Angiography	Pulmonary embolus
Peripheral infusion of chemotherapy	Catheter embolus

Fever or evidence of sepsis prior to institution of TPN does not necessarily contraindicate the use of the technique. In a postoperative, debilitated, immunosuppressed, or critically ill patient, sepsis often accompanies the primary problem and accentuates the nutritional requirements. If, however, the clinician suspects that the infectious course of the patient might be caused or aggravated by the central venous feeding catheter, it should be removed, cultured promptly, and replaced.

Although multiple lumen (double, triple) catheters have recently gained popularity and rather extensive use, their use has been associated with a significant increase in catheter-related sepsis. Accordingly, every reasonable attempt must be made to avoid or minimize the use of multiple lumen catheters for TPN, and the indication for their continued use should be reevaluated on a daily basis. Additionally, it is important to promptly remove or replace a multiple lumen catheter whenever one of the ports or lumens is clotted in order to avoid or minimize catheter-related sepsis. Finally, it should be emphasized that before infusion is started via a multiple lumen central venous catheter, easy aspiration of blood should be obtained from all ports to insure that all lumens of the catheter are within the lumen of the central vein in order to avoid extravasation of hypertonic solutions or medications into the chest and other perivascular tissues.

Although development of thrombophlebitis is always possible with the use of long-term indwelling central venous feeding catheters and infusion of hypertonic nutrient solutions, superior vena cava thrombosis has been observed clinically only rarely. Under ordinary conditions in an adequately hydrated patient, the high rate of blood flow in the large diameter vessel assures prompt dilution of the hypertonic fluid and minimizes the risk of chemical phlebitis. Attention to sterility has practically eliminated infectious thrombophlebitis, although occasional incidences of thrombosis have occurred in patients when the catheter tips were misdirected into or malpositioned in a jugular, internal mammary, intercostal, azygos, hemiazygos, or axillary vein. Other central venous catheter-related hazards, such as inadvertent air embolism or catheter embolism, can be easily avoided by adherence to the principles and techniques of safe central venous catheterization previously discussed. A thorough knowledge of anatomy combined with common sense and strict adherence to established principles and techniques should minimize the potential technical hazards of percutaneous central venous catheterization.

The potential metabolic complications associated with TPN can be classified according to glucose, amino acid, lipid, vitamin, and mineral metabolism and are summarized in Table 5.[75]

One of the most serious metabolic complications is hyperosmolar coma, which can be precipitated acutely by rapid infusion of the hypertonic solution, causing severe osmotic diuresis, serum and urine electrolyte aberrations, dehydration, and malfunction of the central nervous system. A chronic form of this syndrome can occur surreptitiously when impaired glucose tolerance is not promptly recognized, particularly in the presence of diabetes mellitus, after extensive burns or major trauma, or after intracranial operations or trauma.

If blood and urine sugar levels are not conscientiously measured in such patients, hyperglycemia may occur with markedly elevated blood sugar levels, accompanied by weakness, listlessness, and coma. If the condition is not recognized and corrected promptly, permanent neurologic damage or even death can result. Treatment of this syndrome consists of prompt infusion of isotonic or half-strength solutions of saline or dextrose together with insulin and potassium, while frequent measurements of fluid losses, central venous pressure, electrolytes, blood sugar, and serum osmolality are obtained. A thorough assessment and understanding of the patient's disease and metabolic status and rigid adherence to the established principles and techniques of TPN will prevent a great majority of these complications.

X. FUTURE FRONTIERS

In the past, most clinicians have been interested primarily in nutrition of the body as a whole. It was of highest priority to achieve basic nutritional goals, such as growth and development of infants or weight gain to ideal body weight in adults; nitrogen equilibrium or positive nitrogen balance; increased strength and sense of well-being; improved function and activity; decreased morbidity and mortality rates; improved risk:benefit ratio; improved recovery, convalescence, and rehabilitation; decreased hospital stay; and improved cost:benefit ratio. These were general, but very important, aims of the early endeavors to provide and improve nutritional support.[80]

Today, interest in these broad clinical objectives continues; however, TPN support has undergone spectacularly great advancement and growth during the past 3 decades compared with all of the previous centuries of interest in this area.[81] The same considerations and concerns that have existed through the years continue to be addressed, although recently, efforts are increasingly directed toward improving the materials and methods for assessing and providing nutritional support. Subsequently, the substrates for TPN and enteral nutrition have been greatly improved and expanded. The basic and clinical investigations with fat emulsions; essential and nonessential fatty acids; short-, medium-, and long-chain triglycerides; and lipoproteins and other lipid substrates continue to progress and will require much more work in the future. Energy substrates in addition to the fats include glucose, fructose, sorbitol, xylitol, carbohydrate polymers, glycerol, ethanol, and many other biochemical compounds that might be considered as fuel sources in future formulations. The major electrolyte and mineral investigations must continue, especially

TABLE 5
Potential Metabolic Complications of Total Parenteral Nutrition

Complication	Etiology	Indicated action
Glucose metabolism		
Hyperglycemic glycosuria, osmotic diuresis, non-ketotic hyperosmolar dehydration, and coma	Excessive total dose or rate of infusion of dextrose; inadequate endogenous insulin; glucocorticoids; sepsis	Reduce amount of glucose infused; increase insulin; administer a portion of calories as fat emulsion; temporarily stop TPN
Ketoacidosis of diabetes mellitus	Inadequate endogenous insulin response; inadequate exogenous insulin therapy	Administer insulin and potassium; reduce glucose concentration and total dose; increase water ration
Postinfusion (rebound) hypoglycemia	Persistence of endogenous insulin production secondary to prolonged stimulation of islet cells by high-carbohydrate infusion	Administer 5–10% dextrose in a taper mode before stopping infusion
Respiratory acidosis with hypercarbia	Excessive dextrose administration	Decrease concentration and total dose of dextrose; infuse bicarbonate; substitute fat calories for dextrose
Amino acid metabolism		
Hyperchloremic metabolic acidosis	Excessive chloride and monohydrochloride content of crystalline amino acid solutions	Administer Na$^+$ and K$^+$ as acetate salts instead of chloride salts
Serum amino acid imbalance	Unphysiologic amino acid profile of the nutrient solutions; different amino acid utilization with various disorders	Change amino acid solution to more favorable formulation
Hyperammonemia	Excessive ammonia in solutions; deficiencies of arginine, ornithine, aspartic acid and/or glutamic acid in crystalline amino acid solutions; primary hepatic disorder	Reduce total amino acid intake; administer branched-chain amino acid solutions; administer neomycin and lactulose, if possible
Prerenal azotemia	Excessive total dose or rate of infusion of amino acid solution	Reduce amino acid intake; increase non-protein calories
Lipid Metabolism		
Hyperlipidemia	Excessive total dose or rate of administration of fat emulsion	Decrease rate of infusion; allow serum lipid clearance before infusion; administer IV heparin
Pyrogenic reaction	Fat emulsion idiosyncracy	Exclude other causes of fever; stop emulsion; switch fat emulsion
Hyperbilirubinemia	Excessive dose or rate of administration of fat emulsion	Decrease rate of infusion; allow serum lipid clearance
Hypoxia	Interstitial lipoid pneumonitis with alveolar capillary block	Discontinue fat infusion
Serum deficiencies of phospholipid linoleic and/or arachidonic acids; elevations of 5, 8, 11-eicosatrienoic acid	Inadequate essential fatty acid administration; inadequate vitamin E administration	Administer essential fatty acids in doses of 4% of total calories
Other impaired liver function tests	Fat emulsion or underlying disease process	Exclude other causes of hepatic dysfunction; correct EFAD; stop emulsion

TABLE 5 (continued).
Potential Metabolic Complications of Total Parenteral Nutrition

Complication	Etiology	Indicated action
Calcium and phosphorus metabolism		
Hypophosphatemia Decreased erythrocyte 2, 3-diphosphoglycerate; Increased affinity of hemoglobin for oxygen; Aberrations of erythrocyte intermediary metabolites	Inadequate phosphorus administration; redistribution of serum phosphorus into cells and/or bone; excessive phosphate excretion	Administer phosphorus (20mEq potassium dihydrogen phosphate/ 1000 cal); evaluate antacid or calcium administration or both
Hypocalcemia	Inadequate calcium administration; reciprocal response to phosphorus repletion without simultaneous calcium infusion; hypoalbuminemia	Increase calcium dose; correct hypoalbuminemia
Hypercalcemia	Excessive calcium administration with or without high doses of albumin; excessive vitamin D administration	Decrease calcium and/or vitamin D administration
Vitamin D deficiency; hypervitaminosis D	Inadequate or excessive vitamin D administration	Alter vitamin D administration appropriately
Miscellaneous		
Hypokalemia	Inadequate potassium intake relative to increased requirements for protein anabolism; diuresis	Confirm adequate renal function, increase potassium administration
Hyperkalemia	Excessive potassium administration, especially in metabolic acidosis; renal decompensation	Reduce or stop exogenous potassium; if EKG changes are present, treat with Ca gluconate, insulin, diuretics
Hypomagnesemia	Inadequate magnesium administration relative to increased requirements for protein anabolism and glucose metabolism	Increase magnesium administration (15–20 mEq Mg/1000 cal)
Hypermagnesemia	Excessive magnesium administration; renal decompensation or failure	Decrease or stop magnesium administration; increase calcium dose; dialysis for renal failure
Anemia	Iron deficiency and/or deficiencies of folic acid vitamin B_{12}, copper, protein; other deficiencies	Supplement deficient substrate; transfusion of packed red blood cells
Bleeding	Vitamin K deficiency	Administer vitamin K
Hypervitaminosis A	Excessive vitamin A administration	Withhold exogenous vitamin A
Elevations in SGOT, SGPT, and serum alkaline phosphatase	Enzyme induction secondary to amino acid imbalance; excessive glycogen and/or fat deposition in the liver; EFAD; cholestasis; cholelithiasis	Exclude primary liver disorders; correct dehydration; decrease calorie:nitrogen ratio; alter fat emulsion administration (triene:tetraene ratio)

those concerned with trace element imbalances and deficiencies. The precise requirements for both fat- and water-soluble vitamins must also be determined under various conditions, even while integrating these micronutrients with the major components of enteral and parenteral nutrition.

Future pathophysiologic interest of clinicians should be directed primarily toward disease-specific nutritional support.[82] A fundamental concern and responsibility of all physicians, regardless of their specialty, must be the orientation and dedication of their efforts to maintain optimal function of the maximum number of cells in the body cell mass of the patient at all times to ensure optimal organ and system function.

Because nutrition appears to play a significant role in the development of atherosclerosis and subsequent cardiac morbidity and death, it is imperative that investigations continue into the cause, prevention, and reversal of heart disease. Rudimentary attempts have been made, and require sophisticated refinement, to nourish the myocardium optimally after an attack of ischemia or infarction so that the heart muscle can heal as much as possible with maximum return of function and to avert replacement of the infarcted myocardial mass with scar tissue. The development of special substrate formulas for improving cardiac function in various myocardiopathies will continue to challenge biochemists, nutritionists, cardiologists, and surgeons. Attempting to use intermediary myocardial metabolites as sources of energy and function rather than the standard types of amino acid, fatty acid, and carbohydrate mixtures that have been used for general enteral or parenteral nutrition will remain a major challenge. The nutritional support of heart-transplant patients has been helpful in allowing acquisition of knowledge of heart function in a clinical investigational setting. However, a major problem exists to balance optimum nutrition of patients with heart transplants having other problems, such as cardiac cachexia and myocardial failure, while using specifically tailored immunosuppression formulas to minimize rejection and immunoaugmentation formulas to minimize infection. Maximum endeavors must be made to maintain optimal heart function from a substrate standpoint in order to sustain optimal quality and longevity of life.

The advantage of using a totally i.v. diet to stimulate reduction of plasma cholesterol levels is that the components of the diet can be precisely defined and administered directly into the circulation, where they can immediately become involved in appropriate biochemical reactions. The cholesterol reduction effect of an optimal mixture of amino acids occurs rapidly to effect 40 to 70% reductions, which are unprecedented with any other single form of anticholesterol therapy.[83] This technique allows the application of clinical biochemistry directly to the management of a complex metabolic disorder, with gratifying early biochemical and clinical results, and also allows a degree of control of the myriad biochemical processes of the body that is impossible to achieve currently with oral and enteral regimens.

The pancreas has been a subject of focal or organ concern, and many special formulas have been studied in attempts to reduce the ravages of acute and chronic pancreatitis, cystic fibrosis, and diabetes, or to increase the efficacy of both the exocrine and the endocrine cells of the pancreas selectively by manipulating specific substrates by mouth or by vein. This is a most stimulating area of endeavor that will require much investigation, especially considering the array and variety of endocrine, exocrine, and paracrine cells crowded into this organ and responsible for many important and highly specialized functions.

In managing respiratory failure, problems have been encountered with high-carbohydrate diets in some patients. Great progress has been made in manipulating the substrates in such patients in order to maximize the effects of ventilator support and to minimize the problems of weaning patients from ventilators while accomplishing normal ventilatory and respiratory function. The role of fat emulsions as a major source of nonprotein calories in patients requiring lung support is a timely topic that must be studied further in the future. The use of branched-chain amino acids has also been advocated in these patients and may prove to be beneficial in their management.[84]

The kidney has been studied from the standpoint of the advantage of low-protein oral diets for many decades and from the inception of TPN with multiple renal failure formulas based on multiple etiologies and the severity of renal decompensation. Because there are many types and causes of renal failure, the therapy of each individual patient with impaired renal function secondary to a different pathological process will probably require some modification in formula composition in order to provide optimal nutritional support. Donor kidney perfusion with special nutrient formulations designed to prolong the quality and duration of preservation prior to transplantation is another fruitful area for future work. Refinement of the keto acid concept for recycling urea and the development of other nitrogenous substrate support for renal transplant patients that might act as adjuncts to both the nutritional and the immunosuppressive requirements for success in this vital area will continue to stimulate the ingenuity of surgeons, nephrologists, and immunologists.

Regarding specific organ nutrition, the liver presents the most difficult challenge because of its multiple and complex functions. From a clinical standpoint, there has been great interest in some of the general biochemical activities of the liver which include protein synthesis, especially of albumin, globulins, and other specialized proteins; enzyme synthesis and function in the various metabolic pathways; energy metabolism; cholesterol synthesis, breakdown, and excretion; bile composition, secretion, and stasis; and gallstone formation. Hepatic encephalopathy has been shown to respond to specific nutritional manipulation by increasing the branched-chain amino acids and decreasing the aromatic amino acids in the ration, and clinical investigation is likely to continue in this area. Judicious use of intermediary metabolites as nutrient substrates in order to achieve results better than those now possible with the use of the common amino acid, fatty acid, and dextrose substrates will continue to test the ingenuity of surgical and medical hepatologists in the future.

Diets must be perfected to insure maximum absorption of all required nutrients in order to maximize adaptation of the short bowel, to support future bowel transplantation, and to maintain the mucosal barrier and integrity against invasion by pathological microorganisms. Much work has already been done in this area, with the demonstration of the importance of glutamine as a major intestinal nutrient, but much more study and work are indicated if this deceptively simple, but actually complex, tubular organ responsible for many complex functions is to be understood fully.[85–87] Furthermore, the role of various types of fiber and other substrates given by tube or by mouth in the genesis of adenocarcinoma and other malignancies, atherosclerosis, bowel motility disorders, and other disorders must be addressed and identified.

As nutritional investigative work progresses to the cellular and subcellular level, the potential for developing nutrient regimens specifically tailored to inhibit the growth and division of cancer cells or to render the malignant cells more susceptible to antineoplastic agents should be more readily exploited. Currently, parenteral feeding of cancer patients has reduced the ravages and morbidity of starvation but has not uniformly been of obvious benefit in altering mortality rates. Studies of the general effects that feeding cancer patients with enteral or parenteral arginine-enriched diets and the effects on improving the capacity of the body's immune system to contain, or even kill, the malignant cells are already underway.[88] The reversal and treatment with specific nutrients of other conditions, such as multiple systems organ failure, hematopoietic disorders, and brain and central nervous system disorders remain great challenges of the future for clinicians and investigators. The current strategies of nutritional support of the whole organism and of the key organ systems must proceed and advance to the cellular level of nutritional support if the ultimate goal of providing optimal nutrition for all patients under all conditions at all times is to be realized. The relationships between nutrient substrates and the human genome are myriad, and their identification, classification and beneficial exploitation in the management of patients in all likelihood will open new frontiers for clinical nutrition in the next century.[89]

XI. CONCLUSION

In 1968, corroborative and integrated laboratory and clinical investigations demonstrated unequivocally for the first time that all essential nutrient substrates can be administered intravenously for long periods of time to support normal growth and development in infants and to achieve or maintain a state of anabolism in nutritionally debilitated adults.[44] This resulted in positive nitrogen balance, wound healing, and rehabilitation and demonstrated the clear-cut positive impact of nutrition support. Since that time, the methodology and technology for providing safe and effective long-term supplemental or total parenteral feeding have been modified and improved steadily as a result of numerous scientific developments and clinical applications in this rapidly advancing field of endeavor. Furthermore, the dramatic results of the technique, coupled with acquired expertise in catheter insertion, solution formulation and preparation, and safe delivery, resulted in the widespread acceptance and application of central venous nutrient infusion. Today, it is possible for patients with inadequate or compromised GI tract function, who would otherwise succumb directly or indirectly to starvation or malnutrition, to be maintained practically for prolonged or indefinite periods of time with various i.v. feeding regimens and techniques. Indeed, not only have the vast majority of such patients recovered dramatically from their critically impaired states of health, but they have also been discharged from the hospital to return to productive roles in society. Of those less fortunate individuals whose nutrient requirements cannot be obtained solely by the alimentary tract, most can be nourished successfully by ambulatory continuous or intermittent home parenteral nutrition techniques. These and other exciting and innovative forms of lifesaving nutritional and metabolic support have significantly influenced the clinical management of critically ill patients, have improved the capacity for restoring previously hopeless patients to normal or near normal function, and promise to revolutionize further the concepts and delivery of TPN in the future.

REFERENCES

1. **Harvey, W.** *Exercitatio Anatomica de Motu Cordis et Sanguinis in Animalibus.* Francofurti, Guilielmi Fitzeri, 1628.
2. **Fortescue-Brickdale, JM.** A contribution to the history of the intravenous injection of drugs; together with an account of some experiments on animals with antiseptics, and a bibliography. *Guy's Hosp Rep,* 58:15–80, 1904.
3. **Wretlind, A.** Recollections of pioneers in nutrition: landmarks in the development of parenteral nutrition. *J Am Col Nutr,* 11:366–373, 1992.
4. **Sanderson, I, Basi, S, and Deitel, M.** History of nutrition in surgery. In: *Nutrition in Clinical Surgery, 2nd ed.,* Deitel, M, Ed. Williams & Wilkins, Baltimore, 1985, 3–13.
5. **Courten, W.** Experiments and observations of the effects of several sorts of poisons upon animals made at Montpellier in the years 1678 and 1679 by the late William Courten. *Philos Trans R Soc Lond,* 27:485–500, 1710–1712.

6. **Escholtz, J.** *Clysmatica Nova, Sive Ratio qua in Venam Sectam Medicamenta Immitti Possint.* Amsterdam, Berolini, 1665.
7. **Latta, T.** Relative to the treatment of cholera by the copious injection of aqueous and saline fluids into the veins. *Lancet,* 2:274–277, 1831.
8. **Bernard, C.** *Lecons sur les Proprietes Physiologiques et les Alterations Pathologiques des Liquides de l'Organisme.* Vol. 2, J B Bailliere, Paris, 1859, 459.
9. **Hodder, E.** Transfusion of milk in cholera. *Practitioner,* 10:14–16, 1873.
10. **Rhoads, JE, Dudrick, SJ, and Vars, HM.** History of intravenous nutrition. In: *Clinical Nutrition, Vol. 2, Parenteral Nutrition,* Rombeau, JL and Caldwell, MD, Eds. W.B. Saunders, Philadelphia, 1986, 1–8.
11. **Lister, J.** On the effects of the antiseptic system of treatment upon the salubrity of a surgical hospital. *Lancet,* 1:4–6, 40–42, 1870.
12. **Pasteur, L and Joubert JV.** Charbon et septicemie compte V, Hebd Seave. *Acad Sci Paris,* 85:101–115, 1877.
13. **Landerer, A.** Ueber tranfusion und infusion. *Arch Klin Chir,* 34:807–812, 1887.
14. **Matas, RM.** A clinical report on intravenous saline infusion in the Charity Hospital, New Orleans (1881–1891). *New Orleans Med Surg J,* 14:88–83, 1891.
15. **Matas, RM.** The continued intravenous "drip". *Ann Surg,* 79:643–661, 1924.
16. **Starling, EH.** On the absorption of fluids from the connective tissue spaces. *J Physiol,* 19:312–326, 1895.
17. **Biedl, A and Kraus R.** Ueber intravenose traubenzucker infusionen an menschen. *Wien Klin Wochenschr,* 9:55–58, 1896.
18. **Folin, O.** Laws governing the chemical composition of urine. *Am J Physiol,* 13:66–115, 1905.
19. **Folin, O.** A theory of protein metabolism. *Am J Physiol,* 13:117–138, 1905.
20. **Kausch, W.** Ueber intravenose und subkutane ernahrung mit traubenzucker. *Deutsche Med Wochenschr,* 37: 8, 1911.
21. **Henriques, V and Andersen, AC.** Ueber parenterale ernahrung durch intravenose injecktion. *Z Physiol Chem,* 88:357–369, 1913.
22. **Funk, C.** The etiology of the deficiency disease. *J State Med,* 20:341–368, 1912.
23. **Murlin, JR, and Riche JA.** Blood fat in relation to depth of narcosis. *Proc Soc Exp Biol Med,* 13:7–8, 1915.
24. **Woodyatt, RT, Sansum, WD, and Wilder, RM.** Prolonged and accurately timed intravenous injections of sugar. *JAMA,* 65:2067–2070, 1915.
25. **Yamakawa, S.** Zur frage der emulgierten fetten. *Nippon Naika Gakkai Zasshi,* 17:122, 1920.
26. **Seibert, FD.** Fever producing substance found in some distilled waters. *Am J Physiol,* 67:90–104, 1923.
27. **Cuthbertson, DP.** Observations on the disturbance of metabolism produced by injury to the limbs. *Q J Med* 25:233–246, 1932.
28. **Cuthbertson, DP.** Further observations on the disturbance of metabolism caused by injury, with particular reference to the dietary requirements of fracture cases. *Br J Surg,* 23:505–520, 1936.
29. **Cuthbertson, DP.** Historical background to parenteral nutrition. *Acta Chir Scand, Suppl,* 498:1–11, 1980.
30. **Rose, WC.** The significance of amino acids in nutrition. *Harvey Lect,* 30:45–65, 1934.
31. **Rose, WC.** Nutritional significance of amino acids. *Physiol Rev,* 18:109–136, 1938.
32. **Holt, LE, Tidwell, HC, and Scott, TFM.** The intravenous alimentation of fat. A practical therapeutic procedure. *J Pediatr,* 6:151–160, 1935.
33. **Elman, R.** Amino acid content of blood following intravenous injection of hydrolysed casein. *Proc Soc Exp Biol Med,* 37:437–440, 1937.
34. **Elman, R and Weiner, DO.** Intravenous alimentation with specific reference to protein (amino acid) metabolism. *JAMA,* 112:796–802, 1939.
35. **Shohl, AT and Blackfan, KD.** Intravenous administration of crystalline amino acids to infants. *J Nutr,* 20:305–316, 1940.
36. **Dennis, C.** Preoperative and postoperative care for the bad-risk patient. *Minn Med,* 27:538–543, 1944.
37. **Dennis, C.** Ileostomy and colectomy in chronic ulcerative colitis. *Surgery,* 18:435–452, 1945.
38. **McKibbin, JM, Hegsted, DM, and Stare, FJ.** Parenteral nutrition: studies on fat emmulsion for intravenous alimentation. *J Lab Clin Med,* 30:488–497, 1945.
39. **Zimmerman, B.** Intravenous tubing for parenteral therapy. *Science,* 101:567–568, 1945.
40. **Dennis, C, Eddy, FD, Frykman, HM, et al.** Response to vagotomy in idiopathic ulcerative colitis and reginal enteritis. *Ann Surg,* 128:479–496, 1948.
41. **Dennis, C.** Idiopathic ulcerative colitis. *S Dak J Med Pharm,* 2:83–85, 1949.

42. **Rhode, CM, Parkins, WM, and Vars, HM.** Nitrogen balances of dogs continuously infused with 50% glucose and protein preparation. *Am J Physiol,* 159:415–425, 1949.

43. **Aubaniac, R.** L'Injection intraveineuse sous claviculaire: avantages et techniques. *Presse Med,* 60: 1456, 1952.

44. **Dudrick, SJ, Wilmore, DW, Vars, HM, and Rhoads JE.** Long-term total parenteral nutrition with growth, development and positive nitrogen balance. *Surgery,* 64:134–142, 1968.

45. **Wilmore, DW and Dudrick SJ.** Safe long-term venous catheterization. *Arch Surg,* 98:256–258, 1969.

46. **Dudrick, SJ, Wilmore, DW, and Vars HM.** Long-term venous catheterization: an adjunct to surgical care and study. *Curr Top Surg Res,* 1:325–340, 1969.

47. **Moore, F.** *Metabolic Care of the Surgical Patient,* W.B. Saunders, Philadelphia, 1959.

48. **Geyer, RP.** Parenteral nutrition. *Physiol Rev,* 40:150–186, 1960.

49. **Shuberth O and Wretlind, A.** Intravenous infusion of fat emulsions, phosphatides and emulsifying agents. *Acta Chir Scand, Suppl,* 278:1–21, 1961.

50. **Dudrick, SJ.** The genesis of intravenous hyperalimentation. *JPEN,* 1:23–29, 1977.

51. **Rhoads, JE.** Diuretics as an adjuvant in disposing of extra water employed as a vehicle in parenteral hyperalimentation. *Fed Proc,* 21:389, 1962.

52. **Rhoads, JE, Rawnsley, HM, Vars, HM, et al.** The use of diuretics as an adjunct in parenteral hyperalimentation for surgical patients with prolonged disability of the gastrointestinal tract. *Bull Soc Int Chir,* 24:59–70, 1965.

53. **Lehr, HB, Rhoads, JE, Rosenthal, O, and Blakemore, WS.** The use of intravenous fat emulsions in surgical patients. *JAMA,* 181:745–749, 1962.

54. **Dudrick, SJ, Steiger, E, Wilmore, DW, and Vars, HM.** Continous long-term intravenous infusion in unrestrained animals. *Lab Anim Care,* 20:521–529, 1970.

55. **Dudrick, SJ, Vars, HM, and Rhoads, JE.** Growth of puppies receiving all nutritional requirements by vein. In: *Fortschritte der Parenteralen Ernahrung.* Symposion der International Society of Parenteral Nutrition 1966, Pallas Verlag, Lochham bei Munchen, 1967, 1–4.

56. **Dudrick, SJ, Wilmore, DW, and Vars, HM.** Long-term total parenteral nutrition with growth in puppies and positive nitrogen balance in patients. *Surg Forum,* 18:356–357, 1967.

57. **Wilmore, DW and Dudrick, SJ.** Growth and development of an infant receiving all nutrients by vein. *JAMA* 203:860–864, 1968.

58. **Dudrick, SJ, Groff, DB, and Wilmore, DW.** Long-term venous catheterization in infants. *Surg Gynecol Obstet,* 129:805–808, 1969.

59. **Dudrick, SJ, Wilmore, DW, Vars, HM, and Rhoads, JE.** Can intravenous feeding as the sole means of nutrition support growth in the child and restore weight loss in an adult: an affirmative answer. *Ann Surg,* 169:974–984, 1969.

60. **Wilmore, DW, Groff, DB, Bishop, HC, and Dudrick, SJ.** Total parenteral nutrition in infants with catastrophic gastrointestinal anomalies. *J Ped Surg,* 4:181–189, 1969.

61. **Wilson, JN, Grow, JB, Demong, CV, et al.** Central venous pressure in optimal blood volume maintenance. *Arch Surg,* 85:563–578, 1962.

62. **Mogil, RA, DeLaurentis, DA, and Rosemond, GP.** The infraclavicular venipuncture. *Arch Surg,* 95:320–324, 1967.

63. **Dudrick, SJ, Long, JM, Steiger, E, and Rhoads, JE.** Intravenous hyperalimentation. *Med Clin N Am,* 54:577–589, 1970.

64. **Dudrick, SJ.** Long-term total parenteral nutrition. *Phila Med,* 67:45–55, 1971.

65. **Dudrick, SJ.** Past, present and future of nutritional support. *Surg Clin N Am,* 71:439–448, 1991.

66. **Daly, JM, Dudrick, SJ, and Copeland, EM.** Total parenteral nutrition: techniques and indications. In: *Integrated Medicine: A Comparison to the Life Sciences.* Day, SB, Ed. Van Nostrand Reinhold, New York, 1981, 566–579.

67. **Dudrick, SJ.** Parenteral nutrition. In: *Manual of Preoperative and Postoperative Care.* Dudrick, SJ, Baue, AE, Eiseman, B, et al. Eds. W.B. Saunders, Philadelphia, 1983, 86–105.

68. **Buzby, GP, Williford, WO, Peterson, OL, et al.** A randomized clinical trial of total parenteral nutrition in malnourished surgical patients: The rationale and impact of previous clinical trials and pilot study on protocol design. *Am J Clin Nutr,* 47:357–365, 1988.

69. **Jensen, TG, Englert, DM, and Dudrick, SJ.** *Manual of Nutritional Assessment.* Appleton-Century-Crofts, Norwalk, CT, 1983.

70. **Dudrick, SJ, Latifi, R, and Fosnocht, D.** Management of the Short Bowel Syndrome. *Surg Clin N Am,* 71:625–643, 1991.

71. **Dudrick, SJ, and O'Donnell, JJ.** Central venous lines: inserting them safely and minimizing complications. *Contemp Ob/Gyn,* 3:95–103, 1983.

72. **O'Donnell, JJ, Clague, MB, and Dudrick, SJ.** Percutaneous insertion of a cuffed catheter with a long subcutaneous tunnel for intravenous hyperalimentation. *South Med J,* 11:1344–1348, 1983.

73. **Dudrick, SJ, O'Donnell, JJ, and Englert, DM.** Ambulatory home parenteral nutrition for short-bowel syndrome and other diseases. In: *Nutrition in Clinical Surgery,* 2nd ed., Deitel, M, Ed., Williams & Wilkins, Baltimore. 1985, 276–287.

74. **Dudrick, SJ and Latifi, R.** Total parenteral nutrition. Part I: Indications and techniques. *Pract Gastroenterol,* 16(6):21–29, 1992.

75. **Dudrick, SJ and Latifi R.** Total parenteral nutrition. Part II: Administration, monitoring and complications. *Pract Gastroenterol,* 16(7):29–38, 1992.

76. **Wilmore, DW and Dudrick, SJ.** Treatment of acute renal failure with intravenous essential L-amino acids. *Arch Surg,* 99:669–673, 1969.

77. **Hiyama, DT and Fischer, JE.** Nutritional support in hepatic failure: the current role of disease-specific therapy. In: *Total Parenteral Nutrition,* 2nd ed., Fischer, JE, Ed., Little, Brown, Boston, 1991, 263–278.

78. **Baue, AE.** Nutrition and metabolism in sepsis and multisystem organ failure. *Surg Clin N Am,* 71:549–565, 1991.

79. **Mascioli, EA, Bistrian, BR, and Babayan, VK,** et al. Medium chain triglycerides and structured lipids as unique nonglucose energy sources in hyperalimentation. *Lipids,* 22:417–420, 1987.

80. **Dudrick, SJ.** Past, present and future of nutritional support: the inevitable evolution of total parenteral nutrition. In: *Nutritional Support in Organ Failure,* Tanaka T and Okada, A, Eds. Elsevier, Amsterdam, 1990, XIX–XXV.

81. **Dudrick, SJ.** Past, present and future of nutritional support. *Surg Clin N Am,* 71:439–448, 1991.

82. **Dudrick, SJ and Latifi R.** Total parenteral nutrition in surgery—current status. *Contemp Surg,* 41:41–48, 1992.

83. **Dudrick, SJ.** Regression of atherosclerosis by the intravenous infusion of specific biochemical nutrient substrates in animals and man. *Ann Surg,* 206:296–315, 1987.

84. **Manner, T, Wiese, S, and Katz, DP,** et al. Branched-chain amino acids and respiration. *Nutrition,* 8:311–315, 1992.

85. **Souba, WW, Scott, TE, and Wilmore, DW.** Intestinal consumption of intravenously administered fuels. *JPEN,* 9:18–22, 1985.

86. **Souba, WW, Smith, RJ, and Wilmore, DW.** Glutamine metabolism by the intestinal tract. *JPEN,* 9:608–617,1985.

87. **Dudrick, PS, and Souba, WW.** Amino acids in surgical nutrition: principles and practice. *Surg Clin N Am,* 71:459–476, 1991.

88. **Daly, JM, Lieberman, MD, Goldfine, J, et al.** Enteral nutrition as supplemental arginine, RNA, and omega-3-fatty acids in patients after operation: immunologic, metabolic, and clinical outcome. *Surgery,* 112:56–67, 1992.

89. **Wair, PP.** Nutrients and human genome: new frontiers for the next century. *Fed Am Soc Exp Biol,* 7:501–502, 1993.

Chapter 9

NUTRITION IN SURGICAL PATIENTS

Rifat Latifi and Stanley J. Dudrick

TABLE OF CONTENTS

0-8493-7847-8/94/$0.00+$.50

I. INTRODUCTION

Malnutrition, as defined by anthropometric and serum albumin measurements, has been estimated to be present in up to 50% of surgical patients, especially among indigents and patients in intensive care units. Although most of the patients are malnourished upon admission as a result of disease-induced poor food intake, others become malnourished subsequently secondary to hypercatabolism associated with trauma, infection, surgical intervention, or other forms of stress. Malnutrition occurs secondary to many complex interacting biologic and social factors. Alterations in host defense may be different when protein deficiency dominates, compared with combined protein-calorie malnutrition or with single-nutrient deficiency states. Although a clear demonstration of cause and effect in malnutrition and diminished host resistance to sepsis is lacking, it is most likely that malnutrition and sepsis predispose to each other, and/or coexist in a vicious cycle with other factors. From the therapeutic point of view, this does not make much difference, because the objective is to improve patient survival with combined nutritional repletion and immunologic restoration.

The relationship between B-cell function, T-cell function, and malnutrition has been described in Chapter 5 of this volume and elsewhere in detail.[1] Other non-specific immunologic changes occur with malnutrition as well. For example, the activation of circulating polymorphonuclear neutrophils seems to be altered adversely. Protein-malnourished children, as well as laboratory animals, have demonstrated reduced phagocytic cell delivery to inflammatory lesions in both the number of delivered cells and the kinetics of the cellular influx.[2,3] The failure of a prompt recruitment of phagocytic cells into a focus of infection allows establishment of local sepsis, which may eventually disseminate systemically. The primary function of the complement system is to mediate some aspects of inflammation and to facilitate ingestion of pathogens by phagocytes. Although this action is nonspecific only in the immunologic sense, the biochemical steps that constitute the sequence of complement interactions are highly specific.

Noticeable differences in the immune responses of young vs. elderly surgical patients are clear cut and dramatic. The major age-related changes in the immune system are attributed to thymic involution. A significant reduction in the size of the thymus gland occurs during growth and development. This decline becomes apparent during adulthood, and by middle age the remaining thymic tissue is vestigial.[4] Consequent reduction in the secretion of a family of polypeptide thymic hormones is apparent. The total number of the T lymphocytes does not change with age; however, the proportion of the T cell subpopulation is altered, with a higher number of immature T cells in the blood of the elderly. There is also a relative increase in the number of T-suppressor cells and a reduction in the T-lymphoid cell number. This alteration in the distribution of T cells is thought to account for the increased prevalence of many diseases that accompany the aging process.

It is apparent that malnutrition contributes significantly to sepsis-related complications, and nutritional support in the form of i.v. hyperalimentation can restore humoral, cellular, and phagocytic functions in previously malnourished subjects.[5] Thus, it is clear that nutritional support in the form of parenteral or enteral feeding can improve protein-sparing and can decrease infection and mortality rates in malnourished surgical patients.

The clinical indices that have proved valuable in assessing the nutritional status of surgical patients include (1) a history of unintentional or unexplained weight loss of 10 pounds or 10% of body weight during the previous 2 months, (2) a serum albumin concentration of less than 3.4 g/dl, (3) impaired immunocompetence as determined by a standard battery of skin tests or *in vitro* immunologic tests, and (4) an abnormally low total lymphocyte count (less than 1200/mm^3). These are the fundamental clinical criteria by which decisions can be made virtually by any clinician to employ special techniques and substrates for nutritional support, especially of elderly surgical patients. Furthermore, these criteria are particularly important in establishing the nutritional status of a patient who is a candidate for an elective or semi-elective major operative procedure because of the well-known adverse positive correlation between the degree of preoperative malnutrition and the incidence of postoperative complications and death.

II. SPECIFIC SURGICAL INDICATIONS FOR NUTRITION SUPPORT

A. SHORT-BOWEL SYNDROME

The most fundamental and obvious requirement for specific nutritional support is in the management of patients with short-bowel syndrome. The detailed nutritional management of this complex condition has been addressed comprehensively in this volume Chapter 12. Suffice it to reiterate here that following massive small-bowel resection, TPN has made it possible to provide all necessary nutrient substrates from the time of operation until maximal bowel adaptation is achieved, thus significantly reducing the morbidity and mortality of the short-bowel syndrome both in children and adults.

B. INFLAMMATORY BOWEL DISEASE

Patients with inflammatory bowel disease (Crohn's disease) experience frequent exacerbations of signs and symptoms which vary, depending upon the location and extent of the disease. This unpleasant, chronic, granulomatous inflammation may affect any part of the alimentary tract from the mouth to the anus, but predominantly involves the terminal ileum and colon.[6,7]

The majority of patients with Crohn's disease weigh approximately 10% below their ideal body weight when first examined, especially if the ileum is extensively involved. Protein-calorie malnutrition is the most common deficiency in patients with inflammatory disease; however, a wide variety of specific nutritional deficiencies have been reported including anemia, hypoalbuminemia, hypomagnesemia, hypophosphatemia, hypocalcemia, folic acid deficiency, and deficiencies of niacin, vitamin B_{12}, vitamin C, vitamin A, vitamin D, iron, zinc, copper, and selenium.[8–18] Frequent exacerbations and/or prolonged periods of active inflammatory bowel disease can induce profound catabolism and cachexia, together with debilitating abdominal pain and diarrhea. Significant nutritional deficiencies that can occur in patients with Crohn's disease may be prevented or counteracted by various specially formulated enteral and total parenteral diets. The use of TPN and total bowel rest in these patients promotes positive nitrogen balance, allows substantial amelioration of diarrhea and pain, and also allows active disease to become quiescent without the concomitant use of sulfasalazine, corticosteroids, azathioprine, and other drug therapies.[19,20] The general indications for long-term total parenteral feeding in these patients include (1) prolonged periods of active disease with significant associated catabolism, (2) periods of perioperative support, (3) incomplete intestinal obstruction, (4) short-bowel syndrome, (5) indolent wounds, (6) gastrointestinal fistulas, and (7) adjunctive therapy during an acute exacerbation of the disease.[19]

The impairment of nutritional status can be highly significant, particularly in the pediatric age group in whom inadequate protein and calorie intake is the primary cause of growth retardation.[21–23] To compound matters further, oral feeding often initiates or aggravates abdominal pain, nausea, and diarrhea. Although malnutrition can occur regardless of the location of Crohn's disease in the alimentary tract, it is more common in patients with involvement of proximal segments of the small intestine. Additionally, incomplete mechanical small-bowel obstruction or lactose intolerance is often associated with acute postprandial cramping pain, vomiting, and diarrhea. Iatrogenic dietary restrictions aimed at reducing the severity of adverse symptoms of the inflammation can further reduce the quantity and quality of nutritional support.

The mechanism for clinical remission following treatment with TPN or enteral diets is unknown and has generally been ascribed to "total bowel rest" rather than to any beneficial effect of avoiding specific foods. The use of TPN or enteral feeding as primary therapy for inflammatory bowel disease, although widely practiced, is not "curative", but can be beneficial in preventing malnutrition or rehabilitating nutritionally depleted patients with this devastating disorder. Accordingly, parenteral nutritional support has become a major component of the management of patients with Crohn's disease or ulcerative colitis and has been directed primarily toward correcting malnutrition in the adult and growth retardation in children.

Total parenteral nutrition has had not only a profound effect on the management of patients with inflammatory bowel disease, but also served as an innovative tool in promoting the rapid progression of a wide variety of sophisticated and diverse techniques for nutritional support.[24]

The total length of bowel involved with the inflammatory process is crucial in determining the severity of an acute attack, the degree to which nutrients can be assimilated enterally, and the likelihood of successful remission with conservative management. Secondary to multiple-bowel resections for recurrent exacerbations and/or fistulas, the short-bowel syndrome with its attendant complications can result, particularly in patients with Crohn's disease.

Intestinal fistulas that are a frequent complication of Crohn's disease result from a chronic inflammatory mucosal reaction and transmural progression, ulceration, and eventually adherence or penetration of visceral and parietal peritoneal surfaces. Although internal or external fistulas can occur *de novo* in patients with inflammatory bowel disease, external fistulas more commonly arise at a previous operative site. Postoperative fistulas arising in the region of resected bowel usually close with adequate periods of total parenteral nutrition and bowel rest, whereas fistulas present in areas of active bowel disease rarely close spontaneously, often recur if they do close, and usually require definitive operative therapy.[25] In general, up to 70% of GI tract fistulas in which the primary mode of treatment consists of total bowel rest and TPN closed spontaneously overall.[25,26]

Although the natural course of inflammatory bowel disease frequently includes recurrence of symptoms, the use of total bowel rest and TPN can provide the required nutritional support, while allowing optimal conditions for spontaneous remission of an acute exacerbation without operation, corticosteroids, or immunosuppressive drugs. Moreover, the judicious use of TPN and total bowel rest can accelerate wound healing and tissue repair and reduce morbidity and mortality rates.

The demonstration of the effectiveness of TPN in controlling the activities and complications of Crohn's disease has increased the interest of clinicians in diet as a primary therapy. Symptomatic, nutritional, and radiographic improvement has been documented in patients treated exclusively with an elemental diet.[27] Several uncontrolled studies have suggested further that clinical remissions of Crohn's disease could be achieved if patients were treated with an elemental diet.[28–30]

Major advantages of using an elemental diet to induce remission of Crohn's disease include the virtual absence of significant side effects, avoidance of, or reduction in, the use of drugs, and improved growth in children.[31,32] Furthermore, elemental diets are less expensive and allegedly simpler and safer to use than TPN. Their major disadvantage is unpalatability, which can be overcome to some extent by nasogastric infusion, but which introduces another group of potential problems. Finally, elemental diets can be administered at home at night without necessitating lengthy hospitalization and can, thereby, allow early return to work, school, or other full daytime activities.

As much as nutritional therapy with elemental diets or TPN has been shown to be an effective method of inducing remission in Crohn's disease, the role of effective nutritional support in the maintenance of long-term remission is not known. Most reports indicate that the majority of patients receiving TPN relapse when they return to a normal diet. On the other hand, controlled randomized trial revealed that the efficacy of TPN (71%) was not superior statistically to an elemental diet (58%) in steroid-resistant forms of Crohn's disease,[33] whereas an uncontrolled study of TPN in particularly severe, steroid-resistant Crohn's disease patients demonstrated a rapid and highly efficacious improvement in 90% of the cases.[34] In patients that eventually require elective or semi-elective surgery, aggressive nutritional therapy, whether elemental diet or TPN, can be very useful in perioperative management.

C. ALIMENTARY TRACT FISTULAS

Patients with enterocutaneous fistulas commonly present with malnutrition, electrolyte imbalance, and sepsis. The most frequent causes of enterocutaneous fistula are direct operative injury to the small bowel, disruption of an anastomosis, or a perianastomotic abscess. Other causes include sharp or blunt trauma that result in fistula formation by direct penetration, compression, ischemia, or necrosis of the bowel; benign and malignant neoplasms of the bowel; inflammatory diseases of the bowel (Crohn's disease, tuberculosis, amebiasis, etc.); vascular disorders (collagen diseases, low-flow states, mesenteric artery embolus, thrombosis, or plaque); and foreign body or radiation injury.[35] The majority of fistulas that originate in the upper small bowel are classified as high-output fistulas and initially may drain as much as 4000 ml or more of fluid daily. The problems presented by such massive losses of water, electrolytes, and nutrients are formidable, and management is frequently complicated by sepsis secondary to one or more intrabdominal abscesses. A high-output fistula is defined as one with more than 500 ml fluid loss per 24 h and is virtually uniformly associated with severe malnutrition. A significant but lesser degree of malnutrition is associated with moderate-output fistulas, which drain between 200 and 500 ml/d. Low-output fistulas with fluid losses of less than 200 ml/d have a much lower incidence of associated malnutrition.

The main objective in nonoperative fistula management is to minimize fluid output. Absolutely nothing should be allowed by mouth, not even ice chips. Gastric acid secretion and intestinal or pancreatic secretions are initially inhibited maximally by intravenous H_2 receptor blockers and i.v. or subcutaneous somatostatin, respectively. After stabilizing the patient with an enterocutaneous fistula and correcting the blood volume and electrolyte and clotting deficits, TPN is initiated through a central venous catheter that is inserted into the superior vena cava percutaneously via one of the subclavian veins.[35] Infusion of the nutrient solution is begun at levels to provide water requirements (35 to 45 ml/kg body weight per day). Although the final caloric intake is calculated at 30 to 40 kcal/kg body weight per day, usually only one third to one half of the caloric ration is given as dextrose on the first day. After tolerance and utilization of the dextrose are established, the concentration and dosage are gradually increased over the next few days to meet full caloric requirements. Fat emulsion of 20% concentration is infused in 250 ml doses two to three times a week, primarily to prevent essential fatty acid deficiency. However, in patients with diabetes mellitus, congestive heart failure, or severe obstructive pulmonary disease, it is sometimes infused daily in 500 ml doses to provide high-density fat calories, thus reducing the dextrose and water in the ration and reducing the carbon dioxide produced subsequently by oxidation of the dextrose.

In addition to hypertonic dextrose and standard amino acid solutions (4.25 to 15%), the crystalloid nutrient formulation is specifically tailored to provide the electrolytes, trace elements, and vitamins for each patient individually. Supplemental albumin, insulin, and H-2 receptor blockers can be added directly to the solution as desired.

Although it is often difficult or impossible to provide adequate enteral nutrition in the presence of an enterocutaneous fistula because of sepsis, ileus, and/or inadequate absorptive capacity, spontaneous fistula closure can be accomplished in selected patients. If at least 4 ft of functioning small bowel exist between the ligament of Treitz and the fistula, nasogastric or nasoduodenal tube feedings of highly absorbable, low-residue nutrients can be administered with reasonable results. Sometimes a small, soft tube can be passed into the bowel below a high fistula for continuous enteral feeding by pump. The volume and concentration of tube feedings initially must be low, and subsequently increased incrementally to full volume and strength, or to tolerance. This process ordinarily takes 5 to 10 days for achievement of caloric and nitrogen balance, during which time the patient should be supplemented concomitantly in decreasing incremental fashion with TPN. A combination of both techniques may be necessary to provide optimal nutrition in some patients.

We do not advocate the insertion of gastrostomy or jejunostomy feeding tubes specifically for the management of enterocutaneous fistulas, as the risks of the operative and postoperative complications are greater than those associated with TPN.

D. LIVER FAILURE

Complex metabolic derangements accompany chronic liver failure (CLF) which reflect the magnitude of the problems associated with insufficiency or decompensation of the liver.[36]

One of the most important metabolic changes in CLF, however, is alteration of plasma amino acid patterns. Insufficiency of liver function and increased muscle breakdown induce an elevation in aromatic amino acids and a reduction in branched-chain amino acid (BCAA) levels. This characteristic profile of amino acid disturbances formed the basis for the initial formulation of an intravenous solution enriched in BCAA as a potentially effective nutritional modality for the treatment of CLF and hepatic encephalopathy.

Advanced liver disease is characterized by protein malnutrition, low plasma albumin and transferrin levels, decreased creatinine-height index, reduced triceps skinfold thickness, and low total lymphocyte count. The most important nutritional indicator, however, is hypoalbuminemia, which is a consequence of decreased albumin synthesis, increased albumin degradation, malnutrition and malabsorption, poor oral intake, and third space losses of albumin in ascitic fluid and elsewhere in the extravascular compartment.

The main objective of nutritional support in liver failure is provision of adequate caloric and protein needs without inducing or aggravating hepatic encephalopathy,[37] thereby insuring the availability of energy substrates for optimal function of the hepatic mitochondria. Nutritional support for a failing liver, even though controversial, should be initiated and actively maintained during the phase in which the arterial blood ketone body ratio (KBR) is decreased.[38] Adequate measures should be taken to increase the KBR or at least to prevent a further decline. Ketone body ratios under 0.4 have ultimately been associated with a poor prognosis and markedly increased mortality.

Patients unable to tolerate oral or enteral feeding should be started on TPN as the only feasible means of providing adequate nutrition support. In those with significant hypoalbuminemia and hypoproteinemia, together with dietary protein intolerance, plasma albumin and total protein levels should be restored promptly intravenously. Safe, effective techniques for accomplishing this important goal include provision of proteins as BCAA in the parenteral nutrition solutions and administration of salt-poor albumin (50 to 75 g/d) in 2 or 3 divided doses intravenously throughout each 24-h period until the plasma protein concentrations are returned to the normal range.

Adequate calories should be given in order to meet or closely approach calculated requirements while maintaining blood glucose levels below 200 mg/dl. Fat emulsions can be given cautiously[39] in dosages sufficient to provide essential fatty acid requirements (usually 250 ml 20% emulsion every other day); however, the plasma bilirubin levels should be monitored closely in jaundiced patients receiving lipids. Vitamin B-complex, vitamin K, and folic acid may require supplementation above usual TPN dosages in patients with liver failure.

In formulating the nutrient solution, the amino acid composition is of primary concern[37] because plasma amino acid levels are frequently abnormal in hepatic failure. Manipulation of the plasma amino acid levels, with correction of the observed abnormalities, should be an important task of physicians involved in the care of these complex patients. Currently, two standard components of therapy in patients with liver failure are oriented toward (1) protein restriction, and (2) decreasing the colonic production of toxic substances that enter the portosystemic circulation. The former may alleviate the hepatic encephalopathy, but will aggravate the already impaired nutritional status. The latter therapeutic goal is achieved by reduction and modification of the colonic bacterial flora with lactulose and related carbohydrates and nonabsorbable antibiotics.[40,41] The main therapeutic controversy concerns the use of specially formulated nutrient solutions enriched in BCAA in patients with hepatic failure.[42]

Various investigators have suggested several justifications and theoretical advantages for the use of BCAA over standard amino acid solutions in the therapy of patients with hepatic encephalopathy or as a preventive measure in patients with liver dysfunction.[37,43,44] These and other studies clearly show that hepatic encephalopathy may be rapidly reversed by using BCAA-enriched solutions.[45,46] Subsequent well-controlled trials have documented that nutritional treatment of liver failure with BCAA is of practical and metabolic importance for promoting clinical improvement of protein malnutrition. The crux of the controversy lies in the fact that although parenteral and/or enteral BCAA-enriched nutrient regimens may relieve the symptoms of hepatic encephalopathy and may improve the protein nutritional status of the patient with liver failure, the beneficial effects in both situations are usually transitory, and the ultimate outcome remains the same.

E. ACUTE PANCREATITIS

Most episodes of acute pancreatitis are short-lived and self-limited, and special nutritional measurements in these patients are rarely indicated. However, in those patients with severe pancreatitis who manifest 2 or more adverse prognostic factors[47] at admission, or develop them subsequently within the first 48 h of hospitalization, TPN support should be started as soon as possible.[48] Aggressive nutritional support is essential to insure optimal provision of nutrient substrates in these patients while maintaining the GI tract and the pancreas "at rest". Several reports have confirmed that administration of all nutrients parenterally has reduced morbidity and mortality substantially.[49-53] Recently, 29 patients with moderate to severe pancreatitis treated with TPN had a mortality rate of 7% compared with 45% in patients receiving conventional intensive therapy without TPN.[54] This and other studies, as well as the vast majority of cumulative clinical experience, has established TPN use in severe acute pancreatitis as the main method of providing nutrition.

Total parental nutrition is administered continuously over 24 h, with appropriate adjustments to infusion rate and to nutrient concentration and composition. Nutritional status of these patients deteriorates very rapidly. In addition, prolonged ileus, respiratory and renal failure, severe metabolic aberrations, and multiple major surgical interventions may interfere with provision of adequate oral or enteral feeding, further complicating or aggravating existing malnutrition. In other collateral clinical conditions such as pancreatic fistulas, pseudocysts, and ascites, nutritional support with TPN has been shown to be a more effective therapy than enteral feeding. Spontaneous closure of pancreatic fistulas has been well documented in patients treated with a regimen of bowel rest and TPN.[55] Similarly, in patients with pancreatic ascites or with pseudocyst formation, TPN reduces morbidity by maintaining nutritional status during the long rehabilitation period.[56,57] Other investigators[54] have concluded that the use of TPN in the treatment of acute severe pancreatitis has decreased complications, has effectively suppressed exocrine secretion, and has been an essential adjunct to conventional intensive care. It appears that TPN reduces pancreatic autodigestion, thereby slowing progression of the pancreatitis. Furthermore, TPN induces reduction of pancreatic secretion either by complete rest of the digestive tract and/or by currently agnogenic direct effects of infusion of the amino acid/dextrose solution. Adequate nutrition provided parenterally not only promotes restoration of damaged pancreatic tissue, but enhances spontaneous closure of pancreatic fistulas.[55] By bypassing cephalic, gastric, and intestinal phases of pancreatic secretion, TPN reduces the pancreatic acinar nuclear volume, acinar cell volume by up to 50% and synthetic activity,[58] and significantly reduces the basal pancreatic proteolytic and bicarbonate secretions.[59,60]

Selection of i.v. nutritional formulations is still somewhat controversial and should be based on the knowledge of the effects that individual nutrient substrates have upon pancreatic secretions. Each nutrient has a different specificity as well as a different potency for stimulating the release of each peptide hormone. Intravenous hypertonic dextrose has been shown to suppress both the water volume and the proteolytic enzyme concentration of pancreatic secretin, actions attributed in part to increased serum osmolality.[61,62] These authors also documented reduced survival rates in patients receiving lipid emulsion combined with dextrose compared with patients who received dextrose as their only energy source in the parenteral nutrition regimen. Their results have indicated clearly that the use of lipid emulsions in acute pancreatitis should be limited, reserving them only for malnourished patients with severe glucose intolerance. However, others have advocated and reported the use of lipid emulsions safely in the management of acute pancreatitis unless the patient had a known dyslipoproteinemia.[63] Contrarily, the i.v. administration of lipids has been shown to increase pancreatic secretions, an obviously undesirable and potentially harmful side effect.[64] Intravenous infusion of 20% dextrose or 30% dextrose and 12% amino acid solution significantly inhibited the secretion of secretin-pancreozymin stimulated pancreatic juice and amylase in dogs with chronic pancreatic fistulas.[65,66] Intravenous administration of some amino acids individually or in combination also had a depressant effect on pancreatic exocrine secretions.[67] Moreover, it is known that free amino acids infused into the duodenum can also decrease pancreatic exocrine secretion. The strongest depressant of pancreatic exocrine secretion, other than somatostatin and glucagon, is the infusion of hypertonic salts and dextrose into the jejunum.[68] On the other hand, hydrochloric acid, meat extracts, antral distension, fat, protein, calcium, and magnesium all increase pancreatic exocrine secretion. From these findings, it appears that the best dietary formulation for patients with severe pancreatitis is a fat-free i.v. solution of crystalline amino acids and hypertonic dextrose to which appropriate daily requirements of electrolytes, vitamins, minerals, and trace elements have been added. Nothing should be ingested orally, and gastric decompression should be maintained to avoid antral distension or duodenal stimulation of pancreatic secretion. Patients with severe acute pancreatitis are metabolically similar to septic patients and have an impairment in their ability to oxidize dextrose[69] with significantly depressed utilization of the exogenous carbohydrate load. Nonetheless, administration of dextrose as the main energy source in acute pancreatitis remains the nutrient therapy of choice. In addition, administration of highly concentrated amino acid solutions, augmented with extra valine, isoleucine, alanine, and arginine, which are significantly decreased in their plasma and tissues, has been recommended in the nutritional support of acute pancreatitis patients.[65,67]

The use of i.v. lipid as an energy source during acute pancreatitis has been controversial. Infusion of lipid emulsions has resulted in a dose-dependent rise in pancreatic secretions that is equal to almost half of the maximal response observed following administration of the synthetic octapeptide of cholecystokinin.[64] Although infusion of i.v. lipid emulsions may appear to be a safe and effective calorie source and may be helpful in the management of acute pancreatitis compounded by severe lung failure accompanied by an elevated pCO_2, each patient must be closely monitored, since fat infusion may aggravate pancreatitis in a significant number of patients.[70-73] Intravenous fat administration has actually been identified and reported as the etiology of pancreatitis in a patient with Crohn's disease being treated with lipid-based TPN.[74] Moreover, patients receiving lipid-based TPN formulations have been known to have significantly higher ($p < 0.05$) elevations of serum AST.[70]

In laboratory animals with severe acute pancreatitis, utilization of the emulsion with production of CO_2 was slightly to moderately depressed, depending on the molecular structure of the fatty acids.[65] Additionally, it has been suggested that excess free fatty acids cause capillary membrane damage with subsequent release of pancreatic enzymes, implying that elevated fatty acid levels may promote pancreatic exocrine secretion.[75] Another clear contraindication to the use of i.v. lipid emulsions as the major energy source is acute pancreatitis associated with a lipid disorder (type I, IV, and V hyperlipoproteinemia).[63,76]

The preferred route of nutritional support depends on the acuteness and severity of the disease, as well as on an understanding of the physiology of pancreatic stimulation. Parenteral nutrition has become a standard component of therapy in the treatment of acute pancreatitis and should be used in the acute phase of the disease whenever possible.[48,76] Enteral feeding may be used as a means of supplying nutrients if the major responses to cephalic, gastric, and intestinal phases of pancreatic stimulation are bypassed by infusion distal to the duodenum.[47] Significant increases in pancreatic secretions and protein output mediated by CCK-PZ stimulation are induced with intraduodenal infusion of elemental diets in dogs.[77] Intrajejunal feeding is the method of choice, if enteral feeding is to be used at all. However, small bowel obstruction, enteritis, entero-enteric and enterocutaneous fistulas, or paralytic ileus often preclude enteral feeding in patients with severe pancreatitis. Maintenance of intestinal mucosal integrity and the gut mucosal barrier has been suggested as a potential benefit of enteral feeding.[78] However, it has been clearly demonstrated that the preferred feeding mode in patients with pancreatic inflammation, abscesses, and fistulas is TPN. Failure to reduce pancreatic stimulation and to reverse malnutrition as a major complication of severe acute pancreatitis may adversely affect survival of these patients. If oral or enteral feedings, especially those containing fat, are accompanied by exacerbations of symptoms or elevations in serum amylase or lipase concentrations, it is advisable to reinstitute TPN. In our clinical experience, stimulation and aggravation of the acutely inflamed pancreas can be minimized by conscientious adherence to the principles of management outlined briefly in Table 1.

F. CHRONIC PANCREATITIS

Pancreatic insufficiency is usually not manifested in chronic pancreatitis until approximately 90% of pancreatic secretory function has been lost.[79] Malnutrition occurs not only secondary to malabsorption but also to decreased oral intake as a result of postprandial

TABLE 1
Principles of Management of Acute Pancreatitis

1. Absolutely nothing by mouth.
   No ice chips; no sips of water.
2. Nasogastric tube decompression.
3. Avoid use of narcotic analgesics.
   If necessary, minimal doses sparingly.
4. Intravenous H-2 receptor blockers.
5. Nutrition preferably by TPN.
   Elemental enteral feedings later.
   Minimize fat in enteral or oral diet.
6. Limit intravenous lipids in TPN regimen.
   Monitor serum amylase and lipase.
   Monitor serum triglycerides.

pain. Initially, nutritional status may be improved by increasing dietary carbohydrates and decreasing fats since the carbohydrates are usually well absorbed, whereas fats require the hydrolytic digestive enzymes produced by the pancreas. Eventually, exogenous pancreatic enzyme administration becomes necessary as significant weight loss occurs and hydrolytic enzyme deficiencies are suspected clinically or confirmed by indirect or direct enzyme functional studies.

A variety of commercially available pancreatic enzyme preparations allow successful supplemental or replacement therapy in pancreatic insufficiency or failure. The major source for these enzymes is pancreatin, which is derived by alcohol extraction from porcine or bovine pancreas. Lipase-augmented pancreatin, generically known as pancrelipase, may reduce steatorrhea more effectively on an equal-weight basis than pancreatin. In addition, a vegetable-derived form of pancreatin is available for use in patients with sensitivities to porcine or bovine protein.

On the basis of normal pancreatic secretion following maximal stimulation with cerulein and secretin, a secretory capacity of 10% corresponds to 100,000 units of lipase activity. Accordingly, effective control of steatorrhea ordinarily will require the administration of at least 100,000 units of lipase/day. In fact, therapeutic success has been documented by a 50% reduction in stool fat with this dosage and a 70% reduction with a dosage of 200,000 units of lipase/day. Rarely, complete restoration of lipid hydrolysis is possible, but requires doses as high as 100,000 units of lipase per meal. However, a high-potency enzyme tablet is available that contains 22,500 units of lipase and 180,000 units each of protease and amylase.

However, the major problem with enzyme preparations is their degradation in an acid environment, especially lipase which is irreversibly denatured at a pH <4. Improved digestive efficiency has been achieved with simultaneous administration of antacids or H-2 receptor blocking agents, substantiating the clinical relevance of acid degradation. Enteric coated preparations are available which release the hydrolytic enzymes at pH >5.5. High enzyme content, rapid-release kinetics, and acid stability are the preferred characteristics of pancreatic extract preparations which have been recently improved, and are likely to improve further as technology advances.

It has been suggested that enzyme preparations relieve pain in chronic pancreatitis.[80,81] The cause of pain in chronic pancreatitis is poorly understood, but is thought to be multifactorial, including ductal hypertension and obstruction, recurrent autodigestion, and progressive nerve infiltration.[82] In several controlled studies, the majority of patients have reportedly experienced a reduction in pain with administration of pancreatic enzyme supplements which increased the levels of intraluminal proteases.[80,81]

Total parenteral nutrition support is indicated and should be administered in exacerbation phases of chronic pancreatitis or in patients undergoing surgical resection of the chronically diseased pancreas. The administration and monitoring of TPN in these patients is essentially the same as that for any other surgical patients requiring this therapy.

G. CANCER PATIENTS

Most oncologic processes have debilitating effects on the body cell mass, and the majority of patients with malignant diseases experience a significant degree of malnutrition. Understanding the interactions of neoplastic disease and specific nutrients and their possible effects on cancer cells has been, and continues to be, a great challenge. For this reason, it is especially important that during the diagnostic phase and later during antineoplastic treatment, the cancer patient should be supported with optimal nutritional therapy in order to achieve the best possible therapeutic results with the lowest morbidity and mortality.

Some cancer patients, especially those with a malignancy of the oral cavity, pharynx, larynx, or cervical esophagus, may present with painful deglutition and progressive difficulty with ingesting and swallowing solid foods. Moreover, patients with cancer of the head and neck often have a history of heavy smoking, excessive alcohol intake, and/or dietary indiscretions which render them protein-calorie malnourished prior to developing malignancies. Surgical treatment of a patient with head and neck cancer often results in diminished oral intake when preoperative, postoperative, or primary radiation therapy induces severe stomatitis, mucositis, and diminished salivary secretions. These adverse symptoms further aggravate the decreased oral intake and increased weight loss of such patients.

Although the reason for malnutrition in patients with cancer is not clearly defined, patients with malignancies present the ultimate challenge to restoration or improvement of nutritional status while receiving primary anticancer therapy. Determining the best method for nourishing the cancer patient depends on three major factors: (1) the patient's nutritional status, (2) the level and degree of residual GI function, and (3) the type and magnitude of antineoplastic therapy. Ideally, adequate voluntary ingestion of food orally is the ultimate goal for all patients. However, most antineoplastic treatment modalities preclude optimal oral intake. Moreover, poor nutritional status results in lassitude and weakness, which further decrease oral ingestion of foodstuffs. If a patient is unable to obtain his daily nutritional requirement voluntarily by oral ingestion of normal nutrients, oral supplementation together with aggressive dietary counseling should be initiated and maintained. Patients should also be encouraged and allowed to make dietary selections of their food preferences whenever feasible. Alert, well-motivated patients should be urged to increase their daily calorie and protein intake through the ingestion of hospital-prepared or commercially formulated supplements before and after surgical intervention, and when possible during other modes of therapy (chemotherapy, radiation, or multimodal). However, some patients are not well-motivated; they have increased nutritional requirements, or they are anorectic secondary to the disease and cannot ingest adequate quantities of nutrients orally. Under these circumstances, tube feeding should be attempted in patients with intact alimentary tract function. Although a functioning alimentary tract provides the best means of assuring normal digestion, absorption, and assimilation of foodstuffs, use of the enteral route is contraindicated in the presence of severe GI dysfunctions, such as intestinal obstruction, upper GI bleeding, and/or intractable vomiting or diarrhea. On the other hand, if the alimentary tract is not available for use, or if rapid precise nutritional repletion is deemed essential, parenteral nutrition should be instituted. Furthermore, TPN should be used in cancer patients as a means of nutritional rehabilitation when such a goal is desirable to maximize the response to chemotherapy and to minimize complications from antineoplastic agents, and when this goal cannot be attained by using the GI tract.

Our group has previously reported a cohort of malnourished patients who required treatment with TPN to complete a planned course of radiation therapy.[83] Anorexia, nausea, and vomiting disappeared during TPN unless the subjects attempted oral feeding, in which case all symptoms recurred. Ninety-five percent of the patients completed their planned courses of radiation therapy and improved symptomatically; 54% of them responded to radiation therapy with a greater than 50% reduction in tumor size. Responding patients gained an average of 5.9 ± 2.9 kg during TPN (average duration of 36.2 days) and radiation therapy (average dose of 3832 rads), whereas nonresponding subjects gained only 2.2 ± 4.9 kg during TPN (average duration of 42.8 days) and radiation therapy (average dose of 3819 rads). Thus, TPN allowed prospectively planned courses of radiation therapy to be delivered to a group of low-risk, malnourished cancer patients; a positive correlation between tumor response and nutritional status was identified; and symptoms of radiation stomatitis and enteritis were reduced or eliminated as long as enteral nutrition was avoided.

It has been shown convincingly, by use of the "prognostic nutritional index" in malnourished cancer patients, that a much higher morbidity and mortality was associated with surgical procedures when nutritional repletion has not been accomplished preoperatively.[84] At the M.D. Anderson Hospital and Tumor Institute, 160 patients who were malnourished or whose treatment would ordinarily result in malnutrition, were tested with a battery of 5 recall skin test antigens at 10- to 14-day intervals throughout antineoplastic therapy and nutritional rehabilitation with TPN. Conclusions derived from this study were (1) among surgical patients with negative skin test reactions, significantly more postoperative morbidity and mortality occurred than among patients with positive skin test reactions, and continued negative skin test reactivity during treatment with TPN was associated with unresolved malnutrition; (2) immune depression attributed to chemotherapy, in part, may be secondary to malnutrition; and (3) skin test reactivity, in general, was depressed during radiation therapy even though nutrition was estimated to be adequate.[85] Other clinical investigators compared 98 patients having surgically resectable GI tract malignancies, treated with TPN pre- and postoperatively, with 94 surgical patients having similar tumors and treated with conventional fluid therapy.[86] In the TPN group, significantly greater weight gain, enhanced nitrogen balance, and improved wound healing were demonstrated. The average hospital stay was 18 days for the TPN group compared with 25 days for the control patients. Similar results have been reported in a group of malnourished patients with upper GI tract cancer who were nutritionally replenished with TPN preoperatively.[87] In another randomized prospective trial, the efficacy of 10 days of TPN in patients with GI tumors was manifested as a significantly lower postoperative morbidity rate in the patients given TPN (17%) than in the control group (32%).[88] Additionally, the mortality rate was significantly lower in the former group (4%) than in the latter group (16%). However, other randomized trials showed no significant advantages of TPN in reducing operative morbidity or mortality.[89] Clearly, severely malnourished patients with cancer of the upper GI tract benefit from preoperative nutrition. The benefit of TPN in less severe cases of malnutrition as an adjunct to oncologic therapy remains to be established.[89]

The efficacy of TPN, postoperatively, has been demonstrated in malnourished subjects with carcinoma of the larynx.[90] Seventy patients received TPN, while an additional 90 patients were fed via nasogastric tubes. Both groups of patients were matched for stage of disease and dose of preoperative radiation therapy. Primary wound healing occurred in 75% of the TPN group vs. 40% of the enteral group. Only 10% of the cases in the parenteral group developed pharyngeal fistulas, compared with 29% of the patients in the enteral group. Those who were given nutrient mixtures by vein, and thereby guaranteed an adequate caloric intake, had significantly better postoperative wound healing than a comparable group fed via the GI tract.

We retrospectively evaluated 100 patients that received TPN as nutritional support. Fifty-two patients underwent extensive curative resections that included abdominoperineal resections, esophagectomies, and total gastrectomies. In those patients who received TPN pre- and postoperatively, weight gain and a rise in serum albumin concentration occurred almost entirely during the preoperative period. Body weight and serum albumin levels were maintained during the postoperative period, but no increase in either occurred. Those patients receiving TPN only postoperatively had usually developed one of the complications of prolonged inanition such a paralytic ileus, wound dehiscence, anastomotic disruption, or wound infection, before TPN was initiated. Weight gain in these cases was difficult to achieve, probably because of increased energy expenditure secondary to the surgical complications. In contrast, those patients who received TPN preoperatively had virtually no postoperative complications and were often eating within 5 to 7 days after bowel resection. Based on data reported by several groups of investigators.[86–89] and data reported by our group,[91] it is obvious that a malnourished patient should be nutritionally replenished preoperatively whenever possible rather than after some catastrophic postoperative complication has occurred.

Malnutrition is common in patients with malignant disease, especially when it involves the GI tract. Regardless of postulated or demonstrated tumor-induced abnormalities in the intermediary metabolism of the host, the predominant factor in the development of cancer cachexia is an imbalance between nutrient intake and host nutrient requirements, which can be treated effectively in severely malnourished patients by enteral or parenteral nutrition, or both. Optimal results from surgical procedures, pharmacologic therapy, chemotherapy, radiotherapy, immunotherapy, respiratory therapy, physical therapy, and other forms of care can only be obtained when the patient is maintained in optimal nutritional condition. Therefore, the ultimate goal in the nutritional management of patients with cancer is the same as with all other human beings—to provide optimal nutrition to all patients under all conditions at all times.

III. CONCLUSION

During the past quarter-century, supportive measures for reducing morbidity and mortality of major operative procedures by improving the nutritional status of patients have expanded greatly from the peripheral i.v. infusion of isotonic carbohydrate and electrolyte solutions to the parenteral and enteral provision of most or all of the nutrient requirements under a wide variety of clinical situations. Primary emphasis has shifted gradually from interest in the body as a whole and in technical aspects of surgical nutrition support to interest in the functions and nutrient requirements of specific organs and systems under normal and pathophysiologic conditions. Efforts have also been directed more recently to the alterations in nutrient requirements induced by specific disease entities and their interaction with the neuroendocrine regulators of metabolism.

Total parenteral nutrition was inaugurated successfully 25 years ago and has evolved into a useful clinical technique. It has been instrumental in saving countless lives and has clearly demonstrated the relevance of providing adequate nutrition in the achievement of optimal clinical results in surgical patients and stimulating the monumental increase in the use of specialized enteral feedings in patients whose oral intakes are inadequate to support normal nutritional status. Today, surgical nutrition is advancing rapidly toward the provision of optimal nutrient substrates to individual cells or tissues, whether normal or abnormal, and represents the practice of clinical biochemistry. In the future, it is likely that parenteral and enteral nutrient formulations will acquire even greater degrees of precision and clinical effectiveness as the molecular biological revolution transforms the practice of medicine and surgery.

REFERENCES

1. **Tellado, JM and Christon, NV.** Nutrition and immunity. In: *Total Parenteral Nutrition,* 2nd ed., Fischer, JE, Ed., Little, Brown, Boston, 1991, 127–139.
2. **Freyre, EA, Chabes, AC, Poemape, O, and Chabes, A.** Abnormal rebuck skin window response in kwashiorkor. *J Pediatr,* 82:523–526, 1973.
3. **Tchervenkov, JI, Latter, DA, Psychogios, J, and Christou, NV.** The influence of long-term protein deprivation on in vivo phagocytic cell delivery to inflammatory lesions. *Surgery,* 103:463–468, 1988.
4. **Lipschitz, DA.** Nutrition, aging, and the immunohematopoietic system. *Clin Geriat Med,* 3:319–328, 1987.
5. **Law, DK, Dudrick, SJ, and Abdou, NI.** The effect of dietary protein depletion on immunocompetence: the importance of nutritional repletion prior to immunologic induction. *Ann Surg,* 179:168–173, 1974.
6. **Dudrick, SJ, Latifi, R, and Schrager, R.** Nutritional management of inflammatory bowel disease. *Surg Clin N Am,* 71:609–623, 1991.
7. **Fischer, JE.** Inflammatory bowel disease. In: *Total Parenteral Nutrition,* 2nd ed., Fischer, JE, Ed. Little, Brown, Boston, 1991, 239–151.
8. **Anderson, DL and Boyce, HW, Jr.** Use of parenteral nutrition in treatment of advanced regional enteritis. *Am J Dig Dis,* 18:633–640, 1973.
9. **Reilly, J, Ryan, JA, Strole, W, et al.** Hyperalimentation in inflammatory bowel disease. *Am J Surg,* 131:192–200, 1976.
10. **Vogel, CM, Corwin, TR, and Baue, AE.** Intravenous hyperalimentation in the treatment of inflammatory diseases of the bowel. *Arch Surg,* 180:460–467, 1974.
11. **Grand, RJ and Colodny, AH.** Increased requirement for magnesium during parenteral therapy for granulomatous colitis. *J Pediatr,* 81:788–790, 1972.
12. **Greig, PP, Deitel, M, and Jirch, DW.** Nutrition in inflammatory bowel disease. In: *Nutrition in Surgery,* 2nd ed., Deitel, M, Ed. Williams & Wilkins, Baltimore, 1985, 320–333.
13. **Denberg, J, Benson, W, Ali, MS, et al.** Megaloblastic anemia in patients receiving TPN without folic acid or vitamin B_{12} supplementation. *Can Med Assoc J,* 117:144–146, 1977.
14. **Elsborg, L and Larsen, L.** Folate deficiency in chronic inflammatory bowel disease. *JPEN,* 3:315, 1979.
15. **Driscoll, RH, Jr., Meredith, SC, Sitrin, M, et al.** Vitamin D deficiency and bone disease in patients with Crohn's disease. *Gastroenterology,* 83:1252–1258, 1982.
16. **Marshall, F, II.** Hyperalimentation as a treatment of Crohn's disease. *Am J Surg,* 128:652–653, 1974.
17. **Takagi, Y, Okada, A, Itakura, T, et al.** Clinical studies on zinc metabolism during TPN as related to zinc deficiency. *JPEN,* 10:195–202, 1986.
18. **Vilter, RW, Bozian, RC, Hess, EV, et al.** Manifestations of copper deficiency in a patient with systemic sclerosis on intravenous hyperalimentation. *N Engl J Med,* 291:188–192, 1974.
19. **Dudrick, SJ, MacFadyen, BV, Jr., and Daly, JM.** Management of inflammatory bowel disease with parenteral hyperalimentation. In: *Gastrointestinal Emergencies,* Clearfield, HR and Dinoso, VP, Jr., Eds. Grune and Stratton, New York, 1967, 193–199.
20. **Steiger, E, Wilmore, DW, Dudrick, SJ, et al.** Total intravenous nutrition in the management of inflammatory disease of the intestinal tract. *Fed Proc,* 28:808, 1969.
21. **Axelsson, C and Jarnum, S.** Assessment of the therapeutic value of an elemental diet in chronic inflammatory bowel disease. *Scand J Gastroenterol,* 77:272–279, 1977.
22. **Belli, DC, Seidman, E, Bouthillier, L, et al.** Chronic intermittent elemental diet improves growth failure in children with Crohn's disease. *Gastroenterology,* 94:603–610, 1988.
23. **Krischner, BS, Klich, JR, Kalman, SS, et al.** Reversal of growth retardation in Crohn's disease with therapy emphasizing oral nutrition restitution. *Gastroenterology,* 80:10–15, 1981.
24. **Dudrick, SJ and Latifi, R.** Total parenteral nutrition-current status. *Contemp Surg,* 41:41–48, 1992.
25. **Schofield, PF.** The natural history and treatment of Crohn's disease. *Ann R Coll Surg Eng,* 36:258–279, 1965.

26. **MacFadyen, BV, Jr., Dudrick, SJ, and Ruberg, RL.** The management of gastrointestinal fistulae with parenteral hyperalimentation. *Surgery,* 74:100–105, 1973.

27. **Shiloni, E, Coronado, E, and Freund, HT.** The role of TPN in the treatment of Crohn's disease. *Am J Surg,* 157:180–187, 1989.

28. **Voitk, AJ, Echave, B, and Feller, JH.** Experience of elemental diets in the treatment of inflammatory bowel disease. Is this primary therapy? *Arch Surg,* 107:329–333, 1973.

29. **Meryn, S.** The role of nutrition in the treatment of inflammatory bowel disease. *Wien Klin Wochenschr,* 94:774–779, 1986.

30. **Navarro, J, Vargus, J, Cezard, JP, et al.** Prolonged constant rate of elemental enteral nutrition in Crohn's disease. *J Pediatr Gastroenterol Nutr,* 1:541–556, 1982.

31. **Sabbah, S and Seidman, E.** Nutritional therapy of children with inflammatory bowel disease. *Can J Gastroenterol,* 2:13A-17A, 1988.

32. **Sanderson, IR, Udeen, S, Davies, PSW, et al.** Remission induced by an elemental diet in small bowel Crohn's disease. *Arch Dis Child,* 71:123–127, 1987.

33. **Greenberg, GR, Fleming, CR, Jeejeebhoy, KN, et al.** Controlled trial of bowel rest and nutritional support in the management of Crohn's disease. *Gut,* 29:1309–1315, 1988.

34. **Lerebours, E, Messing, B, Chevalier, B, et al.** An evaluation of TPN in the management of steroid-dependent and steroid-resistant patients with Crohn's disease. *JPEN,* 10:274–278, 1986.

35. **Dudrick, SJ and Mock, TC.** Enterocutaneous fistula. In: *Current Surgical Therapy,* 3rd ed., Cameron, J, Ed. BC Decker, Philadelphia, 1988, 35–61.

36. **Latifi, R, Killam, R, and Dudrick, SJ.** Nutritional support in liver failure. *Surg Clin N Am,* 3:567–578, 1991.

37. **Fischer, JE.** Hepatic failure. In: *Care of the Surgical Patient, A Publication of The Committee on Pre and Postoperative Care,* Wilmore, DW, Brennan, MF, and Harken, AH, et al., Eds. Scientific American Medicine, New York, 1990, 1–13.

38. **Shimahara, Y, Kiuchi, T, Yamamoto, Y, et al.** Hepatic mitochondrial redox potential and nutritional support in liver insufficiency. In: *Nutritional Support in Organ Failure,* Tanaka, T and Okada, A, Eds. Elsevier Science Publishers, Amsterdam, 1990, 295–308.

39. **Nagayama, M, Takai, T, Okuno, M, et al.** Fat emulsion in surgical patients with liver disorders. *J Surg Res,* 47:59–64, 1989.

40. **Duffy, TE and Plum, F.** Hepatic encephalopathy. In: *The Liver: Biology and Pathobiology,* Arias, I, Popper, D, Schacter, D, and Shafritz DA, Eds. Raven Press, New York, 1982, 693–715.

41. **Okada, A and Kamata, SH.** Hepatic failure (encephalopathy)—acute and chronic. In: *Nutrition in Clinical Surgery,* 2nd ed., Deitel, M, Ed. Williams & Wilkins, Baltimore, 1985, 341–347.

42. **Milikan, WJ and Hooks, MA.** Nutritional support in hepatic failure (editorial), *Nutr Clin Pract,* 3:3, 1988.

43. **Muto, Y, Yoshida, T, and Yamatoh, M.** Nutritional treatment of liver cirrhosis with branched chain amino acids (BCAA). In: *Nutritional Support in Organ Failure,* Tanaka, T and Okada, A, Eds. Elsevier Science Publishers, Amsterdam, 1990, 267–276.

44. **Ogoshi, S, Iwasa, M, Mizobuchi, S, et al.** Effect of a nucleoside and nucleotide mixture on protein metabolism in rats given TPN after 70% hepatectomy. In: *Nutritional Support in Organ Failure,* Tanaka, T and Okada, A, Eds. Elsevier Science Publishers, Amsterdam, 1990, 309–317.

45. **Cerra, FB, Holman, RT, Bankey, PE, and Mazuski, JE.** Hepatic failure in the hypermetabolism organ failure syndrome:nutritional management now and in the future. In: *Nutritional Support in Organ Failure,* Tanaka, T and Okada, A, Eds. Elsevier Science Publishers, Amsterdam, 1990, 287–294.

46. **Egberts, EH, Schomerus, H, Hamster, W, et al.** Effective treatment of latent porto-systemic encephalopathy with oral branched chain amino acids. In: *Hepatic Encephalopathy in Chronic Liver Failure,* Capocaccia, L, Fischer, JE, Rossi-Fanelli, F, Eds. Plenum, New York, 1984, 351–357.

47. **Pisters, PWT and Ranson, JHC.** Nutritional support for acute pancreatitis. *Surg Gynecol Obstet,* 175:275–284, 1992.

48. **Latifi, R, McIntosh, JK, and Dudrick, SJ.** Nutritional management of acute and chronic pancreatitis. *Surg Clin N Am,* 73:579–588, 1991.

49. **Blackburn, GL, Williams, LF, Bistrian, B, et al.** New approaches to the management of severe acute pancreatitis. *Am J Surg,* 131:114–124, 1976.

50. **Copeland, EM and Dudrick, SJ.** Intravenous hyperalimentation in inflammatory bowel disease, pancreatitis and cancer. *Surg Ann,* 12:83–101, 1980.

51. **Goodgame, JT and Fischer, JE.** Parenteral nutrition in the treatment of acute pancreatitis: effect on complications and mortality. *Ann Surg,* 186:651–685, 1977.

52. **Klein, E, Shnebaum, S, Benari, G, and Dreiling, DA.** Effects of TPN on exocrine pancreatic secretion. *Am J Gastroenterol,* 78:31–33, 1983.

53. **Feller, JH, Brown, RA, Toussaint, GPM, et al.** Changing methods in the treatment of severe pancreatitis. *Am J Surg,* 127:196–201, 1974.

54. **Fujita, H, Tanaka, SH, Nakagawara, G, and Miyazaki, I.** Clinical and experimental evaluation of TPN in the treatment of acute pancreatitis. In: *Nutritional Support in Organ Failure,* Tanaka, T and Okada, A, Eds. Elsevier Science Publishers, Amsterdam, 1990, 337–349.

55. **Dudrick, SJ, Wilmore, DW, Steiger, E, et al.** Spontaneous closure of traumatic pancreatoduodenal fistulas with total intravenous nutrition. *J Trauma,* 10:542–553, 1979.

56. **Variyam, FP.** Central vein hyperalimentation in pancreatic ascites. *Am J Gastroenterol,* 78:178–181, 1983.

57. **Variyam, FP, Fuller, RK, Brown, FM, et al.** Effect of parenteral amino acids on human pancreatic exocrine secretion. *Dig Dis Sci,* 30:541–546, 1985.

58. **Paviat, WA, Rodgers, W, and Cameron, JL.** Morphologic analysis of pancreatic acinar cells from orally fed and intravenously fed rats. *J Surg Res,* 19:267–276, 1975.

59. **Johnson, LR, Lichtenberger, LM, Copeland, EM, et al.** Structural and hormonal alterations in the gastrointestinal tract of parenterally fed rats. *Gastroenterology,* 68:1184–1192, 1975.

60. **Johnson, LR, Schanbacher, LM, Dudrick, SJ, et al.** Effect of long-term parenteral feeding on pancreatic secretion and serum secretin. *Am J Physiol,* 233:E524–E529, 1977.

61. **Nakajima, S and Magee, DF.** Inhibition of exocrine pancreatic secretion by glucagon and D-glucose given intravenously. *Can J Physiol Pharmacol,* 48:299–305, 1970.

62. **Pitchumoni, CS, Schele, G, Lee, PC, et al.** Effects of nutrition on the exocrine pancreas. In: *The Exocrine Pancreas: Biology, Pathobiology, and Diseases,* Go, VLW, et al., Eds. Raven Press, New York, 1986, 387–406.

63. **Kirby, DF and Craig, RM.** The value of intensive nutritional support in pancreatitis. *JPEN,* 9:353–357, 1985.

64. **Konturek, SJ, Tasler, J, Cieszkowski, M, et al.** Intravenous amino acids and fat stimulate pancreatic secretion. *Am J Physiol,* 236:E678–E684, 1979.

65. **Ohyanagi, H, Usami, M, Nishimatsu, SH, et al.** Metabolic changes and their management in acute pancreatitis. In: *Nutritional Support in Organ Failure,* Tanaka, T and Okada, A, Eds. Elsevier Science Publishers, Amsterdam, 1990, 351–363.

66. **Saitoh, Y, Tokutake, K, Matsuno, S, et al.** Effects of hypertonic intravenous nutrient solutions on pancreatic exocrine function. *Tohoku J Exp Med,* 124:99–115, 1978.

67. **Saitoh, Y, Honda, T, Matsuno, S, et al.** Effect of eight amino acids on the exocrine and endocrine function. *Tohoku J Exp Med,* 129:257–272, 1979.

68. **Grant, JP.** Use of enteral and parenteral nutrition in acute pancreatitis. In: *Nutritional Support in Organ Failure,* Tanaka, T and Okada, A, Eds. Elsevier Science Publishers, Amsterdam, 1990, 333–336.

69. **Durr, GH, Schaefers, A, Maroske, D, et al.** A controlled study on the use of intravenous fat in patients suffering from acute attacks of pancreatitis. *Infusiontherapie,* 12:128–133, 1985.

70. **Sitzmann, JF, Steinborn, PA, Zinner, MJ, and Cameron, TL.** Total parenteral nutrition and energy substrates in treatment of severe acute pancreatitis. *Surg Gynecol Obstet,* 168:311–317, 1989.

71. **Edelman, K and Valenzuela, JE.** Effect of intravenous lipid on human pancreatic secretion. *Gastroenterology,* 85:1063–1066, 1983.

72. **Goodgame, JT, Lowry, SF and Brennan, MF.** Essential fatty acid deficiency in TPN: time course of development and suggestions for therapy. *Surgery,* 84:271–277, 1978.

73. **Cameron, JL, Capuzzi, DM, Zuidema, GD, et al.** Acute pancreatitis with hyperlipidemia: the incidence of lipid abnormalities in acute pancreatitis. *Ann Surg,* 177:483–489, 1973.

74. **Noseworthy, J, Colodny, AH, and Eraklis, AJ.** Pancreatitis and intravenous fat: an association in patients with inflammatory bowel disease. *J Pediatr Surg,* 18:269–273, 1983.

75. **Havalo, T, Shronts, E, and Cerra, F.** Nutritional support in acute pancreatitis. *Gastroenterol Clin N Am,* 18:525–541, 1989.

76. **Durr, GH-K.** Enteral and parenteral nutrition in acute pancreatitis. In: *Acute Pancreatitis. Research and Clinical Management,* Beger, HG and Buchler, M, Eds. Springer-Verlag, Berlin, 1987, 285–288.

77. **Wolfe, BM, Keltner, RM and Kaminski, DL.** The effect of an intraduodenal elemental diet on pancreatic secretion. *Surg Gynecol Obstet,* 140:241–245, 1975.

78. **Deitch, EA and Bridges, RM.** Effect of stress and trauma on bacterial translocation from the gut. *J Surg Res,* 42:536–542, 1987.

79. **Dimagno, EP, Go, VLM, and Summerskill, WHJ.** Relations between pancreatic enzyme outputs and malabsorption in severe pancreatic insufficiency. *N Engl J Med,* 288:813–815, 1973.

80. **Ihse, I and Permeth, S.** Enzyme supplementation for pain in chronic pancreatitis. In: *Chronic Pancreatitis,* Beger, HG, Buchler, M, Ditschuneit, H, et al., Eds. Springer-Verlag, Berlin, 1990, 354–357.

81. **Isaksson, G and Ihse, I.** Pain reduction by an oral pancreatic enzyme preparation in chronic pancreatitis. *Dig Dis Sci,* 28:97–102, 1983.

82. **Shaff, J, Jacobson, D, Tillman, CR, et al.** Protease-specific suppression of pancreatic exocrine secretion. *Gastroenterology,* 84:44–52, 1984.

83. **Copeland, EM, Souchon, EA, MacFadyen, BV, et al.** Intravenous hyperalimentation as an adjunct to radiation therapy. *Cancer,* 39:609–616, 1977.

84. **Smale, BF, Mullen, JL, Buzby, GP, et al.** The efficiacy of nutritional assessment and support in cancer surgery. *Cancer,* 47:2375–2381, 1981.

85. **Daly, JM, Dudrick, SJ, and Copeland, EM.** Intravenous hyperalimentation: effect on delayed cutaneous hypersensitivity in cancer patients. *Ann Surg,* 192:587–592, 1980.

86. **Dionigi, R, Guaglio, R, Bonera, A, et al.** Clinical-pharmacologic aspects, application and effectiveness of TPN in surgical patients. *Int J Clin Pharmacol Biopharmacol,* 17:107–118, 1979.

87. **Heatley, RV, Williams, R, and Lewis, M.** Preoperative intravenous feeding: a controlled trial. *Postgrad Med J,* 55:541–545, 1979.

88. **Mueller, JM, Brenner, U, Dienst, C, and Pichlmaier, H.** Preoperative parenteral feeding in patients with gastrointestinal carcinoma. *Lancet,* 1:68–71, 1982.

89. **Daly, JM, Redmond, HP, Lieberman, MD, and Jardines, L.** Nutritional support of patients with cancer of the gastrointestinal tract. *Surg Clin N Am,* 71:523–536, 1991.

90. **Senjukov, MV, Khmelevski, IM, Zubov, OG, et al.** Parenteral feeding of patients with cancer of the larynx undergoing combination therapy. *Vestn Otorinolaringol,* 2:660–671, 1978.

91. **Copeland, EM** and **Dudrick, SJ.** Nutritional aspects of cancer. *Curr Probl Cancer,* 1:3–51, 1976

Chapter 10

CARE MANAGEMENT DEVELOPMENT

Randall S. Moore

TABLE OF CONTENTS

0-8493-7847-8/94/$0.00+$.50
© 1994 by CRC Press, Inc.

I. MANAGED CARE FOR HOME NUTRITION SUPPORT PROS AND CONS—IS IT THE WAVE OF THE FUTURE?

A. INTRODUCTION

Depending upon your worldview, we are either facing a health care crisis or the most exciting era of opportunity medicine has ever experienced. Modern health care has focused on the ability of complex technologies to eradicate acute disease states. Policy makers now struggle with the issue of continuing to improve our ability to treat illness, at the same time controlling the associated costs, now in excess of 14% of our gross national product. To meet the health care reform needs of the 1990s, we must develop and advance the tools that will result in the ability to continuously improve our ability to deliver the right care to the right patient at the right time. Nowhere is this more true than for the health professionals involved in the delivery of home nutrition support.

The nutrition support community must expand its responsibility to address issues beyond providing nutrition support resources to the individual patient. The nutrition community has demonstrated its capability of supporting the short-bowel patient outside the hospital, with most patients able to return to a fully functional life. However, gross system deficiencies continue to be present. Individual practice variation is large. There is an information deficit, including a lack of consistently applied standards, practice guidelines, critical pathways, and associated patient outcome and costs. Medical education in home care ranges from limited to nonexistent. Finally, there is not a research structure or environment to facilitate the type of national research that must be done to correct the above deficiencies. The nutrition support community must come together to rectify the current delivery system deficits.

This chapter examines the cultural underpinnings which have significantly shaped the delivery system for home parenteral and enteral nutrition (HPEN). Examination of the issues surrounding HPEN's evolution, current capabilities and practices, as well as the socioeconomic pressures affecting its delivery, will answer the question posed in the title of this chapter. Unlike a traditional medical science text, this chapter doesn't review extensive data because it doesn't exist. Rather, the goal is to challenge you to identify improvements necessary to the delivery of health care. The medical community must refocus its resources and expertise to improve the quality, efficiency, and value of our delivery systems. The sooner changes occur, the better.

1. Traditional Medical Care Delivery Failure in the 1990s

The traditional medical care delivery paradigm is failing. Scientific paradigms help us map out, understand, and explain our view of the world. They provide a frame of reference, a given set of values, rules or thought processes that govern our perception, interpretation, and subsequent intervention addressing a given problem or situation.

Until now, our country's health care paradigm supported the evolution of medicine toward discovery of high-tech, resource-intensive solutions to treating acute disease processes. Cost generally was not a significant factor, as access to the latest technology was a right of everyone covered by health insurance. Medicine was an art as much as a science. The ability and quality of the individual health care professionals or providers was always assumed to be equal. Thus, there was little or no need to demonstrate quality in a measurable, let alone understandable, form.

Because of the absence of measurements of quality, health care providers have been free to add or delete technologies/services as they saw fit. As prices were lowered in a competitive market, providers have lowered costs, or increased units of utilization, to maintain current revenue levels. In essence, health care reimbursement policy has financially rewarded consumption with little regard to outcome or quality of care. By basing compensation on units of treatment purchased, perverse reimbursement mechanisms undermine the point of health care, which is to provide efficacious therapy obtaining the best clinical results as soon as possible.

The result is rapid health care inflation in a setting where the purchasers of health care can no longer afford to pay for it. Attempts to rein in health care costs have been unsuccessful variations on a theme of controlling the price of units of health care. Instead, expanded uses and new technology development have continued to drive health care inflation. The lack of measurement techniques to assess quality appropriateness or value has led to an inability to find out if the increased utilization of current or new health care units produces measurable impact on the health status of our population. In light of a changing cultural expectation, the paradigm which previously governed the delivery of modern health care is rapidly failing.

New paradigms cannot be embraced until we let go of the old. Those who have spent their career working within a paradigm are often unable to change their frame of reference and struggle as they continue to attempt to solve problems and answer questions through the old paradigm that shaped their thinking and careers. Leadership in a nutrition support community must seize the current opportunity to evolve to a new paradigm that reorganizes available resources to develop the necessary patient management tools and systems to move forward.

The art of medicine must be evolved to the science of medicine. Individual practice variations must be controlled through the application of standards, clinical practice guidelines, critical pathways, related outcome data and analysis, and clinical research. Clinical outcome data must be linked to financial data. The medical record must be automated and standardized, such that the same condition, described by two independent practitioners, is described in the same way and that such information is extractable for automated analysis. HPEN patients should have access to centers which can cost efficiently apply the necessary resources to optimize individual patient outcomes while aggregating data for the evolution of care across broader populations. Reimbursement policy must evolve to risk sharing among all parties in the health care system, so financial compensation is tied to the desired outcome, rather than to units of health care consumed. Finally, the new paradigm must support an education system for home care.

The following case presentation and study demonstrates deficiencies within the current delivery system and opportunities for evolving the HPEN delivery system.

a. Case Presentation

A 42-year-old woman was referred to a major teaching institution for surgical takedown of her ileostomy. Despite a 15-year history of Crohn's disease and 7 previous surgeries resulting in 3 ft of remaining small bowel, she was actively employed, supporting her disabled husband and 2 children. Her last surgery, 8 months before admission, resulted in a revision of her ileostomy and an open, nonhealing wound at the site of her previous ileostomy. She was discharged home on a clear liquid diet with instructions to advance to normal feeding as tolerated.

Over the initial 2 months, she was able to advance her diet to what she described as nearly continuous eating. She lost between 6 to 10 L of fluid daily from her ileostomy. Despite a very large caloric intake, she lost 20 lb and showed no evidence of healing her 3×6-in abdominal wound, open to the level of her peritoneum. In addition, she was developing multiple new signs and symptoms of malnutrition with progressive morbidity. Symptoms included an inability to heal wounds, diffuse xerosis, severe alopecia, proximal muscle weakness with deep pain, severe recurrent muscle spasms, decreased night vision, easy bruising, and sore mouth and tongue.

She saw 10 physicians to evaluate her symptoms, emphasizing, ''I think I'm starving to death.'' Only one surgeon recognized that, despite her underlying obesity, she indeed might have short-bowel syndrome resulting in significant malnutrition. He, therefore, started her on a standard total parenteral nutrition formula and sent her home for several weeks of HPN with plans to bring her back for surgical closure of her abdominal wound. Continued weight loss lead to progressively increasing the volume of her HPN, resulting in a final prescription of 3 L daily of A4.25%, D25%, and standard electrolytes and additives, with 500cc 20% lipid TIW.

During her 4.5-month course of HPN, she was hospitalized 3 times. The first hospitalization was unsuccessful in closing her wound. She was hospitalized shortly thereafter for hyperosmolar syndrome with a glucose level of 900, requiring an intensive care admission. She survived this hospitalization only to be admitted 2 weeks later with a candidemia, most likely hyperglycemia-induced complement and leukocyte dysfunction.

Despite continued HPN, progressive disability occurred with health care expenses exceeding $250,000. Consensus at a care conference was that current efforts were futile. HPN was discontinued after a net weight loss of 60 lbs.

Now 8 months after her last bowel resection, 2 months off TPN, an 80-lb weight loss, and a multitude of symptoms, her new internist referred her for potential surgery and further evaluation. A nutrition consult was obtained from an integrated nutrition support team.

Her evaluation revealed severe malnutrition, with multiple specific nutrient deficiencies. In addition to general severe protein-calorie malnutrition, she had clinically significant deficiencies of magnesium, zinc, selenium, chromium, iron, vitamins D, K, A, and several B vitamins. Large baseline nutritional deficits and ongoing ileostomy losses had previously resulted in continued micronutrient deficiencies and lack of response to a standard TPN solution. She was now bedridden and in constant pain, with assistance needed to use the bedside commode to keep her from passing out.

Despite failing 4.5 months of HPN, it was felt that correcting the specific nutrient deficiencies would not only reverse all of her symptoms, but might allow oral or enteral nutrition to be utilized. Within 7 to 10 days of peripheral IV vitamin and mineral replacement, most of her symptoms had resolved, with her 8-month-old open abdominal wound granulating well. The decision to begin HPN was made at that time with plans to reevaluate for possible surgical reanastomosis of her ileum to her colon, granting the patient's main wish to be relieved of her ileostomy.

After 1 month on HPN and a short-bowel diet, the patient returned with marked improvement. On a short-bowel diet and HPN, her ileostomy losses were decreased to 1 to 2 L/d. Functionally improved, she was able to walk about a mile per day. A colonoscopy revealed active Crohn's disease in her proximal colon, necessitating further treatment prior to her surgery. She returned 1 month later and underwent successful reanastomosis of her ileum and colon, closure of all wounds, and stool output decreased to 3 semiformed stools per day. She was able to be discharged on an oral diet with simple vitamin and mineral supplements. She has been able to remain off of TPN for over 3 years, without any rehospitalizations.

b. Case Review

The case points out several issues. *Many physicians lack the ability to recognize or appropriately treat complicated malnutrition.* A complete nutrition support team was able appropriately to recognize, assess, prescribe, monitor response, adjust the prescription to changing needs, and attain an outcome that was both dramatically improved and consumed far fewer health care resources than when the team was not involved. Despite significantly worse malnutrition, the nutrition support trained physician and team rapidly corrected each of her deficiencies. Her prescription was continuously modified, changing individual nutrient amounts to meet her changing needs. Her diet was significantly altered, resulting in much less nutrient loss through her ileostomy. She was closely monitored, with any lack of response resulting in an evaluation and correction. Close contact was maintained at all times to help ensure the very important compliance with her therapy.

Equally obvious from the case is the requirement for further education of the decision makers in the marketplace. Physicians, payers, and case managers had each lacked the knowledge to apply the right resources to the patient to result in an expected and desirable outcome. The people that are determining health care policy must know the resource requirements, demand outcome data, require continuous quality improvement, and change reimbursement policy from paying for consumption to rewarding a desired outcome.

Reimbursement issues warrant further discussion. Before the nutrition support team made the appropriate interventions, over a quarter of a million dollars was paid to providers, which only led to her being discharged home to die. *Ironically, a reimbursement mechanism did not exist for the nutrition support team that reversed her course and led to complete rehabilitation at a small fraction of the previous charges.* The provider and team that provided the better outcome at less overall cost, but higher per day cost, were paid significantly less than the previous providers.

Until the purchasers of health care change their expectations and align their payments with quality outcomes, cases such as this will continue to occur. Beyond case studies, the hospital literature demonstrates the need for expert teams and leveraged revenues. A review of the hospital-based outcomes further demonstrates the value of nutrition support teams.

2. Hospital Studies

Hospital studies provide substantial evidence to support the need for expert teams to avoid the types of complications, costs, and net outcomes as seen in the initial management of the case above. Table 1 reviews hospital-based studies that measured the impact nutrition support teams could have on decreasing complications relating to the delivery of nutrition support in the hospital setting. While each of the studies examined the different issues and team components, there was a uniform decrease (from 35 to 100%) in the frequency of complications encountered. Based on such studies, most hospitals developed nutrition support teams to control or assist in the delivery of hospital-based nutrition support (see Table 1).

Equivalent studies of HPEN patients do not exist. In the 1990s, the complexity of the patients cared for at home parallels that of the patients studies in the previous hospital-based environment. It is unlikely that home-based studies will ever be performed, as historical, ethical, and financial barriers exist.

Taken together, case studies and the published hospital nutrition support team research provide examples of many of the issues confronting HPEN today. The paradigm is showing both its success and failure. The success is in the ability to develop a technology that has the capability of sustaining individuals on HPEN, who previously would have died or been confined to the hospital. Beyond technology development, the paradigm has failed to encourage the development of a delivery system that ensures that the right patient receives the right therapy, managed by competent individuals, at the right time.

3. The Evolution of Home Nutrition Support

Twenty years is a relatively short period of time when one considers the evolution of home nutrition support. The first patients discharged were metabolically stable and mixed

TABLE 1
Nutrition Support Teams Decrease the Percentage of Septic, Mechanical, and Metabolic Complications

	Complication reduction rate		
Study	Septic (%)	Mechanical (%)	Metabolic (%)
Nehme[6]	95	89	72
Ryan[7]	85		
Keohane[8]	88		
Jacobs[9]	100	100	75
Faubian[10]	83		
Hickey[11]	54	35	39
Dalton[12]	45	45	26

their own standard TPN solutions at a cost of under $10,000 annually. Prescriptions were written by university physicians with an active interest in advancing knowledge in nutrition support, while supplies were provided by the respective hospital pharmacy. Geographic proximity to their local academic center allowed patients to be cared for by the nutrition support team and physician. Because total parenteral nutrition (TPN) solutions were standard, these metabolically stable patients were able to mix their own solutions at home.

The commercial development of home nutrition care led to tremendous strides in home nutrition technology, service, and support. No longer was the patient required to live in proximity to the academic center. Restricted standard TPN solutions were replaced by the ability to individually prescribe nutrients tailored for the individual patient needs. Advances in services and support, combined with the health care policy and reimbursement pressures for earlier discharge, led to patients with a higher level of acuity being discharged to home care, earlier in their recovery period, often at a greater distance from the hospital. Responsibility for the clinical care of the HPEN patient was transferred to the local physician and health care team.

While the HPEN community owes a great deal to the commercial industrial developers, we must also recognize that the commercialization followed a developmental path that correlated to reimbursement incentives, rather than a path that optimized clinical care. The academic HPEN community turned much of its attention to the pure science of nutrition and metabolism. Despite the development of patient care standards, the providers of HPEN often failed to meet the minimum standards.

Despite all of our advances, a review of the current state of the art for HPEN shows several areas can be further improved. *First,* we must apply our knowledge and experience to develop standards for practice that are universally recognized and applied. *Second,* education must go beyond the scientific HPEN community and reach the health care purchaser, to ensure an educated, informed, decision-making process for the purchase of HPEN. *Third,* providers of HPEN should be required to participate in data acquisition to enable us continually to revise our standards and evolve clinical guidelines. HPEN should be provided by professionals with advanced training and expertise, utilizing state-of-the-art knowledge and technology, continually refining standards and practice guidelines, to guarantee optimal application of this valuable, but expensive, therapy.

Value must be provided to the HPEN purchaser. Incorporation of national standards, practice guidelines, and resulting severity-adjusted outcome data must be related to the price, and value, of HPEN. In such a setting, the provider who fails to provide necessary services resulting in poor outcome would have an undesirable product. Unlike today, the provider who invests in personnel, systems, quality improvement, patient support, and research can provide enhanced value. Such value could eliminate utilization inefficiencies, decrease complications, and facilitate rehabilitation.

Understanding general consumer/purchaser dynamics can help to underscore how an unintelligent reimbursement system can exist. If a purchaser is in the market for an automobile, performance expectations, maintenance, gas mileage, comfort, etc., are readily understood by the consumer and a purchaser value assigned. Consumer "value" satisfaction results in the success or failure of an automotive company. Depending on purchaser requirements and resources, a new luxury car or a 2-year-old reliable sedan may be desirable purchases. However, a 20-year-old "heap" out of a junkyard would be unacceptable.

While expectations from your automobile are clear and measurable in most consumers' minds, health care is often a black box, and money pours in without appropriate value in return—like a black hole. In many situations, health care quality expectations are either not defined, well understood, or measurable. Sufficient data and information are not available to the consumer to utilize in setting expectations or in measuring provider performance against such expectations. Lacking such information, the market has become very inefficient, allowing the provision of poor care, that is not recognized as substandard, but results in large profits.

4. Window of Opportunity for True Managed Care

Managed care is a health care benefit system that is supposed to control the delivery of health care through setting the rules for utilization, while controlling costs through competitive bidding and optimizing resource utilization. The HMO movement that began in the early 1970s was to be the new model for improving health care status while controlling health care costs. Competing with traditional indemnity insurance, much of the HMO development led to a health care benefit system similar to traditional insurance. Through selective marketing to healthy, young, employed populations, costs were held down through relatively healthy memberships and efforts put on leveraging purchasing power to control costs. In many situations, "primary gatekeepers" were implemented, but intelligent care management systems were not developed.

True managed care must replace "managed costs". Previous focus on controlling the cost per unit of health care delivered has resulted in soaring health care costs through increased unit consumption. Mandating global budgets could, theoretically, limit health care inflation, but would create minimal incentive to improve the quality of care delivered, or increase the health status of our country. In the ideal setting, the managed care program develops the integrated delivery and information management systems that insure appropriate care. Both outcome and cost must be globally assessed in reproducible terms that are easily understood by the consumer.

The managed competition model is the latest attempt to have the market develop a true managed care product. The model requires that the government set the common rules that vertically integrated health care systems must follow, while competing with one another on an equal playing field. The key factors that differentiate this model from previous attempts at managed care are the application of common base rules combined with required outcome data. If successful, the purchaser of health care can leave a position of ignorance and enter into an efficient market, where high-quality, cost-efficient providers will be rewarded.

New market initiatives are already arising in response to the evolving health care quality paradigm. First, there is a rapid proliferation of health care purchaser cooperatives, where large groups of employers are coming together to alter the health care purchaser markets. Combining purchasing power, they are leveraging their ability to purchase *quality* health care at *reasonable* costs. Recognizing the failure of previous costs control attempts, they have turned their focus to quality measures. Previous health policy attempts to control costs have all failed to address the elusive concept of quality and have failed to control health care inflation. Long-term success in business relies on improving quality and value over time. Thus, health care providers are being asked to develop integrated systems that institute total quality improvement, with measurable improvement documented over time.

Reimbursement is being tied to outcome, and the typical 1-year contract is being lengthened to 3 years. The longer contract expands the view of the provider to longer-term outcomes, adding an incentive to provide care today that improves health status 1 to 3 years later.

Longer-term responsibility is another key component for improving care. Acute or chronic disease processes may be best treated by providing health care services in the short term, which may not economically pay off until the longer term. Preventative measures are a classic example. Longer-term contracts will reward providers who invest today to prevent long-term morbidity. Short-term (1 year) contracts can result in a disincentive to provide care components that impact global, longer-term outcome and costs.

The Pennsylvania Coronary Bypass Report[1] represents the ability to collect outcome data and impact the subsequent purchase of health care. All medical centers that perform CABG surgery in Pennsylvania are now required to participate in statewide outcomes data collection. The results of this effort are outlined in a report that gives detailed, risk-adjusted, mortality and cost data by individual surgeon, group, and institution, compared to expected results. This consumer-oriented report reveals a tenfold variation in mortality and with costs ranging from $20,000 to $80,000. More interesting is the association of high-quality outcomes with lower costs. Thus, like many other products, when all costs are considered, quality is often less expensive. There is little doubt that this type of information will alter the consumer savvy and subsequent purchasing decisions for who will deliver what health care.

5. What Is the Impact of Managed Care on HPEN Today?

Like many providers of health care, HPEN providers have been reimbursed on a fee for service based on units of products sent to patients. Initial reimbursement schedules were often based on a discount from the cost of keeping the patient hospitalized. Subsequent efforts have attempted to decrease the cost per unit of therapy, but little attempt has been made to identify the optimal clinical care guidelines that could be utilized to decrease the large variation in care that drives health care costs. With very low barriers to entry, the provider sector rapidly grew, increasing competition, resulting in more competitive bidding between HPEN providers. In an attempt to eliminate paying for wasted products, many payers have switched to per diem reimbursement systems and have aggressively bid out contracts attempting quickly to find the lowest pricing levels that providers will allow.

Accounting for less than 0.5% of the health care dollar, the purchaser of HPEN cannot afford to focus time and resources to attempt to differentiate value among providers. If providers desire purchasing to evolve beyond the cheapest price for the HPEN commodity, then the provider community must demonstrate the broader value of quality HPEN provision.

What factors need to be addressed to assess quality in alternate-site infusion therapy? Donald Berwick is a leading researcher in the area of quality in health services research. He has described four components of quality in health care: (1) efficacy of care practices or knowing what to do, (2) appropriateness of decisions or using what works, (3) execution of care or doing well what works, and (4) purpose of care or clarifying the values that tell us what we wish to do.[2] Quality and cost-effectiveness in health care must find the optimal balance between risks and benefits. In order to maximize quality and cost-effectiveness, the health care community must analyze both the structure and process of care delivery and measure the impact on outcome. For quality and cost-efficiency to be characteristic in the future delivery of alternate-site infusion services, there will need to be fundamental changes to the current delivery system. The current system fails to meet any of the four requirements.

6. Managed Care for Home Nutrition

The delivery system for home nutrition support has made great strides in the development of science and technology of nutrition support. Health care reform demands the HPEN community develop the tools that will tell us how to deliver HPEN optimally, as efficiently as possible, and only to patients that will benefit. Clinical investigators must be supported to focus on HPEN technology assessment for efficacy. New alliances must come together to aggregate patients and resources to ensure safe and effective care delivery.

II. STANDARDS AND GUIDELINES

Measurable improvements in the quality and cost-efficiency will only occur if standards of care are required and quality measurements developed. Stated differently, information on the quality of care and resulting outcomes is necessary to create appropriate and efficient care. The first step to create a system that results in an informed and efficient market is to define the minimum standards that every provider must meet or exceed.

Standards for home nutritional support are available through the American Society of Parenteral and Enteral Nutrition (ASPEN) (Table 2).[3,3a] Despite the fact that ASPEN standards are not rigorous, a very small percentage of the more than 5000 home infusion providers meets these minimal requirements. Even fewer purchasers recognize that the standards exist or incorporate them into their purchasing decisions. It is also important to recall that standards of practice define the minimum level of practice necessary to ensure safe and effective enteral and parenteral nutrition therapy.

Standards that remain internal to a society such as ASPEN do not resolve issues related to the proliferation of substandard care. Standards remain necessary, but not sufficient, to establish universal national minimum standards of practice for all providers and health care professionals. National proliferation will require acceptance and implementation by impartial, accreditation, and standard-setting agencies such as HCFA, JCAHO, CHAP, and other professional societies. Purchasers, in turn, can rely on accreditation for assurance that standards have been met.

Clinical guidelines, critical pathways, or the sequence of processes that a provider should follow in the care of the individual patient must be determined. Initially, based on consensus, expert panels should define what all would agree to be in the care pathways which should govern the application of technology, services, and monitoring for the majority of patients in a particular clinical situation. Guidelines should include, but not be limited to, patient screening, assessment, prescription parameters, monitoring, and expected outcomes. Based on such guidelines, the outcome of patients should be measured and processes evolved to further enhance the quality of care that is delivered to patient populations.

Guidelines and standards should be dynamic, not static, processes. Continuous quality improvement should result from ongoing clinical research to determine the best choice for potential interventions for a given patient at a given time. Outcome parameters must be clinically relevant. Further, providers must agree on common definitions, language, etc., so that the data and information gathered can be analyzed to facilitate the shift in

TABLE 2
American Society for Parenteral and Enteral Nutrition—Standards
for Home Nutrition Support©

Introduction	ASPEN	
Organization standards	Standard 1	Clearly identified and defined roles/responsibilities of Nutrition Support Team (NST), referring physician, and nutrition support person
	Standard 2	Written guidelines/policies/procedures for needs of home patient or patient in transition to home care
	Standard 3	Documentation of home parenteral and enteral nutrition
	Standard 4	Review, evaluation, and updating of home parenteral and enteral nutrition treatment and care plan by NST
Patient selection standard	Standard 5	Indication/contra-indications for home parenteral and enteral nutrition
Treatment plan standards	Standard 6	Determining plan of care for home parenteral or enteral patient and documentation prior to initiation of treatment
	Standard 7	Selection of route(s) to provide assessed home parenteral/enteral nutrition support
	Standard 8	Appropriateness of home parenteral or enteral formula for disease process and compatibility with other drugs/therapies
Implementation standard	Standard 9	Appropriateness of access device and infusion method
	Standard 10	Education of patient/caregiver in preparation and administration of home parenteral and enteral nutrition support
	Standard 11	Education of patient/caregiver in caring for access route
	Standard 12	Education of patient/caregiver in recognition of complications and appropriate responses
Patient monitoring standard	Standard 13	Monitoring patients for therapeutic efficacy, adverse effects, and clinical changes that may influence nutrition support
Termination of therapy standard	Standard 14	Criteria for termination of parenteral or enteral nutrition support

Adapted from the American Society for Parenteral and Enteral Nutrition Standards for Home Nutrition Support, NCP, 1992; 7(2):65–69. ASPEN does not endorse this material in any form other than its entirety. With permission.

practice from the art of medicine to the science of medicine. Additional tools that must be developed include severity scale for risk analysis and health-related quality of life measurements.[4]

The lack of standards and resulting differences in outcome can exist today because of the traditional lack of data on which purchasers could base their decisions for providers. With the exception of the Oasis database, under the direction of Dr. Lyn Howard, essentially no data for outcome research exist. This voluntary national database accounts for only 7% of the home parenteral nutrition patients and is largely skewed toward tertiary care and advance providers.[5] Providing outcome data for patients on home parenteral nutrition should become mandatory.

III. REGIONAL NUTRITION CENTERS

The health care community must come together to aggregate the resources and expertise of the appropriate physicians, provider organizations, purchasers, and patients. If the health care community is to meet the evolving demands of our society, there must be an interdependence that develops. Together, they can create an optimal system based on acceptable and testable standards and guidelines, provide ongoing outcome-oriented research, reward optimal care while discouraging poor care, be accountable for cost-efficiency, and always find better ways to care for patients.

TABLE 3
Network Leveraging

- Intellectual capacity
- Contracts (purchaser and provider)
- Database development
- Data acquisition
- Development of standards, guidelines, critical pathways
- Education support—internal and external
- General administrative functions—legal, regulatory, management information system, credentialling, etc.
- Clinical trials management support

The health care arena has already suggested a mechanism and structure optimally to guide utilization of resources in areas of high cost and/or high risk. The concept of "regional centers of excellence" has been shown to be an efficient structure in the delivery of medical care where wide variation in practice is combined with the requirement for high resource intensity and has associated large cost. Application to areas such as cardiac surgery, transplantation, and mental health have demonstrated changes in outcomes and costs. Through concentration of resources and larger patient experiences, centers of excellence can utilize top-quality information systems, clinical and operational resources, protocols, and personnel to improve patient outcomes continuously and in a cost-efficient manner. Terminology aside, it is more important to identify the components that should be developed for a regional center to care for the home parenteral and enteral nutrition patient populations.

The care of the HPEN patient requires significantly greater levels of professional and technical expertise and the aggregation of patients to maintain clinical care improvement and professional team competence and experience. The patient must remain under the care of an established nutrition support team that includes, at least, a dietitian, nurse, and pharmacist—all under physician leadership—with all team members having requisite expertise in nutrition support. A regional nutrition center clinical team should provide care to the patient, while integrating standards and clinical guidelines with outcomes measurements to continuously improve their care processes.

Standardized processes do not imply the same prescription or formula to each patient. In fact, a team would apply their scientific and clinical knowledge continually to individualize nutrition prescriptions that specifically meet the needs of each patient, based on the patient's pre-existing characteristics, ongoing disease activity, growth and rehabilitative requirements, etc. Integration of the continuous quality improvement process will enable the center's team to evolve clinical protocols. The center should also provide integration of clinical and financial information systems so that cost-efficiency models can be developed. Educational programs must be developed for internal personnel, patients, families, and the local health care community. Patient support group participation should be provided to assist the patient and family in adjusting to the demands of HPEN.

The development of a regional center is a first step to lead to a managed care system for the HPEN patient. However, the development of expert delivery systems will require the application of resources that would be too costly or inefficient to apply at the local level. Table 3 identifies areas that can be leveraged much more efficiently over an integrated network of regional centers.

Intellectual capacity for multiple teams must be leveraged to concentrate the time and specific expertise of a local professional on a specific standard or clinical pathway development. Each team can develop a state-of-the-art approach to a particular disease state. At the same time, that team continues to evolve the care for that particular patient population. If each team is following a common template in their development of their specific standards and guidelines, then those guidelines can be exchanged throughout the network to exponentially drive the knowledge base of each of the teams throughout the network.

Application of modern information technology will facilitate the collection of clinical and financial data that can be analyzed to improve the delivery processes while optimizing cost efficiencies. Centers sharing a common information platform, standards, and clinical pathways can aggregate outcome data that can achieve statistical power to perform clinical research to accelerate the evolution of care excellence. Further, many questions would be incapable of being answered without such aggregation of data. Such an integrated system can also more efficiently examine the development and introduction of new technology and products for patients throughout the network.

Education efforts should be combined to provide a setting to train future professionals in HPEN and related alternate-site health care products. Student externships and postgraduate training would be much more efficient through the aggregation of resources. Similarly, patient and community education could be significantly augmented by tapping into the expertise of professionals dedicated to teaching.

Larger networks could also leverage superior administrative support in areas such as quality assurance, regulatory affairs, purchasing and provider contracting, professional credentialing and ongoing training, operational efficiency teams, and the development of health-related quality of life and severity measurement tools. In an expanded managed care environment, networks might also integrate population-based nutrition care, from patient population screening and prevention to application of TPN.

A. WHAT BENEFITS CAN BE EXPECTED?

The potential benefits that can be expected are significant. Both immediate and long-term enhancements in care will be realized. The immediate benefit will include patient management by a multidisciplinary team, which will optimize patient assessment, therapy prescribing, monitoring, and rehabilitation potential. Ongoing expert management will assure that timely therapeutic changes are made for patients as their nutritional metabolic status evolves. The result will be more efficacious therapy, less product waste, minimization of complications, fewer and shorter hospitalizations, shorter durations of therapy, earlier transition to more cost-effective therapies, and most importantly earlier rehabilitation and return to normal productivity.

The longer-term benefits of a network of regional centers of excellence are even more important. Application of a continuous quality-proven process will assure continuous evolution of the tools available to provide care to the patient populations. Clinical questions can be prioritized and distributed throughout a network to rapidly ascertain the answers to questions that today elude us. No longer will the focus be on how to decrease the cost of providing parenteral nutrition to the HIV or oncology patient. Rather, studies will allow us to answer which patient subpopulations can benefit from the therapy and under what circumstances. In general, factors will be identified that can cause nutrition support to favor the host rather than the underlying disease process. Where current technology is not effective, the system will identify where the application of such technology is futile.

In essence, a network of regional centers can assist us in rapidly moving from the art of medicine to validated scientific clinical pathways. As the process occurs and the individual thought processes of the national experts can be refined and replicated, more of the care can be transferred to local community health care providers. Validated clinical pathways will enhance the quality that the entire medical community can provide while regional centers continue to evolve state-of-the-art care.

IV. SUMMARY

Home parenteral nutrition has undergone a dramatic evolution over a relatively short period of time. It is unfortunate that the current system is barely realizing its potential to enhance patient care while keeping cost reasonable. Although the industry has made the mistake of not demonstrating the importance of quality in the care of patients, third-party reimbursement policy has continued to make an even potentially more critical mistake by rewarding poor quality care systems with higher reimbursement amounts.

Health care purchasers must recognize the provision of product is only a small part of the larger support and service system needed to manage the care of the HPEN patient cost efficiently. The medical community must come together to create a system that leverages the resources available, creates common incentives, and rewards integrated teams that can continuously improve the quality and cost-efficiency of the care of the home nutrition support patient. The development of regional nutrition centers will allow consumers to make intelligent choices in the future application of health care dollars. Working together, the health care purchaser, professional, and provider can gather vital information, optimize patient outcome, and continually improve the care available for the future.

REFERENCES

1. Pennsylvania Health Care Cost Containment Council, *Consumer Guide to Coronary Artery Bypass Graft Surgery.* November 1992.
2. **Berwick, DM.** Health services research and quality of care: assignments for the 1990's. *Med Care,* 27:763–71, 1989.
3. American Society for Parenteral and Enteral Nutrition Guidelines for the Use of Parenteral and Enteral Nutrition in Adult and Pediatric Patients. *JPEN,* 17 (Suppl.):15A–525A, 1993.
3a. Standard for Home Nutrition Support. *ASPEN Nutritional and Clinical Practice,* 7, 65, 1992.
4. **Audet, AM, Greenfield, S, and Field, M.** Medical practice guidelines: current activities and future directions. *Ann Intern Med,* 113:709–714, 1990.
5. *Oasis Annual Report, Home Nutritional Support Patient Registry,* Oley Foundation and ASPEN, 1992.
6. **Nehme, AE.** Nutritional support of the hospitalized patient. *JAMA,* 243:1906–1908, 1980.
7. **Ryan, JA, Jr.** Catheter complications in total parenteral nutrition. *New Engl J Med,* 290:757–761, 1974.
8. **Keohane, PP.** Effect on catheter tunneling and a nutrition nurse on catheter sepsis during parenteral nutrition. *Lancet,* 2:1388–1390, 1983.
9. **Jacobs, DO.** Impact of a nutritional support service on VA surgical patients. *J Am Coll Nutr,* 311–315, 1984.
10. **Faubian, WC, Wesley, J, Khalidi, N, and Silva, J.** Total parenteral nutrition catheter sepsis: impact of the team approach. *JPEN,* 10(6):642–645, 1986.
11. **Hickey, MM.** Parenteral nutrition utilization: evaluation of an educational protocol and consult service. *JPEN,* 3:433–437, 1979.
12. **Dalton, MJ, Schepers, G, Gee, JP, Alberts, CC, Eckhouser, FE, and Kirking, DM.** Consultative total parenteral nutrition team: the effect on the incidence of total parenteral nutrition related complications. *JPEN,* 8(2):146–152, 1984.

Chapter 11

NUTRITION AND RENAL DISEASE

Mark H. DeLegge and Donald F. Kirby

TABLE OF CONTENTS

0-8493-7847-8/94/$0.00+$.50

I. INTRODUCTION

Acute and chronic renal failure are characterized by hypermetabolism, hypercatabolism, and, when prolonged, the development of protein-calorie malnutrition. In a postoperative renal failure patient population, indirect calorimetry energy expenditure measurements of 130 to 190% of predicted values have been documented.[1] Assessing the nutritional status of these patients is often difficult, although important for understanding their degree of malnutrition. Current approaches for the delivery of standard nutritional therapy are often inadequate for this complex patient population.

Historically, dietary modification has provided the focus for nutritional intervention. High-calorie, low-protein diets were developed to maximize caloric intake, yet limit protein breakdown and nitrogenous waste. This therapy was especially important before the development of effective dialysis therapy. High amounts of carbohydrates and fat were administered to patients in "protein-sparing" doses. Unfortunately, these diets were often unpalatable and associated with significant gastrointestinal (GI) symptoms. Diabetes often made serum glucose control difficult. To date, protein restriction still has a role in some patients by preventing the rapid decline of already worsening renal function. However, an adequate protein calorie intake has been found essential in preventing the development of protein-calorie malnutrition and its consequences.

In the 1950s Rose[2] and Giordono[3] published important works concerning the inability to maintain nitrogen balance in renal failure patient without the provision of essential amino acids (EAA). It was also demonstrated that gut bacteria could split urea to ammonia, thus allowing the rebuilding of nonessential amino acids (NEAA) from urea waste. This urea recycling theory led to the development of EAA diets, both orally and parenterally. However, the effectiveness of urea cycling within the body and the clinical effectiveness of an EAA diet has been controversial.[4]

More recently, technical advances have allowed the development of more aggressive nutritional support and intervention. Commercially available products are the standard enteral supplementation. Often, the coexistent anorectic effects of renal failure may require the use of a nasoenteric or percutaneous feeding tube in a properly selected population. Occasionally, co-morbid disease states, especially GI motility disease, may require the use of parenterally administered solutions.

II. MALNUTRITION IN CHRONIC RENAL FAILURE

Malnutrition is best documented in the chronically hemodialyzed population. A recent investigation noted one third of the patients in an Australian dialysis unit to be protein-calorie deficient.[5] Patients in this National Cooperative Kidney Study consumed 37% less calories than recommended and 40% less protein than recommended. In addition, it was estimated that 15 to 20% of these patients had severe muscle wasting. The severity of malnutrition was again noted during the Modification of Diet in Renal Disease study where actual energy intake was far below that prescribed.[6] The risk for malnutrition in this group accelerated as the glomerular filtration rate fell below 10 ml/min. This may be a result of the need for frequent dialysis (a catabolic process), persistent hypermetabolism, and associated anorexia. This universal and devastating problem is even better underscored by Miller et al. who noted that one third of a group of renal failure patients who underwent renal transplantation were below the fifth percentile in midarm muscle circumference preoperatively.[7] It would be unreasonable to expect this group's outcome from surgery to be comparable to a well-nourished control group. Mortality in the chronically hemodialyzed patient with moderate to severe malnutrition can be 100% greater than a population of similar patients with no evidence of significant protein-calorie malnutrition.[8]

The etiology of this malnutrition remains unclear. Multiple metabolic derangements are present; uremia is associated with generalized anorexia. Both uremia and dialysis are catabolic processes which create alterations in nutrient metabolism. These metabolic changes are superimposed on the detrimental effects of other associated, concurrent illnesses. Renal failure leads to alterations in carbohydrate, protein, lipid, mineral, vitamin, and trace element metabolism; these changes worsen with the chronic nature and severity of renal failure.

III. METABOLIC ABNORMALITIES

Urea, a product of protein metabolism, is the major nitrogenous waste produced by the body. Urea is hydrolyzed by intestinal bacteria, converted to ammonia, and converted back to urea by the liver. Urea appearance is the total amount of urea noted in all body fluids as a fraction of the total body urea production.[9] Urea and other nitrogenous wastes accumulate in the face of renal failure. Urea appearance increases as urea clearance decreases. These other nitrogenous wastes are referred to as mid-molecular molecules, which are toxic substances and can interfere with protein metabolism; they have also been postulated to interfere with glucose utilization.[10]

Amino acid patterns in chronic renal failure are similar to other chronic disease states associated with malnutrition. There is often a decreased serum concentration of tyrosine and essential and branched-chain amino acids (leucine, isoleucine, and valine).[11] There is a reduced conversion of phenylalanine to tyrosine, a decrease in phenylalanine clearance, as well as a reduction in histidine synthesis. Kopple et al. documented an improvement in nitrogen balance with histidine supplementation, confirming its essential nature in the chronic renal failure patient.[12]

The total body albumin stores are reduced, both from increased catabolism and decreased protein intake. The recommended daily protein allowance in healthy individuals is 0.8 mg/kg/d. The chronically hemodialyzed patient should receive a minimum of 1.2 g/kg/d of protein to prevent muscle wasting. Protein intake restrictions and restrictive diets complicate adequate oral intake.

Uremia results in a decrease in hepatic production of albumin and other proteins.[13] This reduction in protein synthesis may be a result of altered intrahepatic amino acid transportation secondary to concurrent insulin resistance. Muscle protein degradation is also increased, as a combination of hypermetabolism and reduced oral intake. Furthermore, it is estimated that 6 to 9 g of amino acids are lost with each dialysis treatment.[14] The majority of this protein is derived from the body cell mass (BCM). The BCM accounts for approximately 30 to 38% of total body weight and is a valid indicator of current nutritional state and nutritional health.[15] Reductions in BCM are associated with increased morbidity and mortality. This triad of reduced protein intake, reduced protein synthesis, and increased protein degradation has devastating consequences including infection, generalized weakness, and poor response to medical therapy.

Glucose intolerance is a common finding in chronic renal failure. Fasting hyperglycemia and reduced utilization of glucose in tissues are present secondary to peripheral insulin resistance[16] and increased hepatic glucose production.[17] Maximal glucose uptake and utilization, as measured in the laboratory, increase near the end of a dialysis session, suggesting a small dialyzable protein that interferes with normal glucose metabolism. The inability to utilize glucose effectively for energy usage places further pressure on protein intake to meet energy needs.

Hypertriglyceridemia is often present in chronic renal failure.[18] Triglyceride removal from the bloodstream is reduced, as is insulin-stimulated triglyceride secretion. Impaired hepatic triglyceride lipase activity reduces clearance of exogenous fats.[19] This inability to utilize fats appropriately shifts the emphasis on protein stores for daily energy requirements.

Electrolyte, mineral, and vitamin deficiency are additional complicating features of chronic renal failure. Hyperkalemia and hyperphosphatemia develop as a consequence of acidosis and reduced renal excretion; hypermagnesmia is common.[20] The kidneys are involved in the activation of vitamin D and, therefore, calcium absorption. Due to these factors, there is an increased need for dietary calcium in renal failure. The increase in plasma phosphate levels is also associated with reduced serum calcium levels. Current renal diets are often high in calcium and low in phosphorus. Failure to provide adequate dietary calcium results in hyperparathyroidism and bone destruction as skeletal calcium stores are used. Iron deficiency is common in renal failure because of reduced availability to use available iron stores based on falling erythropoietin serum concentration. The kidney is the principal site of erythropoietin production and is responsible for falling serum levels as functional kidney mass declines. Chronically uremic patients are prone to water-soluble vitamin deficiency, generally B_6, C, and folic acid. This vitamin deficiency is caused by several factors, such as poor cooking methods (boiling or soaking foods), the failing kidney's inability to reabsorb water, and concurrent medication usage interfering with intestinal absorption and metabolism of these vitamins. Prudence must be maintained in prescribing vitamin C, as it is metabolized to oxalate, which cannot be excreted by the kidney. High vitamin C intake may predispose to oxalate formation and deposition in soft tissues. The use of supplemental vitamin A is not recommended, as vitamin A and retinol-binding protein blood levels are elevated in patients with uremia. Persistently high serum vitamin A levels may lead to bone toxicity. Interestingly, zinc deficiency has been noted in some renal failure patients and is associated with sexual dysfunction and dysguesia; supplementation may be helpful, although the evidence supporting this is insufficient. Although decreased tissue levels of other trace elements has been observed in these patients, such as selenium and manganese, observed adverse clinical effects have not been ascribed to these tissue levels, and, therefore, supplementation is not warranted unless symptoms occur.

The actual energy requirements of a renal failure patient are unknown, but estimates for acute renal failure range from 40 to 50 kcal/kg/d. Monteon et al. demonstrated that patients with chronic renal failure have a basal energy requirement of 35 kcal/kg/d in order to maintain neutral nitrogen balance.[21] Dialysis is an active, energy-requiring process, further exacerbating the energy needs of the renal failure patient. Use of glucose-free dialysates causes a significant fall in blood levels of glucose, insulin, and pyruvate and creates increases in acetoacetic acid and beta-hydroxy butyrate, supporting the fact that dialysis is an active, energy-requiring process. In times of inadequate energy intake, the body turns to gluconeogenesis and glucogenolysis to meet its caloric demands. Fats and proteins become main fuel substrates, often at the expense of limited body stores.

IV. NUTRITIONAL ASSESSMENT

The nutritional assessment of the renal failure patient is difficult. Multiple parameters must be used to delineate a complete picture. Our present assessment tools are imperfect, resulting in only an approximation of the patient's nutritional health. We cannot rely upon simple observation to evaluate a patient's nutritional status. Alterations in body composition, consistent with severe lean body mass loss, may occur prior to any change in visible body habitus. A patient may be at severe risk from protein-calorie malnutrition and visually appear well. Most current research of nutritional assessment has been performed in the dialysed renal failure population.

The majority of dialysis patients have weights below normal controls.[21] Patients with weights <90% of their ideal body weight or loss of >10 lb or >10% of usual body weight over a 6-month period are considered abnormal.[22] Determining an individual's dry weight can be difficult because of large variations in dialysis methods and physician recommendation of an appropriate volume status. Trends in weight over time are more likely to define a patient's correct weight status.

Anthropometric measurement of protein muscle mass is the most commonly used tool because of its wide availability and easy applicability at the bedside. Measurements performed with special calipers, such as the triceps skinfold (TSF) and midarm muscle circumference (MAMC), provide an estimation of a patient's fat and protein stores, respectively. For hemodialysis patients, it is customary to take these measurements in the arm without vascular access. In the chronically dialyzed population, TSF measurements are consistently below the 50th percentile.[23] TSF values below the fifth percentile are associated with a protein intake <0.8 g/kg/d. Although not accepted as exact measurements, anthropometry allows a reproducible modality for following a patient's nutritional progress over time.

Serum protein markers, albumin and transferrin, remain difficult to interpret. Marked shifts in intravascular volume status impact on measurements of serum proteins. In addition, the long half-life of serum albumin (21 days) does not allow an accurate assessment of a fluctuating nutritional picture. Transferrin levels in renal failure patients and controls are similar. The reliability of this marker as a measure of nutrition is diminished by its negative correlation with a patient's iron status. Chronically hemodialyzed patients are subject to frequent blood transfusions with dramatic shifts in their total iron stores. Although transferrin's short half-life of 8 days is appealing, it has not correlated well with the "nutritional status" of chronic or critically ill patients.

Immune competence measurements via skin test antigens have been used as a measurement of a patient's nutritional state. However, they are not reliable markers in the renal failure patient.[24] Hypothetically, patients with previous reactive skin tests who develop anergy could be considered malnourished. This becomes very difficult to interpret in the face of multiple concurrent medical problems, such as infection and diabetes. Renal failure patients may also have depressed total lymphocyte counts.[25]

Dietary history has proven a poor indicator of protein-energy intake among the hemodialyzed patients.[26] Patients invariably underestimate their caloric intake when their appetite is good, and overestimate their caloric intake when their appetite is poor. Observing a patient's dietary intake in the hospitalized setting often does not give a clear picture of actual dietary habits, and attempting to train a patient to record diet at home can prove to be difficult and often misleading.

Bioelectric impedance analysis (BIA) provides another parameter for evaluating the nutritional status of the renal failure patient. This method is based on changes in the conduction of an applied electrical stimulus through body tissue. This tissue contains both intra- and extracellular fluids functioning as electrical conductors and cell membranes, which act as electrical capacitors.[27] Lean body tissue contains greater quantities of electrolytes than does fat, allowing estimation of lean body mass (LBM) from assessment of body electrical activity. Several studies have shown that BIA is a more accurate modality for determining lean body mass than those predicted from anthropometric-derived formulas.[28]

Infrared interactance, a principle based on light absorption, reflection, and near-infrared spectroscopy, accurately predicts body fat percentage. Measurements are made by applying a light beam of specific frequency, in the infrared range, to the anterior midline of the biceps, midway between the antecubital fossa and the acromion process. The amount of light absorbed by fat tissue is measurable, therefore providing a reproducible determination of fat content. This method has been compared to deuterium oxide dilution, triceps skinfold, and ultrasound and found to have similar and reproducible results.[29]

There are greater than 200 formulas predicting the energy needs of the individual patient; the Harris-Benedict equation is the most commonly used formula. This traditional equation is often inaccurate when applied to the critically ill patient.[30] This inaccuracy may lead to gross overfeeding or gross underfeeding, both associated with significant complications. Energy expenditure provides important insight into the caloric needs of a patient and can be more accurately determined by indirect calorimetry from data on gas exchange. In the steady state, the amount of oxygen consumed and carbon dioxide released is related quantitatively to the release of energy from the body. Breath analysis may be measured and analyzed via a mouthpiece or bag mask system. Resting energy expenditure may be calculated by the Weir equation $[REE = 3.9 \ (\dot{V}CO_2) + 1.1 \ (\dot{V}O_2)]$.[31]

Accurately determining protein needs is critical to the nutritional health of the renal failure patient. Because these needs may change during the progression of renal disease and the presence of concurrent illnesses, frequent reassessment is required. Nitrogen flux equations are the mainstay of determining nitrogen metabolism. The bulk waste product is urea, and by following urea concentration, we can predict dietary protein intake (DPI), protein needs, and effectiveness of dialysis.

The rise in blood urea nitrogen (BUN) between dialysis treatments is entirely a function of the protein catabolic rate (PCR). Urea is a solute which dissolves in body water and distributes itself evenly in all body compartments, thus allowing kinetic modeling formulations of protein metabolism to be accurate.[32] By standardizing the amount of dialysis treatment given to a patient and plotting the change in BUN between treatments, one can easily calculate the PCR. Manipulations of dietary protein intake can, thus, be adjusted to maximize nutritional status while monitoring the PCR. In addition, urea nitrogen appearance (UNA) formulations can be used to estimate DPI and nitrogen balance (Table 1). This formula complex allows the physician to monitor dietary compliance and understand nitrogen flux.

A comprehensive, standardized nutritional assessment can identify the patient at risk for protein-calorie malnutrition. Relying on simple visual identification for signs of malnutrition, or depending on one or two physical and/or serum protein marker measurements for delineating the patient with malnutrition, will often prove unreliable and may miss the patient with whom aggressive nutritional support would have the greatest impact. Standardizing the approach to nutritional assessment will not only allow improved patient care, but also will provide a frame of reference in which we are able to knowledgeably and scientifically approach interpretation of research specifically dealing with the impact of aggressive nutritional support in the renal failure population.

V. NUTRITIONAL INTERVENTION

A. PROTEIN RESTRICTION

The possibility of a link between diet and renal disease was first postulated in 1932 by Bischoff who concluded that nephrotoxic factors were diet induced.[33] Historically, dietary protein restriction has been used to minimize the symptoms of uremia. Investigators proposed that diet may protect the kidneys from further damage, and that dietary protein increased the workload of the kidney. In the 1970s and 1980s, numerous animal and

TABLE 1
Urea Nitrogen Appearance

1. UNA is utilized to estimate dietary protein intake and nitrogen balance.

$$UNA \ (g/d) = [UUN \ (g/d) + DUN \ (g/d) + CUP \ (g/d)]$$

UNA = Urea nitrogen appearance
UUN = Urine urea nitrogen
DUN = Dialysate urea nitrogen
CUP = Changes in body urea pool

2. CUP is accounted for by changes in the body urea pool and body weight as:

$$CUP \ (g/d) = [CW(kg) - PW(kg) \times 0.4] \times BUN_1 \ (g/L) - [PW(kg) - PW(kg) \times 0.4] \times BUN_2 \ (g/L)$$

CW = Current weight
PW = Previous weight
BUN_1 = Blood urea nitrogen at time of current weight
BUN_2 = Blood urea nitrogen at time of previous weight

3. Nitrogen balance additionally requires the calculation of NUN as:

$$NUN \ (g/d) = CW(kg) \times 0.031$$

4. The dietary protein intake (DPI) can be calculated from the following:

$$DPI \ (g/d) = [6.25 \times UNA(g/d) + NUNB(g/d)]$$

5. Nitrogen balance is subsequently calculated as:

$$NB \ (g/d) = DN \ (g/d) - UNA \ (g/d) - NUN \ (g/d)$$

NB = Nitrogen balance
DN = Dietary nitrogen

human studies were conducted with the belief that dietary protein and phosphate restriction can retard the progression of renal disease.

Zeller et al. studied the effects of a low-protein diet in 35 insulin-dependent diabetics with renal disease. A low-protein (0.6 g/kg/d), low-phosphorus (500 to 100 mg/d) diet was capable of retarding the reduction of creatinine clearance as compared to controls on an unrestricted diet.[34] This concept was confirmed by Brouhard et al. who demonstrated preservation of renal function, a reduction in albuminuria, and maintenance of functional renal reserve in patients placed on a low-protein diet (0.6 g/kg/d) as compared to controls (1.0 g/kg/d).[35] Nutritional parameters, such as dry body weight and mid-arm circumference, were examined and found not to be significantly different between groups. Ihle et al. again found a retardation in the progression of chronic renal failure of a group of patients on a protein-restricted diet as compared to controls.[36] However, a fall in body weight and quality of life in the protein-restricted group was noted. This poses a dilemma for the physician. In a selected group of patients, protein restriction seems to slow down the progression of renal disease; however, this restricted diet does not meet protein needs and may put the patient at risk for the complications of protein-calorie malnutrition. Unfortunately, the nutritional parameters examined in the above-mentioned studies and the size of the study groups do not allow any conclusion in these patient groups concerning the nutritional effects of significant protein restriction. This dilemma has led to the search for alternative methods for providing protein calories to meet minimum daily requirements of protein and caloric needs.

TABLE 2
Essential and Nonessential Amino Acids

Essential amino acids	Nonessential amino acids
Isoleucine[a]	Alanine
Leucine[a]	Arginine
Lysine[a]	Asparagine
Methionine	Aspartic acid
Phenylalanine	Cysteine
Threonine	Glutamic acid
Tryptophan	Glutamine
Valine	Glycine
	Histidine[b]
	Proline
	Serine
	Tyrosine

[a] Branched chain amino acid.
[b] May be essential in renal failure.

B. SPECIALIZED AMINO ACIDS

Essential amino acids (EAA) cannot be synthesized by man and, therefore, are required (Table 2). Nonessential amino acids (NEAA) can be synthesized by man and are not required in the diet. However, a nonessential amino acid may have very important metabolic function. Amino acid losses during dialysis are a combination of EAA and NEAA. Although there has not been shown a demonstrated survival of patients fed glucose plus EAA vs. glucose plus EAA and NEAA, in acute renal failure patients, it is believed that the utilization of a predominately EAA diet would utilize this EAA pool for energy and the formation of required NEAA and, therefore, reduce the urea waste load. This could potentially retard the need for dialysis in a chronic renal failure population. Abel et al. demonstrated a fall in serum potassium, phosphorous, and magnesium levels associated with the use of an EAA formulation in a small group of patients in acute renal failure. This phenomenon would suggest the presence of ongoing anabolism associated with intracellular protein synthesis.[37]

Amino acid patterns and nitrogen balance have been studied in numerous clinical trials. The exclusive use of an EAA solution and glucose as a parenteral mixture resulted in a significant decrease in serum NEAA concentration. Those who gained weight had increased plasma concentrations of valine, histidine, and asparagine, while those who lost weight had higher concentrations of methionine and leucine.[38] Both weight gain[39] and an improved nitrogen balance[40] have been demonstrated in patients receiving a standard amino acid mixture as compared to a restricted essential amino acid mixture. In addition, the exclusive use of an essential amino acid diet results in a significant decrease in serum glutamine levels, an important precursor of NEAA, and necessary for the maintenance of small-bowel mucosa and prevention of bacterial translocation.[41] Previous theories had suggested that the use of an EAA solution would force the production of nonessential amino acids through urea recycling by transamination of ketoacid precursors and a subsequent fall in the blood urea nitrogen and improvement in protein metabolism. This theory has been disputed by Mirtallo[40] who noted no change in the serum BUN with the use of predominately EAA infusions as compared to NEAA infusions and by Varcoe[42] who demonstrated little contribution of this urea pathway to overall protein synthesis. The latest amino acid mixture recommendations of Powers et al. include a combination of EAA and NEAA, with the BCAA containing an increased amount of valine and a decreased amount of phenylalanine and methionine.[43]

C. KETOACIDS

The feasibility of an almost protein-free diet is based on the assumption that ketoacid analogues of certain essential amino acids could be transaminated either by ammonia derived from urea hydrolysis in the gut or by ammonia derived from glutamine in the liver. This reaction would be diagramed as:

$$\alpha\text{-Ketoacid} \xrightarrow{\quad} \text{Amino acid}$$
$$NH_3$$

or

$$\alpha\text{-Ketoglutarate} \xrightarrow{\quad} \text{L-Glutamate}$$
$$NH_3$$

This premise would allow supplementation of protein needs by an almost protein-free diet, decreased production of toxic nitrogenous substances, and reduced intake of potassium and hydrogen ions. In the stressed postoperative population, it has been shown that the use of ornithine-alpha-ketoglutarate as a nutritional supplement resulted in reduced urea nitrogen excretion, improved nitrogen balance, and increased skeletal muscle protein synthesis.[44]

Barsotti et al. supplemented a very low-protein diet with a mixture of keto acids and essential amino acids in a chronic renal failure population.[45] Patients had been maintained on a low-protein (0.6 g/kg/d) diet. The keto acid-supplemented diet resulted in a decline in the rate of loss of renal function. Mitch et al. have also shown that the utilization of keto analogues in a chronic renal failure population who were on a protein-restricted diet reduced blood urea nitrogen (BUN), improved serum albumin, and improved nitrogen balance comparable to a control group on a 40 to 50 g/d protein diet.[46] However, the concept that BUN is reduced via transamination of keto acids with nitrogenous products remains unproven. Most studies have confirmed that the decrease in urea nitrogen excretion exceeded the nitrogen needed to transaminate all the ingested keto acids. Additionally, long-term improvement in morbidity and/or mortality and the clear nutritional effects of a low-protein, keto acid-supplemented diet, such as functional muscle mass, have not been determined.

In a single study comparing three different low-protein regimens, either 0.6 g/kg/d, 20 g protein supplemented with EAA, or 20 g protein supplemented with a keto acid mixture, slowing of renal function loss was seen equally on all three regimens.[47] Again, the impact on morbidity and mortality and the long-term nutritional effects of these regimens were not examined. It would be inappropriate to examine the effects of these specialized diets solely as they pertain to renal status without examining the long-term nutritional ramifications.

D. OTHER DIETARY MODIFICATIONS

Many other dietary and metabolic abnormalities are associated with renal failure. These abnormalities are a direct result of the failing kidney and often may actually contribute to the progression of renal disease. Aggressive dietary management must consider these irregularities when designing nutritional therapy.

Calcium and phosphorus homeostasis is altered as renal disease progresses, mainly secondary to impaired vitamin D metabolism. As the glomerular filtration rate (GFR) falls below 30% of normal, the phosphate excretory ability of the kidney is surpassed, and hyperphosphatemia develops.[48] The combination of elevated serum phosphate levels and reduced serum calcium levels stimulates parathyroid hormone secretion. Reductions of dietary phosphate to less than 1500 mg/d helps to reduce serum phosphate levels.

Low-phosphorus diets have been evaluated independently of protein intake with the premise that calcium-phosphate deposition in renal tissue is reduced on this diet and may reduce progression of renal disease. Results of these studies have been inconclusive. However, as protein in a diet is reduced, phosphorus is reduced and may contribute to the overall improvement in renal function.

The role of lipids in the progression of renal disease is being evaluated. Deposition of lipids in mesangial cells has been postulated as the mechanism of injury. Studies in animals have shown that lowering serum cholesterol may retard the progression of renal disease.[49] In other animal studies, high linolenic acid diets, as a precursor to arachidonic acid and prostaglandins, decrease the progression of renal disease. Prostaglandins affect both blood flow and blood pressure in the glomerulus.

Carnitine, an amino acid necessary for the transport of fatty acids into the mitochondria for oxidation, is suspected in the pathogenesis of hypertriglyceridemia and altered lipid metabolism of renal failure. Patients undergoing dialysis have evidence of carnitine deficiency. During hemodialysis, serum carnitine levels drop by up to 80%.[50] Supplementation with carnitine led to a reduced serum triglyceride level and increased serum and muscle carnitine levels. Bellinghieri et al. orally supplemented L-carnitine (2 g/d) in 14 uremic patients complaining of muscle cramps and weakness and demonstrating rapid muscular fatigue. Oral carnitine supplements increased serum and muscle carnitine levels and reduced the degree and frequency of muscle cramps and weakness.[51]

The failing kidney often has the inability to maintain the normal balance of essential nutrients. Chronic renal failure patients are prone to develop water-soluble vitamin deficiency secondary to dietary restrictions, cooking methods, reduced absorption, and concurrent medication usage, which may interfere with metabolism. Although there has not been a great deal of research on vitamin supplementation in renal failure, certain facts are well known.

Pyridoxine metabolism is abnormal in renal failure patients. Pyridoxal-5′-phosphate (PLP), the active coenzyme form of pyridoxine, has reduced plasma levels secondary to increased plasma clearance.[52] Pyridoxine supplementation of 5 to 10 mg/d effectively normalizes PLP levels. Tissue uptake and utilization of folic acid are altered because competitive inhibition of folic acid transport into cells reduces the availability of it. Also, binding of folic acid to plasma proteins is increased, reducing free folic acid levels. Unfortunately, serum folic acid levels do not accurately reflect the availability of folic acid for the tissues.[53] The combination of these difficulties requires supplementation of folic acid in 1 mg/d doses. Vitamin C is metabolized to oxalate, an insoluble compound, as its urinary excretion is depressed. The use of high doses of vitamin C has the potential for causing calcium-oxalate deposition in body tissue.[54] Vitamin C should be supplemented in the range of 60 to 100 mg/d.

Fat-soluble vitamin abnormalities also exist. Retinol-binding protein and vitamin A plasma levels are elevated secondary to reduced renal clearance and metabolism. Clinical toxicity with vitamin A has been noted even in the absence of supplementation. Toxic levels of vitamin A can cause both bone and neurologic dysfunction. The renal conversion of vitamin D to its biologically active form [$1,25(OH)_2D_3$] is reduced.[55] As a consequence, both bone disease and hyperparathyroidism are common; administration of $1,25(OH)_2D_3$ reduces hyperparathyroidism and hypophosphatemia by increasing calcium absorption. Supplementation with vitamin D must be closely monitored to prevent hypercalcemia with resultant calcium-phosphate precipitation in renal tissue. Table 3 delineates the current recommendations of vitamin supplementation in renal disease.

Blood levels of several trace elements (iron, zinc, chromium, manganese, and copper) are marginal in renal failure patients, and actual deficiencies have been reported. Protein restrictions, specifically for meat intake, limit the heme iron absorption. Concurrent antacid administration reduces iron absorption. Incorporation of iron into red blood cells is reduced because of decreased levels of erythropoietin. Zinc deficiency may be due to

TABLE 3
Vitamin Supplementation in Chronic Renal Failure

Vitamin	Recommended daily amount
Folic acid	1.0 mg/d
Pyridoxine	5–10 mg/d
Niacin	20 mg/d
Riboflavin	1.8–2.0 mg/d
Thiamin	1.5 mg/d
Vitamin A	None
Vitamin B_{12}	3–5 µg/d
Vitamin C	60–100 mg/d
Vitamin D[a]	0.25–1.0 µg/d
Vitamin E	15 IU/d
Vitamin K	None

[a] Generally required in the dialysis patient. Supplementation monitored by serum calcium levels.

dietary insufficiency, as red meats are restricted in favor of foods that have less bio-available zinc. Zinc deficiency is associated with decreased sense of taste, reduced appetite, and sexual dysfunction. Overall, the exact trace element requirement is poorly understood in this population, but recommendations are to meet suggested RDA levels.

Aluminum accumulation in the central nervous system and bony structure of renal failure patients has been reported as the etiology of encephalopathy and osteodystrophy.[56] Although small intestinal absorption of aluminum is intact, renal excretion is reduced. Citrate solubilizes aluminum facilitating its absorption and distribution throughout the body.[57] Dietary aluminum and citrate should be avoided.

Clearly, the dietary needs of each individual renal failure patient will vary. The primary goal of nutritional therapy in renal disease is to control nitrogen intake. Dietary protein restriction attempts to limit nitrogenous wastes and preserve renal function while preventing wasting of lean body mass. Recommendations for protein intake are individualized based on glomerular filtration rate, individual weight, and progression of disease (Table 4).

VI. AGGRESSIVE NUTRITIONAL SUPPORT

Correcting malnutrition and maintaining a normal nutritional state may increase survival and decrease morbidity in the renal failure patient. Poor quality of life attributed to dialysis cachexia may also be significantly improved. Patients with marginal caloric intake and borderline nutritional blood chemistries may be corrected with oral supplements.[58] Allman et al. demonstrated an increase in lean body mass and weight in a group of hemodialysis patients with marginal oral intake who were randomized to the glucose polymer, polycose.[59] This carbohydrate powder supplementation provided approximately 500 additional calories per day.

Enteral nutritional support of the renal failure patient has been hampered by the poor nutritional quality of commercially available specialized enteral formulations. They lack complete vitamin, mineral, and electrolyte fortification, have poor palatability, and are costly. Often, inappropriate quantities of protein, phosphate, and potassium made their long-term, routine use impossible. Second-generation, commercially available products have attempted to correct these deficiencies. Low-protein, calorically dense products are now available. Their caloric content is approximately 50% carbohydrate, 44% fat, and

TABLE 4
Protein Recommendation for the Renal Failure Patient

Glomerular filtration rate (GFR)	Protein restriction
>70 ml/min	None
≤70 ml/min	0.55–0.60 g/kg/d
≤30 ml/min	0.6 g/kg/d
≤20 ml/min	0.45 g/kg/d
≤5 ml/min[a]	0.40 g/kg/d

[a] As GFR falls below 5 ml/min some form of dialysis usually becomes necessary. Because of the catabolic nature of dialysis and the amino acid losses with each dialysis treatment, some form of protein replacement therapy becomes necessary. This changes protein requirements as follows:

Hemodialysis	1.0–1.2 g/kg/d
Peritoneal dialysis	1.2–1.5 g/kg/d

Concurrent medical problems, such as infection, will change both metabolic and catabolic rate, thus altering these protein restrictions.

TABLE 5
Specialized Renal Enteral Supplementation[a]

Vitamins		Minerals		Electrolytes	
Vitamin A	250 IU	Calcium	304 mg	Sodium	186 mg
Vitamin D	20 IU	Phosphorous	173 mg	Potassium	265 mg
Vitamin E	11 IU	Magnesium	100 mg	Chloride	220 mg
Vitamin K	18 μg	Iodine	37.5 μg		
Vitamin C	25 mg	Manganese	1.25 mg	**Other**	
Folic acid	250 μg	Copper	0.5 mg		
Thiamine	0.6 mg	Zinc	5.6 mg	Citrate	0.0
Riboflavin	0.7 mg	Iron	4.5 mg		
Vitamin B$_6$	2.0 μg	Aluminum	0.0		
Niacin	8.0 mg				
Choline	150 mg				
Biotin	120 μg				
Pantothenic acid	4.0 mg				

[a] Per 8 fl oz can.

6% protein. They are lactose and gluten free. Vitamin fortification includes pyridoxine, vitamin D, and folic acid, while other vitamins are provided at RDA requirements. Carnitine and taurine are also supplemented, while aluminum and citrate are avoided. Potassium, sodium, and phosphate levels are reduced, while calcium levels are fortified (Table 5). The palatability of the products has improved, and they are able to provide all of the patient's nutritional needs in approximately one liter per day. Cost remains an important and limiting factor.

The anorectic effect of medications, depression, immobility, anorexia of chronic illness, taste dysfunction, or true GI disease, which prevents nutrient absorption, often precludes enteral supplementation.[60] Altered intestinal absorption of nutrients has been documented in uremia.[61] The placement of a nasogastric tube is poorly tolerated and is

TABLE 6
Sample IDPN Solution

Solution	%	Grams	Volume	kcal
Dextrose	50	100	200 cc	340
Amino acids	10	60	600 cc	240
Lipids	20	40	200 cc	400

Note: Total volume = 1000 cc; total calories = 980 kcal; total protein = 60 gm. Frequent additives: folic acid, sodium chloride, vitamin C, and vitamin B_{12}.

associated with the risk of aspiration. Placement of a percutaneous endoscopic gastrostomy tube (PEG) is contraindicated in the peritoneal dialysis patient. Although there is no contraindication to the use of a PEG in a hemodialysis population, there is no large randomized trial to support its use in the malnourished hemodialysis patient who has failed oral enteral supplementation.

A. INTRADIALYTIC PARENTERAL NUTRITION

Intradialytic parenteral nutrition (IDPN) provides another modality for delivery of nutrients in a manner which bypasses the alimentary tract. IDPN is defined as the infusion of amino acids, glucose, and fats during hemodialysis. Abel et al. first reported increased survival in patients with acute renal failure given total parenteral nutrition (TPN).[62] Heiland and Kult subsequently demonstrated that patients given essential amino acids and carbohydrates over the last 90 min of dialysis significantly increased their levels of total protein, albumin, transferrin, and complement.[63] The efficacy of IDPN has been verified by a >90% retention of infused amino acids, in addition to regained strength and appetite among patients given a dextrose, lipid, and amino acid admixture during dialysis.[64] This amino acid retention was later confirmed by a separate group who infused a dextrose and amino acid mixture to eight end-stage renal failure patients.[38] Olshan et al. also infused a combination of amino acids, dextrose, and fats to a group of 10 end-stage renal failure patients over 6 months. The majority of these patients experienced weight gain and improved appetites. Adverse effects were limited to nausea and flushing with intralipid infusion. No patients experienced significant hyperglycemia, post-transfusional hypoglycemia, or electrolyte imbalance.[65]

IDPN provides only supplemental calories for the patient. With a dialysis regime of 3 times a week, the patient receives, on the average, 430 kcal/d and 26 g protein/d (Table 6). However, anecdotal experience has noted a concurrent increase in the appetite of patients placed on IDPN, perhaps due to their improved well-being from the additional caloric source. IDPN is not appropriate for the patient who has no enteral intake. That particular patient group should be treated with total parenteral nutrition via central access, as they are totally dependent on their parenteral therapy to meet all their caloric and protein needs.[54]

Originally, there were concerns with the use of fats as a caloric source for IDPN. Lipid metabolism is altered in renal failure secondary to an impairment of lipolysis. Parenteral lipid emulsions mainly consist of long-chain triglycerides. Medium-chain triglycerides have theoretical advantage over long-chain triglycerides as an energy source in the renal failure patient, as their transport into the mitochondria is independent of carnitine, a transport protein which is often present in low concentrations in this population. However, recent information has determined that the elimination of long-chain triglycerides is no different from medium-chain triglycerides in the chronic renal failure patient.[66] Experience has proven that the presence of mildly impaired lipid metabolism does not preclude lipid usage in IDPN. In addition, previous concerns that lipids would clog dialysis membranes have proven unfounded. The use of fats as a primary energy source can minimize the complications of carbohydrate infusion, including hyperglycemia and CO_2 production, and provide a significant calorie source in a small volume of fluid.

IDPN solutions are devoid of vitamins. A standard i.v. multivitamin formula is not appropriate for a chronic renal failure patient. Significant losses of the B vitamins, folic acid, and vitamin C occur, and these should be replenished. Vitamin A supplementation is contraindicated, as previously discussed. Concerns with magnesium, calcium, and phosphorus necessitate careful attention. Addition of electrolytes to the IDPN solution is generally avoided, as the dialysis bath can be adjusted to meet the patient's needs.

B. TOTAL PARENTERAL NUTRITION

Total parenteral nutrition (TPN) regimes necessitate careful monitoring of the renal failure patient. A combination of essential and nonessential amino acids should be used in the chronic dialysis population. Hypertonic dextrose solutions (70%) are the preferred source for the bulk of caloric requirement. Glucose intolerance can be treated with addition of insulin to the parenteral solution. Lipid solutions (20%) can be used to administer up to one third of the daily caloric intake. Vitamins and electrolytes have been previously discussed and are tailored to meet the patient's individual needs. The maintenance of fluid balance in the oliguric renal failure patient is important in view of the large volumes of fluid required to meet the patient's caloric and protein needs. Dialysis time may need to be increased, and time between dialysis treatments may need to be reduced. In the intensive care setting, slow continuous ultrafiltration (SCUF) or continuous arterial hemofiltration (CAH) may be utilized to produce a continuous ultrafiltrate across a hemodialysis membrane without utilizing a dialysate; large volumes of fluid can be continuously removed. Paganini administered amino acids via a subclavian catheter to patients receiving SCUF and noted that 90% of the nutrients were retained.[67] Conversely, continuous arteriovenous hemodialysis (CAVHD) does utilize a dialysate. The dialysate is continuously supplied at flow rates of approximately 50 ml/h. This technique permits the administration of nutrients across the dialysis membrane. At low-flow rates, nutrients can be effectively taken up across the dialysis membrane. Feinstein et al. used a 5% dextrose and 0.4% amino acids solution with CAVHD, obtaining 78% absorption of nutrients.[68] CAVHD has been coined "nutritional hemodialysis" or "machineless hemodialysis", as it permits the administration of glucose and amino acids without a central venous catheter.

The ultimate goal is to provide the renal failure patient with the calories and protein required. A stepwise, aggressive nutritional approach should be instituted. This would involve global nutritional assessment, dietary modifications, enteral supplementation, and, if required, parenteral therapy.

VII. PERITONEAL DIALYSIS

Peritoneal dialysis can result in significant protein losses into the dialysate. Stable ambulatory peritoneal dialysis patients may lose 10 to 15 g/d. These losses may accelerate to 40 g/d in the patient with peritonitis. This continual drain on protein sources, combined with the aforementioned difficulties with adequate nutrition in the renal failure population, places the chronic ambulatory peritoneal dialysis (CAPD) patient at risk for the significant complications associated with protein-calorie malnutrition. Dietary protein recommendations are 1.2 to 1.5 g/kg/d, which should be adjusted for additional protein losses associated with episodes of peritonitis or other concurrent illnesses.

The peritoneal dialysate provides significant caloric intake. Patients currently absorb 60 to 80% of the dialysate glucose. This may provide 1000 to 3000 kcal/d.[69] Chronic ambulatory peritoneal dialysis containing 1 to 2% amino acids instead of glucose has been well tolerated.[70] Nutrineal® is a new peritoneal dialysate product, which provides amino acids as the osmotic source. The premise of this formulation is to provide actual protein calories across the peritoneal membrane while reducing peritoneal dialysis protein losses and avoiding the complications of the absorption of a large glucose load. This product is under intense investigation.

VIII. NEPHROTIC SYNDROME

The nutritional effects of nephrotic syndrome are secondary to hypoalbuminemia and hypercholesterolemia. The hypoalbuminemia is secondary to large urinary excretion of albumin based on a change in the charge characteristics of the glomerular membrane. Cholesterol levels are inversely proportional to the albumin levels. Previously, the standard recommendation for patients with nephrotic syndrome was a high-protein diet. Recently, Kaysen evaluated the use of a low-protein diet in this patient population.[71] Although albumin synthesis was less on the low-protein diet, this was more than compensated for by the reduction in albuminuria and albumin catabolism. Recommendations currently are to provide the patient with 0.6 g/kg/d of protein plus 1.0 g/d for each gram of protein lost in the urine.

IX. SUMMARY

Malnutrition is a serious problem for many patients who also suffer from chronic renal failure. Virtually every study that has assessed the nutritional status of these patients has concluded that there is a significant combination of protein depletion and muscle wasting. Assessing these nutritional needs and attempting to delineate who is at risk for protein-calorie malnutrition takes an aggressive, detailed approach to nutritional assessment.

The use of protein restriction retards the progression of renal disease. The utilization of essential amino acids and keto analogues of essential amino acids, as protein sources, may also retard the progression of renal disease. However, there is limited data with any of these dietary modifications with reference to their effect on morbidity, mortality, and long-term nutritional parameters. There are a number of enteral supplements on the commercial market specifically designed for the renal failure patient. These products can often aid in providing additional calories to a borderline malnourished patient. Their use may be limited by palatability and cost.

Dietary regimens and enteral therapy may prove ineffective in correcting malnutrition secondary to patient intolerance or poor absorption and utilization of enteral nutrients. In these patients, IDPN provides a safe and efficient method of providing supplemental nutrients. Significant amounts of proteins, fats, and carbohydrates can be delivered, while fluid overload is prevented by concurrent dialysis. However, the cost/benefit of this therapy has not been adequately assessed. Peritoneal dialysis patients can be supplemented across the peritoneal membrane by dextrose calories, and hopefully in the future, by protein calories.

Appropriate and timely nutritional intervention is extremely important in the renal failure population. Addressing the nutritional needs of individual renal failure patients will provide significant impact on their quality of life, morbidity, and mortality.

REFERENCES

1. **Compher, C, Mullen, JL, and Barker, CF.** Nutritional support in renal failure. *Surg Clin N Am,* 71:597–608, 1991.
2. **Rose, WC, Coon, MJ, and Lambert, GF.** The amino acid requirements of man: the role of lysine, arginine and tryptophan. *J Biol Chem,* 206:421–430, 1954.
3. **Giordono, C.** Use of exogenous and endogenous urea for protein synthesis in normal and uremic subjects. *J Lab Clin Med,* 62:231–246, 1963.
4. **Kopple, JD and Swenseid, M.** Amino acid and keto acid diets for therapy in renal failure. *Nephron,* 18:1–12, 1977.
5. **Shonfield, PY, Henry, RR, Laird, NM, and Roxe, DM.** Assessment of the nutritional status of the national cooperative dialysis study population. *Kidney Int,* 23:580–588, 1983.
6. **Kopple, JD, Berg, R, Houser, H, et al.** Nutritional status of patients with different levels of chronic renal insufficiency. *Kidney Int,* 36:S184–S194, 1989.
7. **Miller, DG, Levine, SE, D'Elia, JA, and Bistrian, BR.** Nutritional status of diabetic and nondiabetic patients after renal transplantation. *Am J Clin Nutr,* 44:66–69, 1986.
8. **Bibrey, GL and Cohen, TL.** Identification and treatment of protein calorie malnutrition in chronic hemodialysis patients. *Dial Transpl,* 18:669–677, 1989.
9. **Bergstrom, J, Assaba, H, and Furst, T.** Middle molecules uremia. In: *Proc 6th Int Cong Nephrol.* Giovannetti, S, Bonomini, V, and D'Amico, G. Eds. New York, 1976, pp 600–611.
10. **Kennedy, A and Burton, J.** Factors affecting prognosis in acute renal failure. *Q J Med,* 42:73–86, 1973.
11. **Furst, P, Alvestrand, A, and Bergstrom, J.** Effects of nutrition and catabolic stress on intracellular amino acid pools in uremia. *Am J Clin Nutr,* 33:1387–1395, 1980.
12. **Kopple, JD and Swenseid, ME.** Evidence that histidine is an essential amino acid in normal and chronically uremic man. *J Clin Invest,* 55:881–891, 1975.
13. **Grossman, SB, Yap, SH, and Shafritz, DA.** Influence of chronic renal failure on protein synthesis and albumin metabolism in the rat liver. *J Clin Invest,* 59:869–878, 1977.
14. **Young, GA and Parsons, FM.** Plasma amino acid imbalance in patients with chronic renal failure on intermittent dialysis. *Clin Chem,* 27:491–496, 1970.
15. **Moore F.** Energy and the maintenance of body cell mass. *JPEN,* 4:228–260, 1980.
16. **Defronzo, RA, Alverstrand, A, Smith, D, et al.** Insulin resistance in uremia. *J Clin Invest,* 67:563–568, 1981.
17. **Wilmore, DW, Goodwin, GW, Aulick, LH, et al.** Effect of injury and infection on visceral metabolism and circulation. *Ann Surg,* 192:490–503, 1980.
18. **Takala J.** Nutrition in acute renal failure. *Crit Care Clin,* 3:155–166, 1987.
19. **Druml, W. Laggner, A, Wildham, K, et al.** Lipid metabolism in acute renal failure. *Kidney Int,* 24:S139–S142, 1983.
20. **Kopple JD.** Nutritional therapy in kidney failure. *Nutr Rev,* 39:193–206, 1981.
21. **Monteon, FJ, Laidlaw, SJ, Shaib, JK, and Kopple, JD.** Energy expenditure in patients with chronic renal failure. *Kidney Int,* 30:741–747, 1986.
22. **Horl, WH, Riegel, W, and Schollmeyer, P.** Mechanisms of abnormal carbohydrate metabolism in uremia. *Contrib Nephrol,* 1:188–202, 1986.
23. **Kopple, JD and Swendseid, ME.** Protein and amino acid metabolism in uremic patients undergoing maintenance hemodialysis. *Kidney Int,* 7:S64–S72, 1975.
24. **Bansal, VK, Popli, S, Pickering, J, and Vertuno, LL.** Protein-calorie malnutrition and cutaneous anergy in hemodialysis maintained patients. *Am J Clin Nutr,* 33:1608–1611, 1980.
25. **Mattern, WD, Hak, LJ, Lamanna, RW, et al.** Malnutrition, altered immune function and the risk of infection in maintenance hemodialysis patients. *Am J Kid Dis,* 1:106–118, 1982.
26. **Fidanza, F.** Sources of error in dietary servings. *Bull Nutr Diet,* 20:108–110, 1974.
27. **Lukaski, HF, Johnson, PE, Bolonchuk, WW, and Lykken, GI.** Assessment of fat-free mass using bioelectric impedance of the human body. *Am J Clin Nutr,* 41:810–817, 1985.
28. **Lukaski, HF, Bolonchuk, WW, Hall, CA, and Spiders, WP.** Estimate of fat-free mass in humans using bioelctric impedance method: a validation study. *J Appl Physiol,* 60:1327–1332, 1986.
29. **Conway, JM, Norris, KH, and Bodwell, CE.** A new approach for the estimation of body composition. Infrared interactance. *Am J Clin Nutr,* 40:1123–1130, 1984.
30. **Makk, LJH, McClave, SA, Creech, PW, et al.** Clinical application of the metabolic cart to the delivery of total parenteral nutrition. *Crit Care Med,* 18:1320–1327, 1990.
31. **Weir, SB.** New methods of calculating metabolic rate with special preference to protein metabolism. *J Physiol,* 109:1–9, 1949.

32. **Sargent, JA.** Kinetic modeling in the guidance of dialysis therapy. *Dial Transpl,* 8:1101–1110, 1979.
33. **Bischoff, F.** The influence of the diet on renal and blood vessel changes. *J Nutr,* 5:431–450, 1932.
34. **Zeller, K, Whittaker, E, Sullivan, L, et al.** Effect of dietary protein on the progression of renal failure in patients with insulin-dependent diabetes mellitus. *N Engl J Med,* 324:78–83, 1991.
35. **Brouhard, BH and Lagrone, L.** Effect of dietary protein restriction on functional renal disease in diabetic nephropathy. *Am J Med,* 89:427–431, 1990.
36. **Ihle, BU, Becker, GJ, Whitworth, JA, et al.** The effect of protein restriction on the progression of renal disease. *N Engl J Med,* 321:1773–1777, 1989.
37. **Able, RM, Abbott, WM, and Fischer, JE.** Intravenous essential L-amino acids and hypertonic dextrose in patients with acute renal failure. *Am J Surg,* 123:632–638, 1972.
38. **Piraino, AS, Firpo, JJ, and Power, DV.** Prolonged hyperalimentation in catabolic chronic dialysis patients. *JPEN,* 5:463–477, 1981.
39. **Young, G, Swanepool, CR, Croft, MR, et al.** Anthropometry and plasma valine, amino acids and proteins in the nutritional assessment of hemodialysis patients. *Kidney Int,* 21:492–499, 1982.
40. **Mirtallo, JM, Schneider, PJ, Mavkok, AJ, and Roberg, RL.** A comparison of essential and general amino acid infusions in the nutritional support of patients with compromised renal function. *JPEN,* 6:108–113, 1982.
41. **Kopple, JD, and Swenseid, ME.** Nitrogen balance and plasma amino acid levels in uremic patients fed an essential amino acid diet. *Am J Clin Nutr,* 24:806–812, 1974.
42. **Varcoe, R, Halliday, D, Carson, ER, et al.** Efficiency of utilization of urea nitrogen for albumin synthesis of chronically uremic and normal man. *Clin Sci Mol Med,* 38:379–390, 1975.
43. **Powers, DV, Jackson, A, and Piriano, AJ.** Prolonged intradialysis hyperalimentation in chronic hemodialysis patients with an amino acid solution (Renamin [amino acid] injection) formulated for renal failure. In: *Perspectives in Clinical Nutrition,* Kinney, JM and Borum, PR, Eds. Urban and Schwarzenberg, Baltimore-Munich, 1989, pp 191–203.
44. **Wernerman, J, Hammarqvist, F, von der Decken, A, and Vinnars, E.** Ornithine-alpha-ketoglutarate improves skeletal muscle protein synthesis as assessed by ribosome analysis and nitrogen use after surgery. *Ann Surg,* 206:674–678, 1987.
45. **Barsotti, G, Guiducci, A, Ciardella, F, and Giovanetti, S.** Effects on renal function of a low-nitrogen diet supplemented with essential amino acids and ketoanalogues of hemodialysis and free protein supply in patients with chronic renal failure. *Nephron,* 19:773–778, 1981.
46. **Mitch, WE, Abras, E, and Walser, M.** Long-term effects of a new ketoacid-amino acid supplement in patients with chronic renal failure. *Kidney Int,* 22:48–53, 1982.
47. **Vetter, K, Froehling, PT, Kashube, I, et al.** Influence of ketoacid treatment on residual renal function in chronic renal insufficiency. *Kidney Int,* 24:S350–S351, 1983.
48. **Bricker, NS.** On the pathogenesis of the uremic state: an exposition of the "trade-off hypothesis." *N Engl J Med,* 286:1093–1099, 1972.
49. **Klar, S, and Harris, K.** Role of dietary lipids and renal eicosanoids on the progression of renal disease. *Kidney Int,* 29:579–587, 1989.
50. **Bertoli, M, Battistella, PA, Vergani, L, et al.** Carnitine deficiency induced during hemodialysis and hyperlipidemia: effect of replacement therapy. *Am J Clin Nutr,* 34:1496–1500, 1981.
51. **Bellinghieri, G, Savica, V, Mallamace, M, and Distefano, C.** Correlation between increased serum and tissue L-carnitine levels and improved muscle symptoms in hemodialysis patients. *Am J Clin Nutr,* 38:521–531, 1983.
52. **Spannuth, CL, Jr., Warnock, LG, Wagner, C, and Stone, WJ.** Increased plasma clearance of pyridoxal-5'-phosphate in vitamin B_6-deficient uremic man. *J Lab Clin Med,* 90:632–637, 1977.
53. **Jennette, JC, and Goldman, JD.** Inhibition of membrane transport of folates by anions retained in uremia. *J Lab Clin Med,* 86:834–843, 1975.
54. **Blacke, P, Schmidt, P, Zazgornik, J, et al.** Ascorbic acid aggravates secondary hyperoxalemia in patients on chronic hemodialysis. *Ann Intern Med,* 101:344–345, 1984.
55. **Baker, LRI, Abrams, SML, Roe, CJ, et al.** $1,25(OH)_2D_3$ administration in moderate renal failure: a prospective double-blind trial. *Kidney Int,* 35:661–669, 1989.
56. **Martin, RB.** The chemistry of aluminum as related to biology and medicine. *Clin Chem,* 32:1797–1806, 1986.
57. **Slanina, P, Frech, W, Ekstrom, L-G, et al.** Dietary citric acid enhances absorption of aluminum in antacids. *Clin Chem,* 32:539–554, 1986.
58. **Evans, RW, Mannisen, DL, Garrison, LP, et al.** The quality of life of patients with end stage renal disease. *N Engl J Med,* 312:553–559, 1985.
59. **Allman, MA, Stewart, PM, Tiller, DJ, et al.** Energy supplementation and the nutritional status of hemodialysis patients. *Am J Clin Nutr,* 51:558–562, 1990.
60. **Foulks, C.** Nutritional evaluation of patients on maintenance dialysis therapy. *ANNA J,* 15:13–17, 1988.

61. **Wizemann, V, Kuhl, LR, and Burgmann, I.** Digestive-absorptive function of the intestinal brush border in uremia. *Am J Clin Nutr,* 31:1642–1646, 1978.

62. **Abel, RM, Beck, CH, Jr., Abbott, WM, et al.** Improved survival and acute renal failure after treatment with L-essential amino acids and glucose. *New Engl J Med,* 288:695–699, 1973.

63. **Heidland, A and Kult, J.** Long term effects of essential amino acid supplementation in patients on regular dialysis treatments. *Clin Nephrol,* 3:234–239, 1975.

64. **Woolfson, M, Jones, M, and Kopple, JD.** Amino acid losses during hemodialysis with infusion of amino acids and glucose. *Kidney Int,* 21:500–506, 1982.

65. **Olshan, AR, Bruce, JB, and Schwartz, AB.** Intradialytic parenteral nutrition administration during outpatient dialysis. *Dial Transplant,* 10:495–496, 1987.

66. **Druml, W, Fischer, M, Sertl, S, et al.** Fat elimination in acute renal failure: long-chain vs. medium-chain triglycerides. *Am J Clin Nutr,* 55:468–472, 1992.

67. **Paganini, EP, O'Hara, P, and Nakamoto, S.** Slow continuous ultrafiltration in hemodialysis-resistant oliguric acute renal failure patients. *Trans Am Soc Artif Int Organs,* 30:173–177, 1984.

68. **Feinstein, EI, Collins, JF, and Blumenkrantz, MJ.** Nutritional hemodialysis. In: *Progress in Artificial Organs,* Atsumi, K, Maekawa, M, and Ota, K. Eds. ISAO Press, Cleveland, 1984, pp 421–427.

69. **Anderson, G, Berquist-Poppen, M, Bergstrom, J, et al.** Glucose absorption from the dialysis fluid during peritoneal dialysis. *Scan J Urol Nephrol,* 5:77–85, 1971.

70. **Arfeen, S, Goodship, T, Kirkwood, A, et al.** The nutritional/metabolic and hormonal effects of 9 weeks continuous ambulatory peritoneal dialysis with 1% amino acid solution. *Clin Nephrol,* 33:192–199, 1990.

71. **Kaysen, GA, Gambertoglio, J, Kimenez, I, et al.** Effect of dietary intake on albumin homeostasis in nephrotic patients. *Kidney Int,* 29:572–577, 1986.

Chapter 12

MANAGEMENT OF PATIENTS WITH SHORT-BOWEL SYNDROME

Stanley J. Dudrick and Rifat Latifi

TABLE OF CONTENTS

I. INTRODUCTION

The short-bowel syndrome is an entity defined not by a specific length of residual functioning small intestine, but rather is a combination of clinical signs and symptoms characterized primarily by intractable diarrhea, steatorrhea, dehydration, weight loss, malnutrition, and malabsorption of fats, vitamins, and other nutrients. Secondary more specific consequences of short-bowel syndrome include hypovolemia, hypoalbuminemia, hypokalemia, hypocalcemia, hypomagnesemia, hypozincemia, hypocupricemia, fatty acid and vitamin deficiencies, anemias, hyperoxaluria, and metabolic acidosis. The clinical presentation of the patient with short-bowel syndrome depends on several factors: (1) the extent of resection; (2) the site of resection; (3) the presence or absence of the ileocecal valve; (4) the residual function of the remaining small bowel, stomach, pancreas, biliary tree, and colon; (5) the capacity for adaptation of the intestinal remnant; (6) the primary disease that precipitated the loss of the small bowel; and (7) the amount and activity of the residual disease in the intestinal remnant.[1-5]

The minimum length of small bowel sufficient for adequate absorption remains controversial because of (1) the variable residual absorptive capacity of the remaining remnant, (2) the wide variation in the length of the normal small intestine, and (3) the difficulty in obtaining reproducible measurements of the length of the remaining bowel following massive resection. Depending upon the contraction or relaxation of the intestine, intraoperative estimates of the length of the normal intact small intestine in the adult vary from 260 to 800 cm (approximately 8 to 26 ft).[6] Mean length of the normal small intestine during life is 350 cm (11 to 12 ft) and post-mortem is 600 cm (20 ft). This great variability renders it difficult to determine the exact length of the remaining small bowel and makes it virtually impossible to estimate the percentage of the total length of small bowel represented by the segment remaining after massive intestinal resection. Moreover, many surgeons only measure the length of the resected small bowel, rather than measuring the length of the remaining intestinal segment, and then fail to describe accurately the nature and extent of the remaining small bowel in the operative record for future reference.

Because of the functional reserve capacity of the small bowel, segmental resections of the small intestine usually do not result in significant problems with digestion and absorption.[7,8] Indeed, resection of as much as 40% of the small intestine is usually well tolerated, provided that the duodenum, the distal half of the ileum, and the ileocecal valve are spared.[9] On the other hand, resection of 50% or more of the small intestine usually results in malabsorption initially, but can be tolerated eventually without specially tailored nutritional support. However, resection of 75% or more of the small intestine usually leaves the patient with 70 to 100 cm (2 to 3 ft) of remaining intestine, resulting in a short-bowel syndrome which can significantly compromise the ability of the patient to maintain normal nutrition and metabolism. This patient will likely require special nutritional care on a long-term or permanent basis, although the presence of the terminal ileum and the ileocecal valve may allow virtually maximal bowel adaptation to occur in time.

Development of safe and efficacious total parenteral nutrition has revolutionized the treatment of patients with the short-bowel syndrome by allowing maintenance of adequate nutrition until the remaining bowel can adapt optimally to oral feeding, thus reducing the morbidity and mortality significantly.[10-15] Prolonged survival has now been achieved in a number of patients having an intact duodenum and 15 cm (6 in) of residual jejunum, with or without the colon.[2-8] If, in addition to the entire duodenum, approximately 60 cm (2 ft) of jejunum or ileum remain functional, survival is the rule rather than the exception. Preservation of the ileocecal valve is of utmost importance during massive small-bowel resection and, by significantly increasing the intestinal transit time, can effectively increase the absorptive capacity of the remaining small bowel to approximately twice that ordinarily anticipated for the same length of small bowel without an intact ileocecal valve. Primarily as a result of mucosal hyperplasia and villous hypertrophy, absorption in the residual intestine of patients with short-bowel syndrome can usually increase as much as fourfold. Therefore, in a patient with an intact ileocecal valve, the total absorptive capacity of the remaining small bowel potentially can be increased maximally eightfold, representing the absorptive equivalent of 200 cm of normal small bowel.

II. PATHOPHYSIOLOGY

The absorption of water, electrolytes, and nutrients is dependent upon the site and extent of the small-bowel resection. The intestinal phase of digestion occurs initially within the duodenum, where pancreatic enzymes and bile acids aid digestion of all nutrients and promote fat absorption. It is uncommon for the duodenum to be resected together with extensive segments of the small bowel; however, total duodenectomy leads to malabsorption of calcium, folic acid, and iron.[1] Proteins, carbohydrates, and fats are absorbed virtually completely in the first 150 cm of the jejunum; therefore, only small quantities of these nutrients ordinarily reach the ileum.[16]

The small intestine receives and processes about 8 L of fluid daily, including dietary ingestion and endogenous secretions. Normally, about 80% of the water transported is absorbed in the small bowel, leaving approximately 1.5 L of fluid to traverse the colon. The colon usually absorbs about 1 to 2 L of fluid with a maximal absorptive capacity of approximately 6 L/d.[17] Because the ileum and colon have a large capacity for absorbing excess fluid and electrolytes, proximal small-bowel resections rarely result in diarrhea. On the other hand, extensive or total ileal resection produces a greater potential for malabsorption and diarrhea. Not only will such resections increase the volume of fluid reaching the colon, but depending upon the length of ileum resected, bile salt diarrhea (cholerrhea) or steatorrhea may ensue with subsequent loss of fat-soluble vitamins. If the ileocecal valve has been resected, transit time may decrease, and bacterial colonization of the small bowel will eventually occur, further aggravating cholerrhea and steatorrhea. As the length of ileal or colonic resections is increased, essential absorptive surface area is lost, resulting in proportionally increased dehydration, hypovolemia, and electrolyte derangements. If the colon remains in continuity with the residual small bowel following massive resection, malabsorbed bile salts can be deconjugated by colonic bacteria, stimulating colonic secretion and further compounding existing diarrhea. With extensive ileal resection, irreversible loss of bile salts results with or without the colon in continuity. Although the excess losses stimulate hepatic synthesis of bile salts, a higher incidence of cholelithiasis occurs in these patients. Because the transit time in the ileum is usually slower than in the jejunum, residual intestinal transit will be slowed, and fecal output will diminish as the length of remaining ileum increases.

Following extensive small-bowel resections, intestinal lactase activity may be decreased leading to lactose intolerance.[18] The unhydrolyzed lactose results in increased hyperosmolality in the intestinal lumen. Moreover, fermentation of the lactose by colonic bacteria produces a large amount of lactic acid that can further aggravate osmotic diarrhea.[1]

The water-soluble vitamins and minerals (vitamin B-complex and C, Ca^{++}, Fe^{+++}, Mg^{++}) are absorbed in the proximal small intestine, whereas magnesium diffuses passively throughout the entire small bowel.[1] The ileum is the only site for absorption of vitamin B_{12} and bile salts. Jejunectomy with preservation of the ileum produces no permanent impairments of protein, carbohydrate, and electrolyte absorption.[19] The ileum can compensate for most absorptive functions, but not for the secretion of jejunal enterohormones. Following jejunal resections, diminished secretion of cholecystokinin and secretin decrease gallbladder contraction and pancreatic secretion. After jejunal resection, gastric hypersecretion is greater than after ileal resection. As a result of the loss of inhibitory hormones, such as gastric inhibitory polypeptide (GIP) and vasoactive intestinal polypeptide (VIP), which are secreted in the jejunum, gastrin levels rise, thus stimulating gastric hypersecretion.[20] Significant gastric hypersecretion can be documented within 24 h postoperatively, and the bowel mucosa can be injured by the high gastric acid output. Subsequently, the high salt load secreted in the stomach, together with the inactivation of digestive enzymes by the low intraluminal pH, serves to compound the other causes of diarrhea associated with short-bowel syndrome.

Ordinarily, the colon is a major site of water and electrolyte absorption. As the ileal effluent increases, the colon may increase its absorptive capacity to 3 to 5 times.[21] Furthermore, the colon has a moderate capacity to absorb other nutrients, and concomitant colon resections can affect the symptomatic and nutritional courses of patients with massive small-bowel resections. Malabsorbed carbohydrates are fermented by bacteria in the colon to yield short-chain fatty acids, principally acetate, butyrate, and propionate.[22,23] The short-chain fatty acids can be absorbed by the colon in quantities up to 500 cal/d and enter the portal circulation to serve as a fuel source.[24,25] Although retention of the colon is highly desirable, its presence can be associated with potential complications. In addition to cholerrheic diarrhea, patients with massive small-bowel resection and an intact colon have a tendency to form calcium oxalate renal stones. These result from the increased absorption of dietary oxalate, which is normally rendered insoluble by calcium in the intestinal lumen and, therefore, ordinarily unabsorbable. However, in patients with short-bowel syndrome and steatorrhea, intestinal calcium is bound preferentially to unabsorbed fatty acids, leading to decreased binding and increased colonic absorption of the oxalate.[6]

Finally, preservation of the ileocecal valve is an important preventive determinant of abnormal metabolic sequelae because the ileocecal valve not only slows intestinal transit but prevents bacterial reflux from the colon into the small bowel. Nutrients which reach the colonic lumen, especially vitamin B_{12}, become substrates for bacterial metabolism rather than being absorbed by the mucosa.[1] Furthermore, bacterial overgrowth in the small bowel in patients with short-bowel syndrome appears to increase the incidence of liver dysfunction.[26]

III. METABOLIC MANAGEMENT

In the metabolic and nutritional management of patients with the short-bowel syndrome, three therapeutic periods having somewhat distinctive characteristics can be identified (Table 1).[27] During the first 2 months, the clinical picture and course are dominated by problems related to fluid and electrolyte balance, adjustment of organ blood flow, especially the portal venous flow, and other effects of the major operative stress and its attendant specific and general complications. During the second period, from about 2 months up to 2 years postoperatively, efforts are directed toward defining maximum oral feeding tolerances for various substrates, encouraging and maximizing intestinal and bowel adaptation, and determining and formulating the most effective individualized feeding regimens. Usually within 2 years, 90 to 95% of the bowel adaptation potential has been realized, and only 5 to 10% additional improvement in absorption and bowel adaptation can be anticipated. The third period constitutes the period after 2 years, by which time nutritional and metabolic stability have usually occurred. At this point, the

TABLE 1
Outline of Short-Bowel Syndrome Management

Immediate postoperative period (First 2 months)	Bowel adaptation period (First 2 years)	Long-term management (After 2 years)
Fluid and electrolyte replacement	Progression of oral diet	Apply previous principles
Lactated Ringer's solution	Water, tea, broth	As indicated individually
Dextrose 5% in water	Simple salt solutions	Ambulatory home TPN
Human serum albumin	Simple sugar solutions	Supplemental or Total;
K^+, Ca^{++}, Mg^{++}	Complex salt/sugar solutions	Continuous, Cyclic, or
supplementation	Dilute chemically defined	Intermittent
Strict intake and output	diets	Surgical management
Daily body weight	High carbohydrate, high	Treat operative complications
Graduated metabolic	protein	Drain abscesses
monitoring	Near-normal, normal diet	Resect fistulas
Antacid therapy	Enteral supplementation	Lyse adhesions
Camalox® suspension	Coconut oil 30 ml po tid	Reduce obstructions
Mylanta® liquid	Safflower oil 30 ml po tid	Restore bowel continuity
Amphogel® suspension	Multiple vitamins 1 ml bid	Probable cholecystectomy
Gelusil® liquid	Ferrous sulfate 1 ml tid	
(30–60 ml via N-G tube	Ca gluconate 6–8 g/d	
q 2 h clamp N-G tube	Na bicarbonate 8–12 g/d	
20 min)	Parenteral supplementation	
Antiulcer therapy	Electrolytes, trace elements	
Sucralfate 1 gm po q 6 h	Divalent cations (Mg,Zn)	
(Clamp N-G tube 30 min)	Vitamin B_{12}, Vitamin K, folic	
Antisecretory/antimotility therapy	acid	
Cimetidine 300 mg IV q 6 h	Albumin, Packed red cells	
Ranitidine 150 mg IV q 12 h	Fat emulsion	
Famotidine 20 mg IV q 12 h	Antisecretory/antimotility	
Codeine 60 mg IM q 4 h	Famotidine 20 mg po q 12 h	
Loperamide 4–16 mg po daily	ProBanthine® 15 mg po	
Lomotil® 20 mg po q 6 h	q 4–6 h	
Somatostatin 50–150 mcg sc	Dicyclomine 20 mg po q 6 h	
q 6 h	Omeprazole 20 mg po q day	
Cholestyramine 4 gm po q 8 h	Deodorized tincture of opium	
Total parenteral nutrition	10–30 gtts q 4 h	
1 L on second post-op day	Codeine 30–60 mg po q 4 h	
Gradually increase dosage as	Paregoric 5–10 ml po q 4 h	
tolerated	(Refer to column one for	
Supplement fluids,	additional agents)	
electrolytes and colloids as		
needed		

patient has either adapted maximally so that nutritional and metabolic homeostasis can be achieved entirely with oral feeding, or the patient is committed to receiving supplemental or complete nutritional support for life, either by ambulatory home TPN and/or specialized enteral or oral feedings.

A. THE IMMEDIATE POST-OPERATIVE PERIOD

During the immediate postoperative period, virtually all nutrients, including water, electrolytes, proteins, carbohydates, fats, all vitamins, and trace elements are absorbed from the GI tract poorly or not at all. Fluid losses from the alimentary tract are greatest during the first few days following massive small intestinal resection, and anal or ostomy effluent frequently reaches volumes in excess of 5 L/24 h. Vigorous fluid and electrolyte replacement therapy must be instituted promptly in order to minimize life-threatening dehydration, hypovolemia, hypotension, and electrolyte imbalances. Frequent vital signs, intake and output, and central venous pressure measurements together with regular hematologic and biochemical indices are essential in monitoring the patient during this period of rapid metabolic change and instability. All patients with short-bowel syndrome will exhibit abnormalities in their liver function, and the vast majority of patients will experience transient hyperbilirubinemia.[28] This is thought by some to be due to the translocation of microorganisms and/or their toxins through the ischemic or gangrenous intestinal mucosa into the portal vein and to the liver.[29,30] Others attribute the jaundice to impaired blood flow to the liver through the portal vein by as much as 40% as a result of the greatly diminished mesenteric venous return following the massive small-bowel resection.[31] Another opinion attributes this phenomenon to a combination of these factors and/or other etiologies.[32] Broad spectrum antibiotic therapy is instituted and maintained for several days to 1 one week following massive intestinal resection.

During this period, typical management efforts are directed toward four primary goals: fluid and electrolyte replacement, antisecretory/antimotility therapy, antacid therapy, and total parenteral nutrition. During the first 24 to 48 h, replacement therapy usually consists of 5% dextrose in lactated Ringer's solution infused intravenously concomitantly with appropriate amounts of potassium chloride and/or acetate, calcium gluconate, magnesium sulfate, and fat- and water-soluble vitamins. Salt-poor human albumin (12.5 to 25 g) usually is added to each liter of crystalloid solution for the first 24 to 48 h postoperatively in order to maintain normal plasma albumin concentration and normal plasma colloid oncotic pressure. In patients with severe diarrhea, zinc losses can increase to as much as 15 mg/d and require appropriate parenteral replacement.[33]

Antacid therapy can reduce the tendency for peptic ulceration, which commonly occurs following massive small-bowel resection. Antacids are given through a nasogastric tube every 2 h in doses of 30 to 60 ml, and the tube is clamped for 20 min after instillation before reapplying suction. Alternatively, or concomitantly, sucralfate can be given by mouth or via the nasogastric tube in a dose of 1 g every 6 h, clamping the tube for 30 min after each dose. To counteract the hypergastrinemia and associated gastric hypersecretion which follows massive small-bowel resection in the majority of patients, an H_2 receptor blocker is given.[34] The i.v. infusion of 300 to 600 mg of cimetidine every 6 h can have a profound effect in reducing gastric acid and intestinal fluid production. Alternatively, ranitidine 150 mg can be given i.v. every 12 h, or famotidine 20 mg can be given i.v. every 12 h. In selected short-bowel patients, somatostatin analog has reduced fecal losses when given in a dosage of 50 to 150 mcg i.v. or subcutaneously every 6 h.[35,36] If diarrhea persists despite these measures, an opiate can be used. Preferably, codeine is given parenterally in doses of 60 mg every 4 h. Improvement in fluid and electrolyte management can also be achieved in selected patients with stomal access to a distal defunctionalized bowel loop by reinfusing the chyme from the proximal ostomy into the distal bowel segment.[37] Later in the course of the postoperative period, when the patient is tolerating liquids by mouth, oral antimotility therapy can be achieved by giving loperamide 4 to 16 mg in divided doses daily, cholestyramine 4 g every 4 to 8 h and/or diphenoxylate 20 mg every 6 h. Codeine 30 to 60 mg, paregoric 5 to 10 ml, or deodorized tincture of opium 10 to 30 drops every 4 h orally can be used to impede bowel motility. The major advantages of giving deodorized tincture of opium are that it is readily absorbed by the upper alimentary tract and that the patient's bowel hypermotility and diarrhea can be titrated to tolerable levels by adjusting the dosage up or down a few drops at a time.

By the second or third postoperative day, the patient's cardiovascular and pulmonary status has usually stabilized sufficiently to allow TPN to be instituted. The average adult patient can usually tolerate an initial ration of 2 L of TPN solution daily administered by central vein. By titrating levels of plasma glucose and glycosuria, the daily nutrient intake can be increased gradually to desired levels or to tolerance. In a patient with diabetes mellitus, or in one who is glucose intolerant, crystalline regular human insulin is added to the TPN solution in doses up to 50 units per 1000 calories. Following an operation of the magnitude of massive small-bowel resection, most patients require 3000 to 4000 ml of TPN solution (3000 to 4000 cal) per day to maintain nutritional and metabolic homeostasis. Supplemental fluid and electrolyte infusions may be necessary for several days or weeks to balance excessive losses as diarrhea. The patient is started on a clear liquid diet as soon as the postoperative condition is stabilized, and fecal output is controlled with antidiarrheal medications. It may take several days to several weeks before the patient is able to relinquish TPN support in favor of oral or enteral feedings. It is essential to provide nutritional supplementation with TPN for as long as the patient requires such support to maintain adequate nutritional status. The TPN ration is reduced gradually in a reciprocal manner as oral intake and intestinal absorption of required nutrients are increased. The patient's diet is advanced slowly and gradually to low-lactose, low-fat, high-protein, high-carbohydrate content according to individual tolerances to the nutrient substrates and to the volume and osmolality of the dietary regimen.[38]

B. THE BOWEL ADAPTATION PERIOD

During the period of bowel adaptation, the patient is allowed to consume increasing quantities of water, simple salt solutions, and simple carbohydrates. Various fruit and other flavorings can be added to 5% dextrose in lactated Ringer's solution as a relatively inexpensive and practical initial oral nutrient solution. Gradually, dilute solutions of chemically defined diets which contain simple amino acids and short-chain peptides are given as tolerated in increasing volumes and concentrations as bowel adaptation progresses. Feeding should progress toward a normal or near-normal diet consisting of high carbohydrate, high protein, and modest fat and comprised of foods most preferred by the patient as the next stage of nutritional rehabilitation. Alternatively, the major nutrients can be provided as required in commercially prepared modular feedings tailored to the needs of individual patients until ordinary food is well tolerated. All essential vitamins, trace elements, essential fatty acids, and minerals are initially supplied in the patient's balanced intravenous nutrient ration. Subsequently, the oral diet may be supplemented most economically by short- and medium-chain triglycerides in the form of 30 ml coconut oil, 2 or 3 times daily; essential fatty acids such as 30 ml safflower oil, 2 or 3 times daily; 1 ml multiple fat- and water-soluble vitamins in pediatric liquid form, twice daily; 1 mg vitamin B_{12}, intramuscularly every 4 weeks; 15 mg folic acid, intramuscularly weekly; and 10 mg vitamin K, intramuscularly weekly. Some patients may require supplemental iron, which may be administered initially by deep intramuscular injection as iron-dextran according to the recommended dosage schedule or as an i.v. infusion after testing the patient for sensitivity. Alternatively, an oral liquid iron preparation can be given 1 to 3 times daily.

The strong tendency for patients with short-bowel syndrome to develop metabolic acidosis usually requires the use of sodium bicarbonate powder, tablets, liquid, or wafers in doses of 8 to 12 g/d for as long as 18 to 24 months, but usually not less than 6 months. It is often helpful to alternate the form of sodium bicarbonate prescribed in order to maximize patient compliance. Because of the difficulty of absorbing adequate dietary calcium, supplemental calcium gluconate should also be prescribed as tablets, wafers, powder, or liquid in doses of 6 to 8 g/d. As bowel adaptation progresses, the dosages of sodium bicarbonate and calcium gluconate can be reduced concomitantly or discontinued; however, such oral supplements may be necessary for as long as 2 years or more in some patients. Occasionally, on the other hand, a patient may become severely acidotic (pH 7 to 7.2), as a result of obviously increased diarrhea, but sometimes more subtly, and may require urgent or emergency infusion of sodium bicarbonate intravenously. Usually the patient responds promptly to the therapy without untoward sequelae. Rarely, calcium gluconate must be given intravenously as a supplement to correct recalcitrant hypocalcemia (<8.0 mEq/dl). Dietary advancement and supplementation must obviously be individualized for each patient. When solid foods are given, they should be dry and followed 1 h later with isotonic fluids to improve nutrient absorption. Lactose intolerance should be anticipated and treated with a low-lactose diet and/or lactase, 125 to 250 mg by mouth as needed. Obviously, milk products should be avoided as much as possible if intolerance persists.

As progress is made during the bowel adaptation period of management of the short-bowel syndrome, fat can be increased in the diet as tolerated, and supplementation with short- and medium-chain triglycerides and essential fatty acids may no longer be necessary. Scrum-free fatty acid levels and triene:tetraene ratios are monitored periodically to determine the need for supplementation and the efficacy of treatment. Contrary to early reports, high-fat diets apparently are comparable to high-carbohydrate diets when evaluated in reference to calories absorbed, blood chemistries, stool or ostomy output, urine output, and electrolyte excretions.[39] However, enteral intake of fat should approach 50 to 100% greater than expected goals to compensate for malabsorbed nutrients.[33] Patients who fail to tolerate a normal oral diet should be given a trial of continuous infusion of an enteral formula. Low-residue, polymeric, chemically defined, or elemental diets offer the theoretical advantage of high absorbability in the short-bowel patient. However, some investigators have recently shown no differences in caloric absorption, stomal output, or electrolyte losses among elemental, polymeric, and normal diets in patients with short-bowel syndrome.[37,40,41]

Depending upon the results of periodic hematologic and biochemical assessments, adjustments are made in the patient's intake of sodium, potassium, chloride, and calcium.[42] In addition, intermittent supplemental infusions of solutions containing magnesium, zinc, and copper may be required. As malabsorption and diarrhea become less troublesome, the vitamin and trace element requirements may be satisfied by multivitamin capsules or tablets containing therapeutic dosages of vitamins and minerals, one capsule or tablet twice daily. Relatively large doses of magnesium, zinc, vitamin C, and the B-complex can be administered in the form of several commercially available therapeutic vitamin and mineral preparations.

In some patients, it may be necessary to correct individual nutrient substrate deficiencies intramuscularly or intravenously for prolonged periods of time. Intermittent infusions of human serum albumin and packed erythrocytes may be required to treat recalcitrant hypoalbuminemia and anemia and to restore the plasma albumin concentration and hematocrit to normal. Cholestyramine can be administered to combat bile salt diarrhea if indicated, but intraluminal cholestyramine itself sometimes causes or aggravates diarrhea. Fatty acid, electrolyte, trace element, vitamin, and acid base imbalances must be corrected enterally or parenterally as required when manifested clinically or by laboratory assessment. The serum vitamin B_{12} levels must be monitored and its deficiency corrected promptly. Hyperoxaluria should be assessed regularly, and if present, foods containing high levels of oxalate such as chocolate, spinach, celery, carrots, tea, and colas, should be restricted.

In patients with severe forms of short-bowel syndrome in which little or no small bowel is present distal to the duodenum, or in which the remaining small bowel has residual disease, hypermotility and recalcitrant or intractable diarrhea may require continuous long-term antimotility/antisecretory treatment with oral and/or parenteral forms and dosages of the previously described pharmacologic agents. Additional medications which have been helpful in selected patients include omeprazole, 20 mg by mouth daily; propantheline bromide, 15 mg by mouth every 4 to 6 h; dicyclomine hydrochloride, 20 to 40 mg by mouth every 6 h.

C. THE LONG-TERM MANAGEMENT PERIOD

Long-term management of the short-bowel syndrome can be accomplished successfully in most patients by conscientious attention to aforementioned principles and practices. However, in a small number of patients who have undergone massive small-bowel resection, total or supplemental parenteral nutrition must be provided in a continuous or cyclic manner for extended periods of time, and sometimes for life.

The metabolic management and nutritional therapy of patients with the short-bowel syndrome must be tailored specifically to each patient, and the clinical responses following massive intestinal resection depend upon many and varied factors. Patients with the short-bowel syndrome pass through several stages of nutritional support during their recovery, convalescence, and rehabilitation. Most of them can ultimately be maintained on a normal or near-normal oral diet. However, depending upon the adaptability of their remaining bowel, they may have to opt for receiving their nutritional requirements via a modified oral diet, an enteral total or supplemental diet, an oral or enteral diet supplemented with intravenous fluid and/or electrolyte replacement, a parenteral nutrition regimen supplemented with a variable oral or enteral diet, or reliance entirely upon total parenteral nutrition.

Virtually all patients with the short-bowel syndrome eventually develop gallstones, usually requiring cholecystectomy within 2 years following massive intestinal resection. Gallstone formation in the common bile duct and elsewhere in the biliary tree is also increased in these patients even after cholecystectomy. Therefore, periodic abdominal ultrasonography may be useful in identifying and monitoring echogenic changes in the gallbladder and biliary tree.

Finally, some otherwise stable patients occasionally develop recalcitrant diarrhea secondary to colonization or bacterial overgrowth of the residual small-bowel segment, requiring stool culture and parenteral treatment with appropriate antibiotics.

IV. CONCLUSION

The patient with short-bowel syndrome represents one of the greatest challenges to gastrointestinal clinicians. Maintaining optimal nutritional and metabolic support until maximum bowel adaptation can occur is the top priority of management. Attempts to ameliorate the untoward effects of the short-bowel syndrome surgically by interposing isoperistaltic or antiperistaltic bowel segments, intestinal valves, or recirculating loops; pacing the intestine electrically; growing new intestinal mucosa; and transplanting small intestine have been of little or no value to date. Therefore, no operative procedure for adjunctive management of the short-bowel syndrome currently is sufficiently safe and effective to recommend its routine use.[27] Long-term parenteral nutrition remains the cornerstone of successful management of the short-bowel syndrome, and its judicious use is recommended for as long and as much as needed to insure maximal gastrointestinal adaptation and nutritional rehabilitation of the patient.

REFERENCES

1. **Allard, J and Jeejeebhoy, K.** Nutritional support and therapy in the short bowel syndrome. *Gastroenterol Clin N Am,* 18:589–601, 1989.
2. **Deitel, M and Wong, KH.** The short bowel syndrome. In: *Nutrition in Clinical Surgery,* 2nd ed, Deitel, M. Ed., Williams & Wilkins, Baltimore, 1985, 255–275.
3. **Dudrick, SJ and Jackson, D.** The short bowel syndrome and total parenteral nutrition. *Heart Lung,* 12:195–201, 1983.
4. **Gouttebel, M, Saint-Aubert, B, Astre, C, and Joyeux, H.** Total parenteral nutrition needs in different types of short bowel syndrome. *Dig Dis Sci,* 31:713–723, 1986.
5. **Weser, E.** Nutritional aspects of malabsorption: short gut adaptation. *Clin Gastroenterol,* 12:443–461, 1983.
6. **Weser, E, Fletcher, JT, and Urban, E.** Short bowel syndrome. *Gastroenterology,* 77:572–579, 1979.
7. **Dudrick, SJ and Englert, DM.** Management of the short bowel syndrome. In: *The Management of Difficult Surgical Problems,* Miller, TA and Dudrick, SJ. Eds., University of Texas Press, Austin, 1981, 225–235.
8. **Dudrick, SJ, O'Donnell, JJ, and Englert, DM.** Ambulatory home parenteral nutrition for short bowel syndrome and other diseases. In: *Nutrition in Clinical Surgery,* 2nd ed, Deitel, M. Ed. Williams & Wilkins, Baltimore, 1985, 276–287.
9. **Trier, JS and Lipsky, M.** The short bowel syndrome. In: *Gastrointestinal Disease: Pathophysiology, Diagnosis, Management.* 4th ed, Sleisenger, MH and Fordtran, JS. Eds. W. B. Saunders, Philadelphia, 1989, 1106–1112.
10. **Conn, HJ, Chavez, CM, and Fain, WR.** The short bowel syndrome. *Ann Surg,* 175:803–814, 1972.
11. **Wilmore, DW, Dudrick, SJ, Daly, JM, et al.** The role of nutrition in the adaptation of the small intestine after massive resection. *Surg Gynecol Obstet,* 132:673–680, 1971.
12. **Wilmore, DW, and Johnson, DJ.** Metabolic effects of small bowel reversal in treatment of the short bowel syndrome. *Arch Surg,* 97:784–91, 1968.
13. **Dudrick, SJ.** A clinical review of nutritional support of the patients. *Am J Clin Nutr,* 34: 1191–1198, 1981.
14. **Sheldon, GF.** Role of parenteral nutrition in patients with short-bowel syndrome. *Med J Aust,* 67:1021–1029, 1979.
15. **Stewart, GR.** Home parenteral nutrition for chronic short-bowel syndrome. *Med J Aust,* 2:317–319, 1979.
16. **Borgstrom, B, Dahlquist, A, Lundh, G, et al.** Studies of intestinal digestion and absorption in the human. *J Clin Invest,* 36:1521–1536, 1957.
17. **Debongnie, J and Philips, S.** Capacity of the human colon to absorb fluid. *Gastroenterology,* 74:698–703, 1978.
18. **Ricotta, J, Zuidema, FD, Gadacz, RT, et al.** Construction of an ileocecal valve and its role in massive resection of the small intestine. *Surg Gynecol Obstet,* 152:310–14, 1981.
19. **Wright, HK and Tilson, MD.** Short gut syndrome: pathophysiology and treatment. *Curr Probl Surg,* 8:1–51, 1971.
20. **Strause, E, Gerson, E, and Yalow, RS.** Hypersecretion of gastrin associated with the short bowel syndrome. *Gastroenterology,* 66:175–180, 1974.
21. **Philips, SF and Giller, J.** The contribution of the colon to electrolyte and water conservation in man. *J Lab Clin Med,* 81:733–746, 1973.
22. **Bond, JH, Currier, BE, Buchwald, H, et al.** Colonic conservation of malabsorbed carbohydrates. *Gastroenterology,* 78:444–447, 1980.
23. **Bond, JH and Levitt, MD.** Fate of soluble carbohydrate in the colon of rats and humans. *J Clin Invest,* 57:1158–1164, 1976.
24. **Haverstad, T.** Studies of short-chain fatty acid absorption in man. *Scand J Gastroenterol,* 21:257–260, 1980.
25. **Pomare, EW, Branch, WJ, and Cummings, JH.** Carbohydrate fermentation in the human colon and its relation to blood acetate concentrations in venous blood. *J Clin Invest,* 75:1148–1154, 1985.
26. **Capron, JP, Gineston, JL, Herve, MA, et al.** Metronidazole in prevention of cholestasis associated with total parenteral nutrition. *Lancet,* 1:446–447, 1983.
27. **Dudrick, SJ, Latifi, R, and Fosnocht, D.** Management of the short bowel syndrome. *Surg Clin N Am,* 71:625–643, 1991.
28. **Dudrick, SJ.** Unpublished data.
29. **Barnett, WO, Oliver, RI, and Elliott, RL.** Elimination of the lethal properties of gangrenous bowel segments. *Ann Surg,* 167:912–919, 1968.

30. **Bounous, G and McArdle, AH.** Release of intestinal enzymes in acute mesenteric ischemia. *J Surg Res,* 9:339–346, 1969.
31. **Ratych, RE and Smith, GW.** Anatomy and physiology of the liver. In: *Shackelford's Surgery of the Alimentary Tract,* 3rd ed, Zuidema, GD. Ed. W. B. Saunders, Philadelphia, 1991, 273–286.
32. **Sarr, MG and Tito, WA.** Intestinal obstruction. In: *Shackelford's Surgery of the Alimentary Tract,* 3rd ed, Zuidema, GD. Ed. W. B. Saunders, Philadelphia, 1991, 372–413.
33. **Woolf, GM, Miller, C, Kurian, R, et al.** Nutritional absorption in short bowel syndrome: evaluation of fluid, calorie, and divalent cation requirements. *Dig Dis Sci,* 32:8–15, 1987.
34. **Cortot, A, Fleming, CR, and Malagelada, JR.** Improved nutrient absorption after cimetidine in short-bowel syndrome with gastric hypersecretion. *N Engl J Med.* 300:79–80. 1979.
35. **Ladefoged, K, Christensen, K, Hegnhoj, J, and Jarnum, S.** Effect of long acting somatostatin analogue SMS 201–995 on jejunostomy effluents in patients with severe short bowel syndrome. *Gut,* 30:943–949, 1989.
36. **Nightingale, J, Walker, E, Burnham, W, et al.** Short bowel syndrome. *Digestion,* 45(Suppl. 1):77–83, 1990.
37. **Levy, E, Frileux, P, Sandrucci, S, et al.** Continuous enteral nutrition during the early adaptive stage of the short bowel syndrome. *Br J Surg,* 75:549–553, 1988.
38. **Ovesen, L, Chu, R, and Howard, L.** The influence of dietary fat on jejunostomy output in patients with severe short bowel syndrome. *Am J Clin Nutr,* 38:270–277, 1983.
39. **Woolf, G, Miller, C, Kurian, R, et al.** Diet for patients with a short bowel: High fat or high carbohydrate? *Gastroenterology,* 84:823–828, 1983.
40. **McIntrye, P.** The short bowel. *Br J Surg,* 72:S93–S99, 1985.
41. **McIntrye, P, Fitchew, M, and Lennard-Jones, J.** Patients with a high jejunostomy do not need a special diet. *Gastroenterology,* 91:25–33, 1986.
42. **Ladefoged, K.** Intestinal and renal loss of infused minerals in patients with severe short bowel syndrome. *Am J Clin Nutr,* 36:59–67, 1982.

Chapter 13

DIET AND CANCER PREVENTION: PUZZLES YET UNSOLVED

William L. Banks, Jr. and Richard B. Brandt

TABLE OF CONTENTS

I. OVERVIEW AND LIMITATIONS

Attempts at defining the putative roles of various dietary components, both nutrient and non-nutrient, in the etiology of human cancer have been the subject of very intense investigation in recent years. An expanded focus of research effort in the area of diet, nutrition, and cancer has occurred since the publication in 1982 of a seminal compendium of nutrition and cancer relationships from research findings that spanned the previous half-century.[1] Shortly before that review was published, the National Cancer Institute (NCI) launched a major funding initiative, the "Diet, Nutrition, and Cancer Program", that supported investigations ranging from elucidation of dietary factors involved in the etiology of cancer to defining the role of nutrients in the therapy of cancer patients. The picture that has emerged at this juncture is far from complete, and the relationships between dietary factors and human cancer is in a constant state of flux as new results, spawned from the NCI initiative and other subsequent research programs by the American Cancer Society (ACS) and other agencies worldwide, are published.

One might describe the current state of our knowledge about the role of diet in cancer etiology in terms of a jigsaw puzzle which has different pictures on both sides of the pieces. Part of the edge of the puzzle is in place; other areas of the picture have some pieces linked together, which hint at relationships. However, to which picture, front or back, they belong is not at all clear. This view implies that apparently contradictory published findings are mostly valid, but that the relationships between them are yet to be developed because of missing pieces. Some investigators, however, espouse the notion that when the eventual connections are made between the pieces of the puzzle, only then can we validate whether some of the pieces (findings) are bogus and do not belong at all to either picture.

Moreover, is the etiology of the cancer picture related to the role of nutrients in cancer therapy, or are they independent of one another in some fundamental way? Or are there some similarities between the roles(s) of specific nutrients in cancer etiology and their role(s) in the complex of cancer-host interactions? What is clear is that the absolute certainty of the completeness of any area of these puzzles is not possible at present, for some very basic reasons. The greatest volume of reports regarding research findings in the etiology of human cancer are derived from the epidemiological literature. These studies provide direction for mechanistic studies, but no insight into the precise role(s) of specific nutrients with respect to the stages and mechanism(s) of carcinogenesis. On the other hand, the findings evolved from experimental animal models may give insight into the mechanistic process of carcinogenesis resulting in cancer growth, but may or may not directly correlate with the various human epidemiologic findings. Moreover, these different views of the truth exist within the overall framework of the lack of clarity with respect to the precise mechanisms of carcinogenesis, especially for human cancers. Thus, the subtitle: "Puzzles Yet Unsolved".

This review will concern itself primarily with dietary components for which there is some relatively consistent scientific evidence that they may play a role in the etiology of human cancer(s). The degree to which diet is related to cancer deaths was estimated by Doll and Peto[2] to be 35% with a remarkable wide range of 10 to 70% as the possible contribution of dietary factors. Specifically, the chapter will focus attention on the experimental evidence that has led to the consistent dietary recommendations that have been promulgated by the American Cancer Society,[3-5] the National Cancer Institute,[6] the Surgeon General,[7] and more recently, the National Research Council.[8]

In this chapter, there are aspects of food preparation and manmade or natural additive constituents which will not be addressed, since they might each constitute the subjects of

TABLE 1
Dietary Recommendations

1. Avoid obesity by decreasing caloric intake to caloric expenditures.
2. Decrease overall fat intake to 30% or less of total energy intake.
3. Increase dietary fiber intake to approximately 20 to 35 g/d.
4. Increase the intake of fruits and vegetables which will result in an increased intake of foods containing vitamin C, carotenoids, and also include foods from the cruciferous or cabbage family group of vegetables.

reviews themselves. Excluded will be cooking methods, preservatives, and additives involved in agriculture and the processing of foods for market. Further, we will not deal with dietary supplementation, whether or not the supplements are the same or are derivatives of endogenous constituents in foods. Thus, we have excluded discussion of work which involves pharmacologic doses of specific vitamins, provitamins, or minerals that have been reported to be beneficial in cancer prevention. Although this latter issue is of considerable import, the crossover area between levels of constituents in foods to those same chemicals provided in pharmacological doses transcends the focus of dietary factors per se and is best considered by viewing results of clinical drug trials or human intervention studies which are currently underway in another discussion format. Finally, we will not address the issue of secondary and tertiary prevention, that is, which nutrients are involved in therapy to prevent recurrence or metastasis of diagnosed disease following detection and treatment. This review will deal with the rationale for the various recommendations that relate to aspects of primary prevention of human cancer. We will focus our attention on the evidence relating various public health recommendations and attempt to identify the degree of scientific strengths for each.

Before we examine the issue of diet and cancer, we will briefly review the current model for the mechanism of carcinogenesis. As a result of studies using animal model systems, it was popular to describe the "two-step" mechanism leading to cancer in these systems.[9] This concept involved two distinct events, one called "initiation", which involved an alteration in the cell's genetic material, such as a mutation, followed by another series of insults termed "promotion". These two stages were obliged to take place in this order for a cancer cell to form. Various agents have been indicted as ones that may cause initiation, and these often differ from agents or insults that are involved in promotion in various animal test systems. Recently, as our knowledge of the process grows, identification of distinct biochemical changes in the later stages of promotion have been redefined as the "conversion" stage. The process subsequent to promotion and conversion has been termed "progression".[7] Thus, the two-stage mechanism has evolved into at least four stages for the purpose of a mechanistic model to which we can relate in the subsequent discussion of the roles of dietary factors in the etiology and prevention of cancer. The sequence of stages is as follows: initiation, promotion, conversion, and progression.

II. RECOMMENDATIONS FOR CANCER PREVENTION

Presently, there are four generally recognized recommendations regarding dietary factors and cancer prevention that fall within the scope of this review: (1) avoid obesity, (2) decrease fat calories, (3) increase dietary fiber intakes, and (4) increase consumption of fruits and vegetables (Table 1). These, of course, are not the only recommendations regarding dietary factors and cancer, but they seem to be generally agreed upon by the scientific mainstream groups identified above that have promulgated dietary recommendations and guidelines. The details may vary somewhat between groups, but the recommendations are essentially the same, which should not be surprising since they are derived from the same published scientific research findings.

From a public health perspective, none of these recommendations has been shown to be detrimental to health, and there is at least some scientific support for each, however incomplete. Even the most vociferous critics of the details of these recommendations usually end up conceding that they are the best we have at present and no apparent harm should befall those who follow them. We will examine each of them in terms of the scientific information from which they are derived.

A. AVOID OBESITY

Obesity is the accumulation of excess body fat and results when energy balance is positive over a period of time and has been related to various health problems, including cancers.[10] Biochemically, triglyceride stores in adipocytes provide a selective advantage for humans, both lean and obese, to survive during periods when food is scarce. However, in modern industrialized societies, caloric abundance is most often the case, as the typical "Western" diet tends to contain far more caloric content than our non-agrarian lifestyle can easily expend. The results from the American Cancer Society Cancer Prevention Study I,[11,12] involving a very large cohort sample in the U.S., provided epidemiologic evidence that the risk of certain forms of cancer was significantly elevated in both men (33%) and women (55%) when the body weight exceeded 40% of the "ideal" body weight as defined by gender and height/weight tables. This excess body weight relationship resulting in obesity correlated for cancers of the gallbladder, kidney, stomach, colon, breast, and endometrium.[4] Other studies, described in the Surgeon General's report,[7] consistently noted that body weight or body mass index were associated with reported increased risks for thyroid, kidney, and endometrial cancers and in breast cancer of post-menopausal women, whereas no significant differences in relative body weight were noted for prostate and colorectal cancers in case-controlled studies. Excess body weight resulting from a positive energy balance may very well be related to the etiology of only specific cancers.

The reports that excess caloric intake favors the growth of certain tumors, as described above, are balanced by research results that demonstrate that underfeeding, especially in energy content, compromises tumor growth. In the now-classic studies of Tannenbaum et al.,[13,14] animals that were underfed, especially during early developmental stages, showed a lowered incidence of spontaneous and chemically induced cancers, whereas obese animals demonstrated a higher incidence of tumors.[15] Kritchevsky and Klurfeld at the Wistar Institute have addressed this issue in animal models involving mammary tumor induction using a rat mammary tumor model.[16] By manipulating rat diets using graded caloric restriction through various energy levels, they were able to alter the number and size of the tumors, with the lowest caloric intakes corresponding to smaller tumor burdens. Excess calories alone, from whatever source, predispose the induction of experimental cancers, which may be different for each tumor type. Moreover, the energy balance equation may be altered by increased exercise. Kritchevsky[17] notes that colon cancer risk is increased in "sedentary men," whereas college athletes have lowered cancer risk, especially of cancers of the reproductive system.[18] Finally, excess alcohol intake in any form is thought to exert at least part of its effect as a factor in the formation of cancer, as a result of the excess energy (calories) it provides.

There are several questions that derive from the area of over- and underfeeding. What is the mechanism of this effect? Does this effect of excess calories occur as a result of high fat diets? After all, the greatest dietary caloric density is obtained from fat in the diet, so it could be expected that the correlation of obesity and cancers could be due to consumption of diets high in fat (see discussion below). Moreover, with the notable exception of colon carcinoma, the same cancers are not found in obese or high fat fed animals as they are in the human epidemiological experience cited above. This disparity may be as much a result of the lack of appropriate animal model systems than a "real" difference in mechanism. It is certainly possible that a common factor, such as hormonal imbalance, could predispose an individual to accumulate excess body fat (i.e., obesity) and foster a specific type of cancer growth as well.

B. REDUCE FAT IN THE DIET TO 30% OR LESS OF TOTAL CALORIES

There have been many studies that have specifically addressed the issue of dietary fat as a "carcinogen" in the etiology of cancer. From the perspective of epidemiologic considerations, examination of total fat consumption by various populations reveals that "Western" industrialized countries that consume high levels of fat in the diet have a greater incidence of colon and breast cancers.[19,20] These studies identified a positive correlation between dietary fat consumption and the incidence of these two major cancers. In general, those countries which are industrialized with "Western style" diets had a higher incidence of cancers than those that were more agrarian and less affluent. The consumption of meat seemed to some to be the determinant factor in elevated cancer incidence. Migratory population studies also correlated higher fat intakes and colon cancer incidence.[21] Wynder and Reddy[22] described the results of animal models and groups of laboratory investigators who analyzed fecal samples for sterol contents in patients with and without a history of colon cancer. The human studies found a greater concentration of secondary fecal sterol concentrations in those population groups that consumed greater amounts of dietary fat than those groups, such as Seventh Day Adventist vegetarians, who did not consume the "typical American high fat" regime. These findings focused attention on possible mechanisms of the effect of dietary fat content and the etiology of various forms of human cancers.[23]

Several mechanistic approaches have been fruitful and perhaps begin to reveal a possible mechanism for human colon carcinogenesis.[24] High fat diets tend to produce an increase in fecal sterols, whose pattern favors the formation of secondary bile acids derived in the gut via the action of the intestinal bacterial flora. The appearance of secondary bile acids correlates with the incidence of colon carcinoma and has been suggested to play a role in tumor promotion using the carcinogenic scheme described earlier.[25] Studies of the gut anaerobic flora suggest that at least some strains isolated in fecal samples from various population groups and colon cancer patients may be responsible for formation of mutagens involved in the carcinogenic process. Further study of this class of intestinal bacteria has revealed some unique metabolic aspects. In fact, Bruce and colleagues in Toronto have identified a fecal mutagen whose presence was affected by the level of dietary fat.[26] They subsequently found an intermediate in the pathway of conversion of primary to secondary bile acids by a strain of anaerobic colon bacteria that had carcinogenic properties.[27] An interesting scenario that could describe the role of fat in colon carcinogenesis involves a lengthy consumption of a high fat diet, leading to enhanced secretion of bile acids, which are processed in the gut by anaerobic bacteria via a route that produces tumor "promoters". Thus, one can envision a long-term assault resulting in colon cancer formation from cells that had been initiated by another mechanism, perhaps also prompted by high fat diets, or genetic predisposition to colon cancer, as in familial adenocarcinoma.

When a prospective approach was employed to examine a variety of lifestyle factors, including dietary fat, using a group of approximately 90,000 nurses as subjects, the results did not coincide with those from animal model studies for breast cancer,[28,29] although fat intake and colon cancer were associated in this group.[30] The association with colon cancer incidence and dietary fat has been noted in many epidemiological studies, although there are a distressing number of studies that show no or negative associations with reported fat intake.[31] Nevertheless, there is at least some concordance between epidemiologic and laboratory animal model studies with respect to the etiology of colon cancer. Prostate cancer has also been cited as associated with high fat in the diet, a relationship that is very tentative since both positive and negative associations have been reported.[7,17] Whether these associations are due to excess caloric intake by individuals consuming high fat diets remains a salient issue, in view of the preceding discussion relating to caloric excess and cancer etiology.

Furthermore, calcium in the diet appears to also play a role in colon cancer, perhaps by interfering with the effects of bile acids and/or free fatty acids on the colonic epithelia.[32] An interesting hypothesis by Garland and Garland relates to the worldwide incidence of colon carcinoma often being greatest in populations in the higher latitudes.[33-35] Thus, the exposure to annual sunlight in these populations is lower than their counterparts who live at latitudes nearer to the equator. Colder mean temperatures as well as a differential in sunlight results in less exposure of skin and a marked decrease in endogenous vitamin D production. Calcium absorption from the diet is dependent upon the hormonal action of a 1,25 dihydroxyl derivative of vitamin D and is possibly decreased in northern-dwelling populations. A few additional factors need to be addressed as this line of thought is followed. Exogenous levels of vitamin D via fortification of dairy products is often the major source of this vitamin/hormone in the "Westernized" diet. However, adult consumption of dairy products may, in fact, be reduced, especially in aged populations, who also may lack adequate sun exposure. Further, those populations that live in the higher latitudes tend to consume less fresh fruits and vegetables, which presumably contain anticarcinogens.

With regard to mechanistic considerations relating to dietary fat and cancer, recent animal studies suggest that linoleic acid plays a growth-stimulating role in cancer oncogenesis process.[17,32] This unsaturated fatty acid is found in all balanced diets. Its metabolism may result, in part, in the formation of hydroperoxide and hydroxyl-derived epoxides which may explain its role in one of the stages of carcinogenesis, presumably the promotion stage. When a similar structure, conjugated dienoic acid derivatives of linoleic acid (CLA), is provided under the same circumstances to animals, it becomes an anticarcinogen. Thus, the balance of carcinogen and anticarcinogen in food is an important concept that provides a confusing overlay to the entire picture of the relationship of food components to the etiology or protection from cancer.[36] This confounding variable would be sufficient to thoroughly confuse the situation by itself, but the relationships are further complicated by other lifestyle factors, such as smoking, which promotes a xenobiotic response in humans. In addition, the relationship of fat to dietary fiber and its impact on the carcinogenic process must be considered. Diets that are intrinsically high in fat are, in fact, low in fiber. Those diets that are high in fiber are naturally low in fat, and, thus, there is a dietary interrelationship if not a carcinogenic relationship between fat and fiber.

Finally, we cannot ignore the contribution of the genetic factors in colon carcinogenesis, so elegantly described by the work of Vogelstein and White and their colleagues.[37] The accumulation of mutations of several tumor suppressors plus the K-*ras* proto-oncogene were identified. By cloning cells in various stages of the long-term transition from precancerous adenomatous polyps to adenocarcinoma, they were able to identify alterations that are required in the formation of human colon cancer. How this genetic component relates to the possible roles of fat, bile acid derivatives, calcium status, fiber and/or dietary linoleic acid is presently not very clear, but is likely to be understood in the next few years. They may all be pieces in the same area of the puzzle.

C. INCREASE INTAKE OF FOODS CONTAINING FIBER

Since the initial observations of Burkitt regarding the lower incidence of colon cancer among the Bantus in Africa, who consume very large quantities of plant foods containing

TABLE 2
Dietary Fiber Composition

Nature	Substance	Food sources
Insoluble	Cellulose	Bran, whole wheat, root vegetables
	Hemicellulose	Bran, cereals, whole grains
	Lignin	Wheat
Soluble	Hemicellulose	Bran, cereals, whole grains
	Pectin	Apples, citrus fruits, berries
	Gums and mucilages	Beans, legumes, oatmeal
	Algal polysaccharide	Algae, seaweed (carageenan)

fiber, there has been the implication that dietary fiber interferes with the carcinogenic process in the large bowel.[38] Recently, the epidemiologic literature dealing with fiber and colon cancer has been reviewed with the revelation that there is little clear support for fiber as an unequivocal protective factor in the diet for colorectal cancer.[39] This conclusion is a result of Ausman's review of eight correlational, twenty case-control, and two cohort studies reported from 1973 to 1990. One half of the studies showed a negative association, eleven of thirty showed essentially no association, and two studies resulted in a positive association between fiber and colorectal cancer.

The difficulty in assessing the role of fiber is that it is a functional category and not a chemically related group of food constituents. There are at least five major subcategories of dietary fiber, and plant-derived foods contain varying proportions of each (Table 2). The most likely category to play a role in the colon cancer/fiber story is the insoluble lignins, celluloses, and perhaps hemicellulose. The feature that connects the heterogenous "fiber" category of food constituents is their lack of digestibility and absorption. Thus, they are relatively unprocessed in the digestive tract and are, therefore, non-nutrients. They are found as sizeable components of cereal grains as well as fruits and vegetables in a typical balanced diet. Physiologically, fiber's action involves dilution of the colonic lumenal contents due to water extraction from cells of the digestive tract. This hydraulic effect tends to decrease the stool transit time and increase the stool bulk, thus diluting the fecal material.

Burkitt noted that the Bantus produced huge amounts of "watery" fecal material per day in as many as 10 to 12 bowel movements, as compared to their "Western" diet-eating contemporaries. It was assumed that since diets high in fiber would be decidedly low in fat content, then carcinogens produced by fat in the digestive tract may be effectively diluted in the colon by the action of insoluble fibers. Moreover, a low fat/high fiber diet, such as the Bantus and other vegetarians consume, would be expected to produce a diminished concentration of potentially carcinogenic materials. However, it is extremely difficult to factor out the effect of fiber, independent of the dietary fat and other contents that may play a role in human cancer etiology in Western cultures. In addition, it is generally accepted that not all components of dietary fiber are equally beneficial in the modulation of colon carcinogenesis. When the 27 epidemiologic studies that differentiated between the types of plant-derived food sources (i.e., cereals, vegetables, and fruits) were computed, 16 studies showed a negative association, 6 showed no association, 2 gave purely a positive association, and 3 gave a mixed positive and negative association for the different types of foodstuffs. Thus, a beneficial effect of one constituent of this heterogeneous dietary component fiber could be obscured by the amount of other components, which are not involved but present in the total dietary fiber measured. This could very well account for the marked variability in results from a whole host of epidemiologic studies.[40] When meta-analysis was performed by combining 13 case-control studies for the risk of fiber and colorectal cancer, then it became clear that as fiber intake increases, risk decreases.[41] This age-adjusted result is independent of tumor location in the lower GI tract and the food sources of fiber. Dwyer[40] indicated that if this relationship identified by Howe[41] withstands the test of time, then "colorectal cancer risk among Americans could be reduced approximately 31% if fiber intakes from food sources were increased by 13 g/d—the amount of fiber in an average-sized apple and one half cup of cooked legumes". The meta-analysis cited above also corrected for ascorbic acid and carotenoid intake, which will be discussed in the next section of this review.

The range of recommended fiber intakes varies between 20 and 35 g. These figures represent "guesstimates," based upon the typical American diet containing 8 to 17 g of total fiber.[39] The amount of the fiber that may be beneficial for colon cancer prevention could be much smaller if only a single component, such as lignin, were effective. Considerably more investigation needs to take place regarding the amount and type of fiber intake that should be recommended.

Since fiber is only found in plant materials, along with other possible anticarcinogens, the independent assessment of the benefit of any single nutrient or of fiber will require new types of dietary analyses or approaches to identify the specific "active ingredients" that have displayed at least some benefit in ameliorating the effects of various putative carcinogens. Carcinogenesis is a complex process, as briefly described previously, and when imprecise dietary component analyses are applied to attempt to ascertain the precise role of dietary factors in the process, it becomes a situation ripe for expansive speculation. It is certainly difficult to tease out the contribution of dietary fiber alone, independent of other plant constituents, much less ascribe a clear benefit to a specific type of fiber source at present. Nonetheless, there is evidence for some benefit at least in ingesting cereal grains, vegetables, and fruits that contain fiber and are incidentally low in fat before and during preparation.

D. INCREASE THE INTAKE OF FRUITS AND VEGETABLES

The least controversial recommendation is to increase the daily intake of fruits and vegetables. In fact, it has been popular to recommend the "Five-A-Day Plan", which promotes the consumption of five servings of fruits and/or vegetables per day. This "educational marketing" approach was developed in California, has been promoted by various groups concerned with nutrition and public health, and is listed in the U.S. Department of Health and Human Services, Healthy People 2000 Program.[42] This recommendation evolved from a multitude of epidemiologic studies, which were comprehensively reviewed recently by Block et al.[43] The conclusion that these scientists reached from nearly 200 studies is that, for most types of cancer studied, frequent consumption of fruits and vegetables tended to be associated with lowered cancer risk when compared to diets in which few of these categories of foods were consumed. A lower relative risk was found for lung, head and neck, colorectal, pancreatic, gastric, bladder, ovarian, uterine, and breast cancers. Only prostate cancer results were ambiguous with respect to the potential protective effects of dietary fruits and vegetables. In fact, some studies showed an increased risk of prostate cancer associated with fruit and vegetable consumption.

Vegetables and fruits are particularly rich sources of a number of nutrients that have been shown to affect the process of cancer etiology in laboratory and animal model systems.[7] As foods, plants are complex and contain fiber of various compositions as described earlier, as well as many nutrient components. Even though there is general agreement that fruits and vegetables in the diet are beneficial in a cancer prevention sense, which component(s) of these foods are the "active ingredients" and the mechanisms by which they work is unclear. In fact, various components of fruits and vegetables have been identified as candidates, such as the antioxidants vitamin C, β-carotene, vitamin E, and selenium, as well as various forms of fiber, vitamin B_6, folacin, and riboflavin.[44] In addition, some have suggested that their role(s) simply involve lowering the caloric and/or the fat content of the diet by substitution for relatively high fat foods. A number of epidemiologic studies have linked dietary assessment of some of the above nutrients to a beneficial effect with respect to various cancers.[45,46]

Although the strongest epidemiological data supported beneficial roles for fruits and vegetables, investigators have sought to identify the specific components of those food categories that might play roles as anticarcinogens. One category that was nominated for a major role was the carotenoids and retinoids.[47] These were identified by noting the nature of the foods in the fruit and vegetable categories that related to lower incidences of human cancers, coupled with β-carotene's antioxidant properties as identified using biochemical model systems. The degree of concordance between epidemiological and laboratory findings has recently been reviewed by Byers and Perry,[48] and the mechanisms of these antioxidant nutrients and their roles in carcinogenesis have been summarized by Mirvish[49] and Sies et al.[50] Other mechanisms of action may include effects on enhancing immune surveillance[51] or the conversion to vitamin A due to its effect on cellular differentiation.[48]

The initiation stage of carcinogenesis is thought to take place with an attack on a cell's DNA by an agent that may involve chemical-free radicals generated by oxidation processes. Thus, the role of antioxidants would be to suppress the formation of spurious agents that may serve to initiate this process. Vitamin C, for example, is a powerful reducing agent that in the laboratory can convert potentially carcinogenic nitrites to a benign product, especially in an acidic environment.[49] This action of vitamin C could be involved in the steady decline in primary stomach cancer in the U.S. in the past 30 to 40 years.[52] Since foods containing this vitamin are more available in the current food supply than they previously were, and the acidic environment of the stomach could potentiate the reduction of nitrites that are found endogenously in vegetables or used as preservatives for processed meats, then the vitamin C may suppress the formation of carcinogenic compounds. Of course, this scenario is speculative, but provides a consistent thread linking the epidemiology with laboratory chemical findings. Vitamin C by its various roles, such as free radical scavenging, protection against lipid peroxidation, vitamin E sparing, immune function modulation, and maintaining tissue integrity, may inhibit or protect against cancer at various stages of the carcinogenic process by different mechanisms.[53] Epidemiological evidence from diet analysis on case control and prospective studies showed risk reduction in 6 of 7 studies on oral cancer with increasing dietary vitamin C or fruit intakes.[53] Similar findings for esophageal cancer were reported, but again these studies do not clearly discriminate between fruit and vitamin C intake. For many cancers, including lung, pancreatic, cervical, colon, and breast, there were consistent findings of lowered risk reduction with increasing dietary vitamin C. Dietary fat has an important interaction with statistical analysis of the vitamin C effect on risk reduction. For ovarian or prostate cancer, no risk reduction was observed due to dietary vitamin C. Studies that show risk reduction for green leafy vegetables that were assumed to be the action of β-carotene may also show a vitamin C risk reduction effect, since these foods frequently are high in vitamin C also. Indeed, by statistical treatment, where dietary β-carotene levels or risk factors were controlled, the vitamin C analysis still accounted for a risk reduction effect.

β-carotene is the most prevalent member of all the carotenoids in foods. It has been noted to possess the biochemical property in the laboratory of trapping free radicals and modulating other destructive oxidative metabolic processes. Inhibition of initiation and promotion may occur with β-carotene, due to its multimetabolic roles. β-carotene has been targeted as a prime compound found in the diet, in part, due to the publication of a summary of its role as a potential protection against cancer.[54] Recently, Ziegler et al. asked the question, "Does β-carotene explain the reduced cancer risk associated with vegetable and fruit intake?"[55] The transition from the suggestion of earlier literature that vitamin A could reduce the risk of cancer was, in part, based upon the β-carotene being both the most abundant carotenoid in fruits and vegetables and the most effectively converted to vitamin A. The protective role of β-carotene was also shown in epidemiological studies. β-carotene serum levels are maintained by physiological control within a specific range for all but extreme levels of intake. In prospective studies, where dietary information or blood samples were collected from subjects free from disease and who were followed over time, eventual diagnoses of cancer were compared to matched controls from the cohort. Seven prospective studies worldwide have been published. Only three actually determined carotenoids, and a variety of cancers were assessed. Three of five studies showed a risk reduction in all types of cancers that correlated with both fruits and vegetables as well as carotenoids. The greatest effect appeared to be on reduction of lung cancer in five of six studies. Prospective studies on blood carotenoid levels again showed in five of six studies an association of elevated blood levels of carotenoids with lower lung cancer rates. Stomach cancer was lower in three of four studies showing β-carotene protection. Variable findings occur for some other cancers. Plasma vitamin C was not strongly associated with risk reduction for lung cancer, but was associated with stomach cancer. In retrospective studies on carotenoids, patients with a particular cancer are paired with control subjects. Fourteen of fifteen studies of lung cancer showed a decreased risk with increased intake of carotenoids or green and yellow-orange vegetables.[55] The obvious overlap with the vegetables complicates the interpretation. Are other carotenoids than β-carotene involved, or are other constituents of vegetables and fruits involved? Are there other dietary practices among people who frequently ingest vegetables and fruit that contribute to an anti-cancer effect?

In addition, vitamin E has also been suggested as an anticarcinogen for its free radical trapping and antioxidant properties noted in the laboratory.[48] Animal studies have shown a vitamin E requirement for optimal immune responses.[56] Finally, the essential mineral, selenium, also has similar biochemical properties, and its role as a human anticarcinogen, like vitamin E, is in the process of being more clearly defined. In the case of vitamin E and selenium, the epidemiologic evaluation has come as a result of the basic laboratory findings and not vice versa.

What all of these nutrients have in common is that epidemiologically the foods that are rich sources for them have been shown to be associated with lowered risk of cancers of several types. In biochemical laboratory model systems, they have demonstrable antioxidant and potentially anticarcinogenic properties, and by providing them in "pharmacologic" doses to animal tumor models have, in some cases, slowed the tumor growth, although not repressed it entirely. This circumstantial evidence is strongest for vitamin C, vitamin E, and β-carotene. Nevertheless, one has to keep in mind that fruits and vegetables are complex mixtures of chemicals and ascribing a cancer-preventive benefit to a single or even a small number of constituents most likely misleads us into neglecting the sophisticated interplay of food constituents and the developing disease process over time.[43] In this regard, the American Cancer Society guidelines that initially included reference to "increasing the intake of foods containing vitamins A and C"[3] has been broadened to "increasing the intake of fruit and vegetables".[5]

Finally, another curious area of interest over the years has been with regard to the anticancer properties noted for vegetables in the plant family, cruciferae.[45] These vegetables, including cabbages, mustards, broccoli, cauliflower, brussels sprouts, kale, kohlrabi, and Swiss chard, have been noted to be consumed by individuals who have lowered relative risks for a variety of human cancers. These vegetables are excellent sources of fiber, vitamin C, carotenoids, and perhaps other ingredients that can interfere with the complex carcinogenic process. Wattenburg has evaluated a number of compounds that might be candidates to induce enzyme processes that result in "blocking" the metabolic formation of carcinogens.[57] Specifically, some pre-carcinogenic substances require "activation", usually by a hydroxylation reaction, to the "ultimate" carcinogenic compound. There are enzymes, glutathione-S-transferase being prominent, that interfere with this activation process. If plant indoles, phenols, and other similar compounds have the ability to increase the amount of the enzyme(s) that interfere with the activation process, then they have the potential to be anticarcinogens. Recently, Zeng et al. at Johns Hopkins have isolated and elucidated the structure of just such a compound from broccoli.[58] Sulforaphane is a potent inducer of the detoxication enzymes quinone reductase and glutathione-S-transferase, in a murine hepatoma cell culture test system. This strengthens the notion that there may be multiple "active" components in fruits and vegetables that could interfere by different mechanisms in the etiology of human cancers and there are not single components that prevent cancer growth. In Table 3, the nutrient analysis of selected fruits, vegetables, cereals, and other foods is listed to amplify this point. This table is not a list of "endorsed foods" necessarily, but rather is presented to illustrate the value of a diet containing a variety of foods in terms of the nutrient, fat, and fiber constituents.

III. SUMMARY AND CONCLUSIONS

By examining the various rationales for the several recommendations put forth regarding dietary factors and cancer, we can agree on four prescriptions that fall within the scope of this review. These are avoid obesity, reduce dietary fat consumption, increase the intake of fiber-containing foods, and increase the intake of fruits and vegetables in the diet. Support for these recommendations comes from the burgeoning studies in cancer epidemiology, biochemical laboratory studies, and tumor animal model systems. One needs to be cautious at this juncture, in ascribing clear-cut mechanisms to the carcinogenic or anticarcinogenic effects of any specific dietary constituent. The puzzle is not at all complete, but some of the areas seem to fit together.

Avoiding obesity, by balancing caloric intake with caloric output, is clearly beneficial. Excess body weight correlates with certain forms of cancer, and undernutrition, at least in animal tumor model systems, delays the growth of cancers. Obesity can result from a high fat diet more easily than by other routes. Thus, it is not clear whether fat, per se, in the diet predisposes to cancer by a mechanism independent of its provision of calories, or by reducing fat in the diet concomitantly lessens the caloric density of the diet. Perhaps a constituent of dietary fat, linoleic acid, which has tumor growth-promoting action in various test systems is responsible for the effects of fat in the etiology of cancer. Certainly, possible fat-related metabolites may also play roles, especially in the development of colon carcinoma. Lowering fat in our dietary regimen can only benefit our population, but how the pieces in that area of the puzzle fit together is yet to be ascertained. A case in point, the question of the possible role of dietary calcium in cancer, is provocative and deserves continued appraisal, but does it relate at all to fat?

Cereals, fruits, and vegetables are also noted to be beneficial. Data for the NHANES II Survey reveals that many Americans tend to consume too few servings of fruits and vegetables.[59] Some pieces in the puzzle can be linked together to show how dietary fiber, vitamin C, β-carotene, vitamin E, and cruciferous vegetables may exert anticancer properties at different points in the carcinogenic scheme. However, we again must be cautious in ascribing an exclusive and decisive mechanism for the effects of specific food constituents since the best associations that have been reported involve foods and specific cancers, rather than specific nutrients. The latter, however, can be determined secondarily

TABLE 3
Nutrient Analysis[a] of Selected Parameters for Representative Foods

Food	Serving size as consumed	Energy (cal)	Fat calories (%)	Fiber (gm)	Vitamin C (mg)	Vitamin E (mg)	Carotenoids (RE)[b]	Selenium (μg)	Calcium (mg)
Orange juice	1 cup	111	4	1	124	0.8	50	0.5	27
Broccoli	1 cup	24	11	3	82	0.6	136	0.2	42
Brussels sprouts	1 cup	38	6	4	75	0.8	77	8.1	36
Carrots	1 cup	70	4	5	4	1.4	3830	1.8	48
Beans (Navy)	1 cup	259	4	16	2	2.1	0.3	5.0	128
Bran cereal	1 cup	178	17	20	63	2.7	0	6.2	46
Whole wheat bread	1 slice	86	16	3	0	0	0	19.3	25
Peanuts (dried)	1 cup	827	78	13	0	14.6	0	10.8	85
Milk (2%)	1 cup	121	36	0	2	0.1	5	6.4	297
Milk (skim)	1 cup	86	5	0	2	0	0	6.6	302
Cheese (American processed)	1 oz	106	75	0	0	0.2	10	2.5	174
Egg	1 each	75	60	0	0	0.4	0	12.4	25
Mayonnaise	1 tbs	35	77	0	0	2.7	0	—	0
Recommendations[c]			30%	20–35 g	60 mg	15 mg		70 μg	800 mg

a   Database used from Food Processor II computer program. ESHA Research, P. O. Box 13028, Salem, OR 97309.

b   Expressed as retinol equivalents.

c   For vitamin C, vitamin E, calcium and selenium from 1989 RDA Tables, for males, 25 to 30 age group, fiber and fat percentage recommendations.

from the food consumption data using various food/nutrient databases. Since most "Westernized" diets involve foods which contain an abundance of all essential nutrients, identification of specific nutrients as being involved in cancer etiology and/or protection leaves out a number of components of food composition. This is easily seen in the example of citrus fruit consumption, where we might ascribe effects to ascorbic acid, when, in fact, other nutrients such as potassium, carotenoids, carbohydrate, and fiber are also consistently present in this group of foods. Thus, it is important that the identification of the risk and protective factors be based upon the concordance of epidemiological findings with other scientific results, preferably in man. The latter condition is difficult to achieve, since prospective studies over a long period are scientifically difficult and prohibitively costly to perform with human populations. So, we are most often left with attempting to correlate animal studies with the findings from various types of epidemiologic research, knowing full well that rats and mice are not humans. This is painfully apparent in studies involving vitamin C, which cannot be performed in rodents that synthesize endogenous vitamin C. For example, most animals other than higher primates synthesize vitamin C. However, guinea pigs have been used for vitamin C research, but less information is available regarding cancer for this animal model.

A confounding variable that is beginning to emerge in importance as we learn more specifics is the genetic background of the human populations. As we learn more and more about nutrition, we note an increasing identification of differences that can be ascribed to genetic factors and the processing or interaction with nutrients and foods. Are there susceptible individuals or populations to different carcinogens and anticarcinogens? If some nutrients are anticarcinogens, is their effect mediated via genetically derived capabilities? This is neither a fact nor fallacy, but rather it is our scientific ignorance of all of the genetic and environmental factors that lead to cancer.

Another concern for future research is that these recommendations, or ones similar, have been promulgated by many agencies in the U.S. and abroad. To what extent have the populations in the industrialized nations changed their diets due to effective marketing of these public health messages? If the diets have changed, then we may begin to see a confusing epidemiologic picture emerging over the next decade, since the various sample groups have been "contaminated" with diet-health information relating to a set of chronic diseases that may fail to occur a decade or two hence. In our experience, using the NCI "Diet and Health Habits Questionnaire" with incoming medical students, the percent of fat calories that several classes reported dropped over a 4-year period from 36 to 32%.[60] What are to be the control groups of the near-term future if these health messages are received and are basically correct? From a public health perspective, it doesn't matter since the goal was achieved even though the mechanism is not yet defined. Scientifically, however, we may have lost the ability to conduct further meaningful population studies. If, however, the message—or part of it—is incorrect, then the effect of altered dietary practices on the development of cancer will be further confused, but we'll have to wait and see.

Finally, we must keep in mind that there are really not "good" or "bad" foods, but the whole diet, lifestyle, and genetic factors are important. Especially compelling for future exploration is the potential interrelationship between genetic mutations and diet in human cancer. Young and Richardson[61] cautioned us regarding food-related fallacies, since historically the area of diet and disease has been fraught with fads and fallacies. We must complete some of this puzzle, especially in the area of mechanisms, before we can be content that the science is clear and the public health recommendations can be more well defined. The prescriptions listed above, however, can be supported by epidemiologic and laboratory cancer research findings.

ACKNOWLEDGMENT

The authors wish to thank Mrs. Carole Justice for her contributions in preparing the manuscript, and Ms. Belle Jones for her help in researching references. This chapter was supported in part by grants CA-22032 and DE-09523.

REFERENCES

1. **National Research Council.** *Diet, Nutrition and Cancer,* National Academy of Sciences, Washington, D.C., 1982.
2. **Doll, R, and Peto, R.** The causes of cancer, quantitative estimates of available risks of cancer in the United States today. *JNCI,* 66:1191–1308, 1981.
3. **American Cancer Society.** Causation and prevention: an American Cancer Society special report. *Cancer,* 34:121–126, 1984.
4. **Nixon, DW.** Nutrition and cancer: American Cancer Society guidelines, programs and institutions. *Cancer,* 40:71–75, 1990.
5. **American Cancer Society.** Guidelines on diet, nutrition and cancer. *Cancer,* 41:334–338, 1992.
6. **National Cancer Institute.** Cancer control objectives for the nation: 1985–2000. *NCI Monogr.,* 2:1–93, 1986.
7. **U.S. Department of Health and Human Services.** The Surgeon General's Report on Nutrition and Health, U.S. Govt. Printing Office, Washington, D.C., Publication PHS 88–50210, 1988.
8. **National Research Council.** Cancer. In: *Diet and Health: Implications for Reducing Chronic Disease Risk.* National Academy Press, Washington, D.C., 1989.
9. **Boutwell, RK.** Anticarcinogenesis in the mouse skin two-stage model. *Cancer Res,* 43:2465S–2468S, 1983.
10. **NIH Consensus Development Conference Statement.** Health implications of obesity. *Ann Intern Med,* 103:147–151, 1985.
11. **Lew, EA, and Garfinkel, L.** Variations in mortality by weight among 750,000 men and women. *J Chronic Dis,* 32:563–576, 1979.
12. **Garfinkel, L.** Nutrition and cancer. *Cancer,* 41:325–327, 1991.
13. **Tannenbaum, A.** The initiation and growth of tumors: introduction I. Effects of underfeeding. *Am J Cancer,* 38:335–350, 1940.
14. **Tannenbaum, A.** Relationship of body weight to cancer incidence. *Arch Pathol,* 30:509–517, 1940.
15. **Wolff, GL.** Body weight and cancer. *Am J Clin Nutr,* 45:168–179, 1987.
16. **Kritchevsky, D, and Klurfeld, DM.** Caloric effects in experimental mammary tumorigenesis. *Am J Clin Nutr,* 45:236–242, 1987.
17. **Kritchevsky, D.** Diet and nutrition. *Cancer,* 41:328–333, 1992.
18. **Frisch, RE, Wyshak, G, Albright, NL, et al.** Lower lifetime occurrence of breast cancer and cancers of the reproductive system among former college athletes. *Am J Clin Nutr,* 45:328–335, 1987.
19. **Wynder, EL, Rose, DP, and Cohen, LA.** Diet and breast cancer causation and therapy. *Cancer,* 58:1804–1813, 1986.
20. **Carroll, KK, Braden, LM, Bell, JA, and Kalameghan, R.** Fat and cancer. *Cancer,* 58:1818–1829, 1986.
21. **Marks, PA.** Nutrition and the cancer problem: an overview. In: *Nutrition and Cancer.* Winick, M, Ed., Wiley & Sons, New York, 1977.
22. **Wynder, EL and Reddy, BS.** Diet and cancer of the colon. In: *Nutrition and Cancer.* Winick, M, Ed., Wiley & Sons, New York, 1977.
23. **Wynder, EL.** Dietary habits and cancer epidemiology. *Cancer,* 43:1955–1961, 1979.
24. **Greenwald, P, Kramer, B, and Weed, D.** Expanding horizons in breast and prostate cancer prevention and early detection. *J Cancer Ed,* 8:91–107, 1993.
25. **Reddy, RS.** Dietary fat and its relationship to large bowel cancer. *Cancer Res,* 41:3700–3709, 1981.
26. **Bruce, WR, Varghese, AJ, Furrer, A, and Lad, PC.** A mutagen in the feces of normal humans. In: *Origins of Human Cancer.* Hiatt, HH, Watson, JD, and Winstein, JA, Eds., Cold Spring Harbor Laboratory, New York, 1977.
27. **Bruce, WR.** Recent hypotheses for the origin of colon cancer. *Cancer Res,* 47:4237–4242, 1987.
28. **Willet, WC, Stampfer, MJ, Colditz, GA, et al.** Dietary fat and the risk of breast cancer. *N Eng J Med,* 316:22–28, 1987.

29. **Willet, WC, Hunter, DJ, Stampfer, MJ et al.,** Dietary fat and fiber in relation to breast cancer—an 8-year follow-up. *JAMA,* 268:2037–2044, 1992.

30. **Willett, WC, Stampfer, MJ, Colditz, GA, et al.** Relation of fat, fiber and meat intake to colon cancer risk in a prospective study among women. *N Eng J Med,* 323:1664–1672, 1990.

31. **Kolonel, LN.** Fat and colon cancer: how firm is the epidemiological evidence. *Am J Clin Nutr,* 45:336–341, 1987.

32. **Pariza, M.** Dietary fat and cancer risk: evidence and research needs. *Ann Rev Nutr,* 8:167–183, 1988.

33. **Garland, CF and Garland, FC.** Do sunlight and vitamin D reduce the likelihood of colon cancer? *Int J Epidemiol,* 9:227–231, 1980.

34. **Garland, CF and Garland, FC.** Calcium and colon cancer. *Clin Nutr,* 5:161–166, 1986.

35. **Garland, CF, Garland, FC, and Gorham, ED.** Can colon incidence and death rates be reduced with calcium and vitamin D? *Am J Clin Nutr,* 54:193S–201S, 1991.

36. **Report of the AMA Council on Scientific Affairs.** *Arch Intern Med,* 153:50–56, 1993.

37. **Fearon, ER and Vogelstein, B.** A genetic model for colorectal tumorigenesis. *Cell,* 61:759–767, 1990.

38. **Burkitt, DF.** Some diseases characteristic of modern western civilization. *Brit Med J,* 1:274–278 (1973).

39. **Ausman, LM.** Fiber and colon cancer: does the current evidence justify a preventive policy? *Nutr Rev,* 51:57–63, 1993.

40. **Dwyer, J.** Dietary fiber and colorectal cancer risk. *Nutr Rev,* 51:147–155, 1993.

41. **Howe, GR, Benito, E, Castelleto, R, et al.** Dietary intake of fiber and decreased risk of cancers of the colon and rectum: evidence from the combined analysis of 13 case-control studies. *JNCI,* 84:1887–1896, 1992.

42. **U.S. Department of Health Services,** Healthy people 2000. *Nutr Today,* 25:29–39, 1990.

43. **Block, G, Patterson, B, and Subar, A.** Fruit, vegetables and cancer prevention: a review of the epidemiological evidence. *Nutr Cancer,* 18:1–29, 1992.

44. **Weisburger, JH.** Nutritional approach to cancer prevention with emphasis on vitamins, antioxidants and carotenoids. *Am J Clin Nutr,* 53:2263–2375, 1991.

45. **Graham, S.** Results of case-control studies of diet and cancer in Buffalo, N.Y. *Cancer Res,* 43:2409–2413, 1983.

46. **Ziegler, RG.** Vegetables, fruits and carotenoids and the risk of cancer. *Am J Clin Nutr,* 53:251S–259S, 1991.

47. **Hennekens, CH, Mayrent, SZ, and Willett, W.** Vitamin A, carotenoids and retinoids, *Cancer,* 58:1837–1841, 1986.

48. **Byers, T and Perry, G.** Dietary carotenes, vitamin C, and vitamin E as protective antioxidants in human cancers. *Ann Rev Nutr,* 12:139–159, 1992.

49. **Mirvish, SS.** Effects of vitamins C and E on N-nitroso compound formation, carcinogenesis and cancer. *Cancer,* 58:1842–1850, 1988.

50. **Sies, H, Stahl, W, and Sundquist, AR.** Antioxidant function of vitamins: vitamins E and C, beta-carotene and other carotenoids. In: *Beyond Deficiency: New Views on the Function and Health Effects of Vitamins.* Sauberlich, HE and Machlin, LJ, Eds., *Ann NY Acad Sci,* 669:7–20, 1992.

51. **Bendich, AB.** Carotenoids and the immune response. *J Nutr,* 199:112–115, 1989.

52. **American Cancer Society,** *Cancer Facts and Figures—1993,* American Cancer Society, Atlanta, GA, 1993, pp. 28.

53. **Block, G.** Vitamin C and cancer prevention: the epidemiologic evidence. *Am J Clin Nutr,* 53:270S–282S, 1991.

54. **Peto, R, Doll, R, Buckley, JD, and Sporn, MB.** Can dietary beta-carotene materially reduce human cancer rates? *Nature,* 290:201–208, 1981.

55. **Ziegler, RG, Subar, AF, Craft, NE, et al.** Does β-carotene explain why reduced cancer risk is associated with vegetable and fruit intake? *Cancer Res,* 52:2060S–2061S, 1992.

56. **Bendich, AB, Gabriel, E, and Machlin, LS.** Dietary vitamin E requirement for optimum minimal response in the rat. *J Nutr,* 116:675–681, 1986.

57. **Wattenberg, LW.** Inhibition of neoplasia by minor dietary constituents. *Cancer Res,* 43:2448S–2453S, 1983.

58. **Zeng, Y, Talalay, P, Cho, C, and Posner, GH.** A major inducer of anticarcinogenic protective enzymes from broccoli: isolation and elucidation of structure. *PNAS (USA),* 89:2399–2403, 1992.

59. **Patterson, BH, Block, G, Resenberger, WF et al.,** Fruit and vegetables in the American diet: data from the NHANES II Survey. *AJPH,* 80:1443–1449, 1990.

60. **Dingles-Sutton, C, Huang, L, Chan, WMY, Brandt, RB, Banks, WL, Jr.** Medical student reported diet practices and the ACS guidelines. *J Cancer,* in press, 1993.

61. **Young, VR and Richardson, DP.** Nutrients, vitamins and minerals, cancer prevention: facts and fallacies. *Cancer,* 43:2125–2136, 1979.

Chapter 14

NUTRITION QUACKERY—FACTS AND FRAUD AND PRACTICAL COUNSELING ADVICE

Donald F. Kirby and Janet V. Starkey

TABLE OF CONTENTS

0-8493-7847-8/94/$0.00+$.50

Quackery has probably existed since man could first barter or buy services and products. The broad definition of quackery actually encompasses both products and people. This includes drugs or food supplements that are promoted with false health benefits, devices or machines that do not perform as claimed, or even people who claim miraculous medical results without accepted scientific data, whether or not they have medical credentials. For any practitioner who believes that his patients do not fall prey to such practices, a recent article in the New England Journal of Medicine reported that approximately one third of Americans have used unproven medical treatment![1] These treatments were most often for long-term ailments such as arthritis, back pain, cancer, and Acquired Immunodeficiency Syndrome (AIDS). It is estimated that $14 billion dollars were spent last year alone on questionable or worthless therapies.

Various levels of nutrition misinformation have existed for centuries. Unfortunately, people will continue to be attracted to and purchase products or services which promise quick and easy solutions to both real and imagined medical problems. This chapter will define what nutrition quackery is, common characteristics of quackery and consumers who are attracted by it, harmful effects resulting from engaging in questionable practices, and finally, recommendations for combating nutrition misinformation and quackery.

I. CURRENT LEGAL IMPLICATIONS

The American College of Physicians defines health quackery as "the promotion and commercialization of unproven and potentially dangerous health products and procedures."[2] It is also known as health "fraud", which can cause harm to consumers nutritionally, economically, psychologically, and medically. Health quackery may be characterized by one or more of the following: direct health hazards, indirect health hazards, and/or economic fraud.[2]

Direct health hazards may be procedures or products that can directly harm an individual. For example, "chelation therapy", which cleans atherosclerotic blood vessels of patients with heart disease, has been associated with severe renal disease and even death.[3] This therapy has never been proven and should be abandoned.

Indirect health hazards may cause patients to forego or to delay seeking more traditional care. The adherence to unsafe diets or use of megadose vitamins to treat an AIDS patient can delay treatment with current therapies that do have proven benefits.

Economic frauds are those that promote worthless or ineffective products or devices that may not cause any detriment to health, but do not perform as promised. These are important to be aware of because people will spend a great deal of money on these products or services. Products that promise complete reversal of baldness but do not are an example.

The main motivation behind these activities is profit. As previously mentioned, about $14 billion dollars were expended on these types of practices last year alone.[1] It would be optimal to redirect these misguided resources into areas that do have proven efficacy or to properly test some of these nontraditional therapies for safety and efficacy. The greatest harm, ironically, is that it can prevent the consumer from attaining optimal health, partially due to the delay in obtaining appropriate treatment from a qualified practitioner. Eisenberg et al. found that among those people who used unconventional therapy for serious medical problems 83% had seen a medical doctor, but 72% did not inform their doctor about their use of alternate forms of therapy.[1]

Consumers must realize that the present laws do not protect them from hearing or reading false, deceptive, or misleading claims about nutrition. The law only requires that these statements do not appear on the label of a product. Table 1 shows which agency has jurisdiction over a particular quackery problem.

TABLE 1
Quackery Jurisdiction

Problem	Agency[a]
Product promoted with misleading or false claims	FDA Office—Regional
Fraudulant mail-order promotion	U.S. Postal Service
False advertising	FTC
Improper treatment	State licensing board/state or local professional
Licensed practitioner	society/local hospital where practitioner is on staff
Unlicensed individual	State Attorney General/local District Attorney

[a] Other agencies can assist with some of these issues on a local basis, and this is not a complete list of all avenues of redress.

Note: FDA = Food and Drug Administration; FTC = Federal Trade Commission.

The Food and Drug Administration (FDA) can only take action when a product is misbranded or includes false or misleading claims on its label. If a product is shown to be harmful or dangerous, then the FDA can have the product seized, obtain an injunction against its sale, seek voluntary compliance with regulations, or undertake legal proceedings.

Two other governmental agencies also provide limited protection to consumers. The U.S. Postal Service (USPS) can act against anyone who uses mail to defraud. When a suspect product, device, or service is brought to the attention of the USPS, they can investigate the case and bring the case to court if need be; however, many cases do not actually go to court because the offending party complies in some manner. This usually does not result in the removal of the focus of the action, so consumers are still at risk from this quackery.

The Federal Trade Commission (FTC) is empowered to act against misleading advertising of health services or nonprescription products by issuing regulations and seeking injunctions. While FTC action against a company or distributor can result in large monetary penalties, these types of cases are a minority with which the FTC concerns itself.

Unfortunately, these agencies are unable to adequately address the quackery issue for many reasons which include limited resources, poor interagency communication, and inadequate legal regulations. Thus, the responsibility to give proper nutritional advice to the consumer should begin with a person's physician. Many physicians are not adequately trained to do this, however, they should know that a Registered Dietitian (R.D.) can assist them in training their patients in proper diets as decided medically prudent by the physician[4,5] (see Appendix III).

In addition to these agencies, it is possible to take direct action against an individual or licensed practitioner who is advocating, prescribing, or distributing health quackery. The State Licensing Board or local professional organizations that the practitioner may belong to may take action against a licensed practitioner. For an unlicensed individual, the local district attorney or State Attorney General's offices can be contacted so that inquiries can be made, as well as a number of national and private organizations that watch for consumer fraud.

II. THE CHALLENGE OF MISINFORMATION

Nutrition misinformation lays the groundwork for health fraud and quackery. When presented with deep conviction, misinformation can be quite believable and may held as fact. Sincere testimonials that a product works can be very convincing to the unsuspecting consumer who desires an easy solution to a problem. Also, the promotion of nutrition quackery is not limited to individuals who lack scientific training. Given the right set of circumstances, almost anyone can be vulnerable to becoming a victim of quackery. Those who believe this misinformation fit into three loosely defined categories: those who find it difficult to change their beliefs, even when confronted with scientific evidence to the contrary; those who are more objective and accurate information can help change their behavior; and lastly, those who are so immersed in delusion they are beyond help. For this last group, the level of food faddism becomes a form of food cultism.

Quackery does not need to involve intent to deceive to be considered quackery. Some of its promoters are sincere and well-meaning, yet are misguided individuals who promote questionable goods or services. However, there are others, as in all areas of life, who take advantage of people's vulnerability for selfish economic purposes. Their victims come from all walks of life and educational backgrounds. As long as people want to believe in simple solutions, and that they can gain some control over their destiny, quackery will continue, despite advances in medicine and science, public education, and laws which ensure drug safety and effectiveness.

III. IDENTIFYING NUTRITION QUACKERY

Some forms of quackery are easy to identify, while others are not. The latter may be based upon some medical report which sounds impressive. According to the Department of Health and Human Services,[6] some of the more common characteristics of quackery include the following:

- A "special", "secret", "ancient", or "foreign" formula, available only through the mail and only from one supplier.
- Testimonials or case histories from satisfied users as the only proof that the product works.
- A single product is effective for a wide variety of ailments.
- A scientific "breakthrough" or "miracle cure" that has been held back or overlooked by the medical community.

It is easy to see why a quick and painless cure to a long-standing problem such as being overweight or obese has appeal. The fact is, if the remedy sounds too good to be true, it probably is. "Special" or "secret" ingredients, especially those that are not routinely recommended by established medical practices, might also have great appeal to some who want to feel exotic or special.

Testimonials are a source of great pressure and are used in convincing potential consumers especially when there are no supporting medical studies. Testimonials that report fantastic or incredible results may reflect the power of suggestion or the placebo effect. This is why scientific studies are needed to help establish whether or not a purported remedy actually works; yet, many consumers are not aware that some remedies work solely because people want them to work. In many disorders, about one third of patients will show signs of improvement with the use of a placebo.[7] Confidence in the treatment or in the practitioner makes it more likely that a positive effect will occur. Many physical symptoms that are experienced have a psychological component that can account for the subsequent relief that is experienced. What many consumers do not know is that the body will heal itself in many instances with or without special treatment. Many times, improvements could be due to the psychological effects of taking something or to the recuperative abilities of the body. Few remedies will be fully accepted by the medical community unless there is a comparison of the remedy with some accepted treatment or compared to a placebo control group.

''Quacks'' are often familiar with current scientific advice and recent studies, and they may alter the meanings to their advertising advantage. For example, the National Academy of Sciences reported that fruits and vegetables high in vitamins C and beta carotene could reduce the incidence of certain cancers. The supplement industry began marketing tablets containing these vitamins because the consumer was led to believe that taking them could reduce the risk of cancer. However, the National Academy of Sciences was careful to state that eating foods rich in these nutrients was advised, not the taking of supplements. One of the reasons for this stance is that it is not known whether other components of these foods are also responsible for reducing cancer risk. Those individuals looking for a ''quick fix'' are more willing to ingest supplements than to stop smoking, to lose weight, or to exercise more, which might offer a healthier lifestyle and alleviation or amelioration of certain diseases.

IV. DISTORTION OF SCIENTIFIC DATA

Distortion of scientific facts also promotes nutrition misinformation and quackery. The public is generally not familiar with scientific terms such as ''enzymes'', ''free radicals'', or the processes of digestion and absorption well enough to know what they really mean. Most consumers have a limited understanding of how the body works and fall prey to erroneous information regarding metabolism, anatomy, and physiology. They also do not know exactly how vitamins regulate and facilitate metabolic functions by acting as co-enzymes to form metabolically active enzymes that catalyze chemical reactions in the body. An example of a product sold in health food stores and nutrition catalogs is SOD (superoxide dismutase), which is an intracellular enzyme whose function is to detoxify oxygen free radicals, thereby decreasing cellular damage. What the unsuspecting buyer may not know is that SOD in capsule form is digested similarly to other proteins and rendered useless as an enzyme. Yet some consumers are willing to pay high prices for something they do not understand, but which promises to slow down the aging process.

Exaggerated claims are another way in which nutrition misinformation prospers. No food is perfect or has magical qualities. For example, there is nothing in grapefruit which burns fat, yet grapefruit pills are sold as a weight loss aid. Likewise, wheat grass has been touted to detoxify the system of impurities, yet the chlorophyll, which is the ingredient said to have detoxifying properties, remains unabsorbed by the body. It is true that most consumers have faith that what they purchase must be safe to consume or else it would not be sold, or that actual ingredients match what is written on the label. Unfortunately, this is not usually the case, and consumers really are not adequately protected.

V. SUSCEPTIBLE POPULATIONS

Table 2 lists some groups that appear more susceptible to quackery or nutrition fraud. Major target areas for health quackery include illnesses such as arthritis, cancer, and AIDS, which include both nutritional and non-nutritional remedies. A quick glance at a nutrition mail order catalog will provide one with a cornucopia of products designed to address one's health and appearance concerns.[8] Products are targeted to different audiences, body parts, and medical conditions. Products are designed to ''detoxify'' the system, to improve mental alertness, to increase energy levels, to lose weight, to build muscle, and to grow hair, just to name a few of the purported benefits of purchasing a particular product(s).

Patients with certain cancers and Human Immunodeficiency Virus (HIV) disease may feel that their conditions are hopeless and look for any form of treatment that has the promise of ''help'' or ''cure.'' What is surprising is that it is not necessarily the poorly

TABLE 2
Susceptible Populations for Quackery

Athletes
Certain disease states
    Arthritis
    Cancers
    Human Immunodeficiency
      Virus (HIV) disease
    Obesity
Elderly
People under "stress"
Smokers

educated, lower socioeconomic classes that explore these alternative therapies, but rather the educated, more financially stable patients.[1]

A. CANCER REMEDIES

Cancer patients often turn to unconventional therapy because traditional methods of surgery, chemotherapy, or radiation therapy may have failed to cure or control their disease or because they are afraid of undergoing such treatments. The main problem is that alternative treatments may be available, but rarely have undergone medical scrutiny for safety and efficacy. In the 1970s laetrile was touted as a cancer treatment. This compound came from apricot pits and can produce cyanide, which was supposed to selectively poison tumor cells, but not healthy cells. No scientific evidence has ever been shown to substantiate that theory.[9] Due to political pressures that arose from the U.S. ban on its sale, a multicenter trial was performed which showed that it was an ineffective treatment against cancer.[10] In addition, several of the patients exhibited signs of cyanide poisoning with blood levels approaching the lethal range.

Coffee enemas and restrictive diets have also been offered for the treatment of cancers. Again, documentation of efficacy is not available in a controlled trial. A recent review by Green has critically reviewed the data on the use of coffee enemas and the Gerson theory and diet that suggests this practice.[11] He noted that there is no medical justification to support the theories of these enemas mobilizing and detoxifying the "poisons" from the liver and intestines and that cancer cells will be killed. The diet that accompanies this theory requires that only oatmeal and fresh fruits and vegetables be consumed. The adequacy of this diet is unclear.

Other diets have been suggested for the cancer patient, as well as megadose vitamin therapy. None of these treatments have been tested in controlled trials, and many of the diets can lead to nutritional deficiencies. More patient education is needed to help patients choose appropriate therapy instead of unconventional and sometimes potentially dangerous therapy.

B. HIV DISEASE REMEDIES

One of the most devastating and visible effects of the AIDS virus is progressive weight loss. Ott et al. have recently shown by tetrapolar impedence that the changes in body composition with loss of body cell mass occur early in HIV disease when most patients are asymptomatic and are independent of their body weight.[12] These authors postulated that either there are increased metabolic requirements or a metabolic block permitting utilization of nutrients in these patients, and that dietary intake alone is not the sole problem responsible for the weight loss.

Several studies have shown that patients who are HIV infected have made dietary modifications and many consume more vitamins than they did previously.[13,14] This is

TABLE 3
Unproven Nutritional Therapies and Unconventional
Diets Used by AIDS Patients

Megadoses of nutrients
    Vitamins—A, C, E, B_{12}, and β-carotene
    Minerals—Selenium and zinc
Diet methods
    Dr. Berger's Immune Power Diet[a]
    Gerson Method
    Maximum Immunity Diet[b]
    Macrobiotic Diet
    Kelley Regime
    Yeast Free Diet
Herbal remedies
    Garlic
    Glycyrrhizin
Miscellaneous methods
    AL 721[c]
    Laetrile
    Lecithin
    BHT[d]
    Coenzyme Q (Ubiquinone)

[a] Berger, M., *Dr. Berger's Immune Power Diet*, New York, Avon Books, 1985.
[b] Weiner, M., *Maximum Immunity Diet*, New York, Pocket Books, 1986.
[c] AL 721 = "activated lipids".
[d] BHT = butylated hydroxytoluene.

After Dwyer, J.T., et al., Unproven nutrition therapies for AIDS: what is the evidence? *Nutr. Today,* 1988; 23:25–33. With permission.

usually to help improve their immune status and try to "fight off the disease". Unfortunately, this leads some patients to search for unproven therapies and ingestion of large supplemental doses of nutrients in the hope of helping their disease. Table 3 lists some of the unproven nutritional therapies and unconventional diets that have been used by HIV-infected patients.[15]

In view of the progressive and early nature of nutritional compromise in this population, nutritionists should get involved as soon as possible in the care of the patients. They should encourage HIV-infected individuals to seek medical attention and to participate in therapies that have been shown to be useful or become involved in trials with newer agents that show promise of benefit.

VI. SUPPLEMENTS

Approximately one third of Americans take supplements. This figure is even higher for athletes. Advertisers are good at convincing people they need something even when they do not. People are convinced that they need supplements as a form of nutritional insurance against a fast-paced life, to compensate for "processed" foods, to promote future "superhealth", or to rationalize poor eating habits. It is true that lifestyle habits which deplete vitamin stores, such as excessive alcohol intake or smoking, need to be addressed. Consumers need to be educated that taking supplements will not reverse all of the damage incurred through certain lifestyle habits.

A. AMINO ACIDS

Athletes and body builders are prime targets for nutritional supplements and ergogenic aids. Many body builders take protein supplements in the form of pills and powders in order to gain mass. Amino acid formulas are also available. In reality, excess protein may add excess calories and is not responsible for gains in mass as much as exercise and training are.[16] Also, the safety of using amino acid supplements has not been established.[17] To date, no experimental evidence has been found to suggest that supplements alone enhance athletic performance. To build muscle, one must train and eat adequately.

Ingesting amino acid supplements should theoretically not cause problems, unless patients have medical conditions such as hepatic encephalopathy or renal insufficiency where protein restriction may be indicated for a particular patient. Unfortunately, it has been recognized that eosinophilia-myalgia syndrome is associated with the ingestion of L-tryptophan.[18–21] Patients took the supplement for a number of reasons including premenstrual syndrome (PMS), migraine headaches, insomnia, tinnitus, chronic muscle aches, and appetite suppression. Whether the syndrome results from impurities in the supplements during manufacturing or from a genetic abnormality of tryptophan metabolism is not totally resolved.[22] The number of reported cases has dropped dramatically since the FDA recalled all tryptophan preparations that contained more than 100 mg per daily dose.[23] The most disturbing factor about this syndrome is that while there may be improvement in symptoms over the year after diagnosis and discontinuation of L-tryptophan, only one quarter of affected patients were able to perform their normal daily activities as reported in one population-based cohort study.[24] This, again underscores the importance of not taking megadoses of any "chemical" without better data on potential risks and benefits from treatment. In reality, it has been illegal to sell amino acids as "dietary supplements" since the 1970s when the FDA dropped them from the "generally recognized as safe" (GRAS) list.[25] Unfortunately, a 1992 congressional moratorium on labeling has stopped complete and accurate information from being placed on the labels of these items, again leaving the public uninformed and unprotected.

B. VITAMIN AND MINERAL SUPPLEMENTATION

It is estimated that 60 million Americans take vitamin and/or supplements daily and another 60 million take them occasionally.[25] The income of the supplement industry is estimated to be $3.3 billion dollars annually.

The medical community supports the use of vitamins for specific nutrient deficiencies or to meet particular nutritional needs such as iron supplementation during pregnancy. However, a survey has found that most people do not take them as directed by physicians, but rather to better their sex lives, to prevent hair loss, and to perform better at their jobs.[25]

There is a wide variety of multivitamin/mineral supplements available featuring "scientifically balanced" formulas and "amino acids chelates". Questionable ingredients can be found in a number of these formulas such as alfalfa, rutin, algin, hesperidin complex, bee pollen, and bioflavonoids. Ironically, manufacturers are careful not to include any starch, sugar, artificial flavors or colors in the formula. Due to the Proxmire Amendment, the FDA cannot remove vitamin and mineral supplements from the shelves just because they are considered worthless or offered at a high dose, but it can prevent the packages from carrying health claims.[25]

Generally, the public believes that if something is a nutrient, it must be safe. However, nutrients used in excessive amounts become drugs and in some cases these can be toxic. This is especially true for vitamins A, D, and pyridoxine (vitamin B_6). While a vitamin/mineral supplement at the RDA level will probably do no harm to the majority of people taking them, megadose ingestion over a period of time can potentially have serious side effects. It is unclear how many people have been harmed by vitamin or

TABLE 4
Selected Vitamin Toxicity

Fat soluble vitamins	Doses	Complications
A	Generally safe up to 10,000 IU/day.	>50,000 IU/day—symptoms can include nausea, vomiting, fatigue, anorexia, blurred vision, joint pains. Beware of use during pregnancy since single doses ≥20,000 IU can cause birth defects.
Beta-carotene (Vitamin A precursor)	Generally nontoxic—believed to be safe up to 50 mg/day.	Large doses can cause the palms and soles of feet to appear orange.
D	Safe up to 1000 IU/day—pregnant women should avoid excessive intake of vitamin D.	Can lead to hypercalcemia which may have very nonspecific symptoms such as nausea, vomiting, constipation, fatigue and malaise. Hypertension may be present with the hypercalcemia. Damage to the kidneys and heart has been reported.
E	Safe up to 1000 IU/day.	Doses ≥300 IU/day have caused nausea, diarrhea, intestinal cramps, fatigue, weakness, headache, blurred vision, and gonadal dysfunction. >1200 IU/day an interaction between warfarin has been reported.
Water soluble vitamins		
Thiamin (B$_6$)	Safe maximum dose not known.	≥500 mg/d for extended periods can cause nerve damage that may not be reversible when the vitamin is discontinued.
Niacin	Safe maximum dose not known. Safe maximum dose not set for hyperlipidemia treatment.	Side effects occur at doses used to treat hyperlipidemias, e.g., flushing, tingling, rashes, reactivation of ulcer disease, and liver damage.

mineral supplements because the manufacturers are not required to report any adverse reactions.[18] By examining data from the U.S. Poison Control Centers for 1991, there were approximately 56,000 phone calls from people who were concerned about vitamin and/or mineral pills that they had ingested. Of these calls 1191 had adverse reactions of which 47 were life-threatening. The majority of the 18 deaths were infants or young children who took their mothers' iron supplements. One man died from a large dose of vitamin A taken over 2 weeks for an unknown reason.[25]

Another unfortunate situation is that supplements are not required to conform to any legal standards for quality, potency, purity, or uniformity. This may mean that the ingredients do not contain what the label states and that the supplements are not guaranteed to dissolve so that pills may actually be excreted whole. This is a task for the FDA, but regulations have not been forthcoming. The consumer truly must be wary of *all* supplements because many are untested. Using reference sources such as *Nutrition Action Healthletter* and *Consumer Reports* may provide a less biased view towards individual products compared to other sources which may receive significant advertising revenue from supplement manufacturers.[25]

Table 4 lists the effects of large doses of vitamins known to have potentially toxic side effects. People who are interested in curing insomnia and PMS with vitamin B$_6$, the common cold with vitamin C, heart disease with vitamin E, and cancer with beta carotene are likely to take megadoses of these vitamins with little regard to the consequences. In reality, the daily use of 500 to 6000 mg doses of vitamin B$_6$ for PMS has resulted in neurotoxicity, which may not be completely reversible when the vitamin is discontinued.[26,27]

Excessive intakes of vitamin C provide the individual with no health or medical benefit. Between a level of 250 to 500 mg/day, the body tissue stores become saturated and intestinal absorption becomes limited.[28] In some cases, taking megadoses of vitamin C may reduce the symptoms of a mild cold, but may also cause damage to vitamin B$_{12}$ status by converting B$_{12}$ to anti-B$_{12}$ molecules, among other problems, such as diarrhea.[28,29] Rebound scurvy has occurred when high doses have been discontinued. Though Linus Pauling, who is in his 90s, takes 18 grams of vitamin C each day with 800 IU of vitamin E, he notes that it takes a while to build up the tolerance to take that much.[30] It must be remembered that at higher than RDA levels, these vitamins should be considered drugs since they are being given at doses in excess of that needed to prevent vitamin deficiency.

Among the unproven nutritional therapies used by HIV-infected patients, megadoses of vitamins A, C, E, B$_{12}$, selenium, and zinc have been "recommended" to restore cell-mediated immunity by increasing T-cell activity and number.[31] While it is possible that some of these vitamins and minerals may have some effect on the immune system in the HIV patient, the studies are mostly small and uncontrolled. The studies are also usually short in duration and do not provide significant information on potential toxicity or length of benefit to this population.[31]

C. ANTIOXIDANT VITAMINS AND MINERALS

Studies now suggest that antioxidants such as beta carotene, vitamins A, C, E, copper, zinc, manganese, and selenium may play a role in protection from diseases such as cancer, heart disease, and other problems such as cataracts.[32] It is believed that highly active free radicals can cause damage to cells and their components.[32–34] Also, these vitamins and minerals may inhibit some of their toxic effects.[32] What is not known is which vitamins and/or minerals are most important and what dosage is the minimum effective dose.

Human population studies show that groups eating foods high in these substances tend to have lower rates of those diseases. Some researchers have suggested that higher than normal levels be consumed, which research may bear out some day.[35] Many physicians are concerned about these recommendations because to achieve the higher levels of intake of these micronutrients, it will require supplementation rather than dietary manipulation; while the data is promising, it is not accepted at this point.[25] Currently, it is not wise to recommend megadoses of these nutrients, as optimal levels have not yet been adequately defined. Eating a diet rich in fruits and vegetables will provide more than adequate levels of beta carotene and vitamin C and is associated with decreases in certain cancers, while ingesting supplements have not been proven.[36] Many studies are currently in progress to look at the efficacy of beta carotene in cancer prevention, but the results will not be available for many years.[37]

Higher dietary levels of vitamin E are more difficult to achieve, especially if one is following a low fat diet as well. A firm relationship between the intake of total fat calories and cancers in the postmenopausal breast, pancreas, prostate, distal colon, ovary, and endometrium has been established.[36] Low α-tocopherol levels were associated with a 1.5-fold risk of cancer compared with those patients with higher levels.[38] Thus, most data support a hypothesis that dietary vitamin E protects against some cancers.

Dietary manipulations to ingest more fruits and vegetables would be preferable to oral supplementation because it is still not known what other ingredients in the food may be providing a beneficial effect. However, until more research is done, recommendations for higher dose vitamin intake, and particularly the antioxidants, will need to wait. Health professionals should stay current with this evolving research and be willing to objectively assist patients in choosing supplements, if they insist.

TABLE 5
Selected Mineral Toxicity

	Doses	Complications
Chromium	RDA has not been set at this time. Safe at 200 µg/day.	Toxicity believed to be low with no well-recognized toxicity syndromes in man.
Copper	RDA is 2 mg/day. High doses can decrease zinc absorption.	Excess oral doses (>10–15 mg/day) can cause acute, chronic, or severe problems. Acute: Abdominal pain, nausea, vomiting, diarrhea, hemolysis, jaundice, and renal failure. Chronic: Anemia, diarrhea, and cirrhosis. Severe: Coma and death.
Iron	RDA: 15 mg for women and 10 mg for men. Higher doses recommended for pregnancy and iron deficiency. Safe to approximately 75 mg/day.	>100 mg can interfere with calcium and zinc absorption. Excess iron storage in the liver and heart can lead to cirrhosis and cardiac problems. Adults: lethal dose is between 10,000 to 18,000 mg.
Selenium	RDA: 55 µg for women; 70 µg for men. Safe to 200 µg/day.	Excess (>5000 µg) can cause nail deformities, dental defects, hair loss, and vomiting.
Zinc	RDA: 12 mg for women and 15 mg for men. Safe to 15 mg/day.	>25 mg decreases copper absorption. Prolonged doses of >300 mg can reduce immune responses. ≥2000 mg can cause vomiting.

Note: RDA = recommended daily allowance.

D. MINERALS AND TRACE ELEMENTS

Like vitamins, megadoses of minerals may also be dangerous. Table 5 lists some of the toxicities and interactions of the most common minerals and trace elements. Minerals are elements that are required in amounts greater than 200 mg/day and include sodium, chloride, potassium, magnesium, and phosphorous. "Essential" trace elements are those that are needed in small amounts, but cause a recognizable clinical deficiency state if the substance is not provided, and reversal of the state upon repletion. Essential trace elements include the following: copper, chromium, iodine, iron, manganese, selenium, and zinc. Less is known about other elements and clinical deficiency states have not as yet been identified. An excess of one mineral can be immediately toxic to the body, can interfere with the functioning of other minerals, or can build up to toxic levels over time.[29] Many women take calcium supplements in an effort to prevent osteoporosis. Physicians and patients are usually unaware of the calcium content of nonprescription products, and Milk-Alkali Syndrome has recently been reported in patients presenting with renal failure and hypercalcemia who have been ingesting large doses of calcium and absorbable alkali products.[39]

E. SUPPLEMENT RECOMMENDATIONS

According to the American Dietetic Association,[40] persons who could benefit from supplements include the following:

- Women with excessive menstrual bleeding may need to take iron supplements.
- Women who are pregnant or breast feeding need more of many nutrients, especially iron, folic acid, calcium, and sources of energy. Individual recommendations regarding supplements and diets should come from physicians and registered dietitians.

- People with very low calorie intakes frequently consume diets that do not meet their needs for all nutrients.
- Some vegetarians may not be receiving adequate calcium, iron, zinc, and vitamin B_{12}.

In addition, persons who are lactose intolerant or unable to consume adequate calcium intakes may benefit from taking a calcium supplement to make up the difference between what is consumed and the RDA level. Depending upon the allergy in question, persons with allergies to certain foods or groups of foods may also benefit from the careful use of supplements.

For athletes, it should be known that vitamin and mineral supplementation was found to be without any measurable ergogenic effect, and that it was deemed unnecessary in athletes ingesting a normal diet.[41] In this study no toxic effects of supplementation were found. Another study has shown that vitamin and mineral supplementation have no effect on running performance in trained athletes.[42]

While we have generally been very judicious in our recommendations for vitamin and mineral supplementation, perhaps we should add the elderly to the list. Chandra studied the effect of vitamin and trace element supplementation on immune responses and infection in a group of 95 healthy volunteers over age 65.[43] This was a 1-year randomized, double-blind, placebo controlled trial. The results showed that the supplemented group had less infection-related illness days and fewer nutritional deficiencies than the placebo group. This study did not answer the question of whether supplementation corrected nutritional deficiencies due to poor dietary habits or whether higher doses of vitamin E and beta carotene were needed for the improved results in the supplemented group. While further data is needed, we do not feel that it would be inappropriate to judiciously supplement the elderly.

What options can we offer the public regarding supplements that will not espouse quackery? A recent issue of the *Nutrition Action Healthletter* suggested the following options:[44]

1. Take nothing at all—pay specific attention to dietary intake.
2. Take a standard multivitamin and mineral combination—read the label carefully because they do not provide 100% of all nutrients.
3. Take a standard multivitamin plus E, C, beta carotene, selenium, chromium, and/or calcium and magnesium. This equates to a multivitamin plus an "antioxidant" preparation. For women to get the proper amount of calcium, several pills may be needed.
4. Take only E, C, and beta carotene—pay attention to dietary intake, but this option will provide higher doses of vitamin E which as previously reviewed, are harder to attain from dietary sources alone.
5. Try to get everything from one bottle—this may require several pills each day and generally will be the most expensive option. If your "vitamin plan" costs more than $10/month, then reassess it and reconsider the other options, especially option 3.

VII. HERBAL PRODUCTS

Products made from herbs are another good example of "health" products which are not tested adequately for safety and/or effectiveness. Herbs can be found in various forms; teas and capsules are the most popular. Herbal remedies can occur singly or in combination with any number of other herbs to help "correct" almost any ailment imaginable.

In reality, many medications have plants as their base, such as digitalis, which is used in the treatment of congestive heart failure.[45] Herbal remedies are commonplace in China, where they have been used for centuries. Interestingly, they do not know exactly why or how these remedies work, but continue to administer them as part of medical care. While some herbal remedies have been known to be helpful, few have undergone rigid safety testing or placebo controlled trials. Currently about 250 herbs are available as FDA-approved food additives.

For those interested in herbal products, we recommend the person read about herbs from a source that gives known data about certain products and has not been sponsored by a vitamin or herb company. An example of an unbiased source would be the book *The Honest Herbal: A Sensible Guide to Herbs and Related Remedies*.[46] This source discusses over 100 common herbs and tries to put them into proper perspective. Sources that are more suspect are those on sale in vitamin and health food stores that detail the benefits of herbs in multiple forms and often downplay the potential dangers. One way to help evaluate the information is by examining the references of such works. Often these books are poorly referenced and contain few truly medical comparisons or studies.

Aside from questionable effectiveness, there is the issue of safety. Many plant products have not been tested and their effects on the body are not fully understood. There is no assurance that commercially purchased crude herbs have any particular concentration of active ingredients. Inadequate regulations abound in this area, and consumers must be wary. Several cases of veno-occlusive disease, hepatitis, and cirrhosis have resulted from the use of herbal preparations in the U.S.[46] Many herbal products contain natural toxins; therefore, taking them carries risk.

In view of the reports of serious consequences from ingesting herbal products, Huxtable has suggested the following guidelines:[46]

1. Do not take herbs if pregnant or attempting to become pregnant.
2. Do not take herbs if you are nursing.
3. Do not give herbs to your baby.
4. Do not take a large quantity of any one herbal preparation.
5. Do not take herbs on a daily basis.
6. Buy only preparations when the plants are listed on the packet (no guarantee of safety or correctness).
7. Do not take anything with comfrey (known hepatotoxin banned in Canada, but not in U.S.).

VIII. WEIGHT LOSS AIDS

Many nutritional products are sold which claim to have some positive effect on the human condition. Weight loss is one of the more popular areas in which this is seen. There is no dearth of remedies available to help people shed excess pounds and inches from herbal preparations, special slimming teas, diet powders, special foods, diet plans, gimmicks, gadgets, devices, and prescription drugs. Even with these "aids", most people will regain the weight they lost and try something new. A quick, painless method of losing weight, which does not cause one to significantly alter one's lifestyle, has tremendous appeal, but little long-term success.

While it is beyond the scope of this chapter to discuss all areas of potential nutrition quackery in this area, it is important to recognize that federal agencies again lack the proper support and legislation to help limit quackery and abuse from products that promise quick fixes. *Consumer Reports* surveyed over 95,000 readers to look at what they had done to lose weight over the past 3 years. This also included about 19,000 readers who had used a commercial diet program. The results were interesting in that most programs were not found to be very effective. Table 6 summarizes the results of this survey.[47]

One reason that many weight loss programs fail is that there is little attention to the maintenance phase of weight loss that helps people keep off the weight that they have lost. This results in people gaining and losing weight repeatedly which becomes what has been termed "yo-yo" dieting. The body becomes very efficient with a decrease in calories and can decrease the metabolic rate.[48–50] However, mild to moderate exercise can raise the metabolic rate, whereas vigorous exercise can decrease the metabolic rate.[51–54] It is important to realize that a regular exercise program is key for people to assist in weight loss and maintain weight after goal weight loss is achieved.

A new approach has recently been suggested by Drs. Foreyt and Goodrick which is called "living without dieting".[55] This is a conservative approach that focuses on getting the individual to optimize physical health by concentrating on regular exercise and reduced dietary fat intake without restrictive dieting. Whether this type of program will offer any advantage over other programs is not known, but it aims for a more realistic weight loss of 10%. At that level of reduction medical benefits are known to occur and may provide health benefits without the severe patient frustration of attempting to lose all the excess weight. The five components of the program are as follows:[56]

1. Professional and peer support
2. Ending dieting, normalizing eating
3. Gradually reducing dietary fat
4. Increase in exercise
5. Acceptance of weight achieved

In reality, the best weight control programs are individualized and combine a change in eating, exercise, and attitude. It is best to make changes gradually, allow the use of all food groups, eating moderate portions of all foods in at least three separate meals a day, and balance food choices over time. Increasing the consumption of whole grains, fruits, and vegetables will enhance satiety and provide adequate fiber.

Making healthy eating choices can be confusing to some people. The Food Guide Pyramid,[57] developed by the U.S. Department of Agriculture and supported by the Department of Health and Human Services, can help consumers choose diets which are healthful and which can promote weight loss over time (Figure 1). The pyramid is based upon the following dietary guidelines:[57]

1. Eat a variety of foods.
2. Maintain a healthy weight.
3. Choose a diet low in fat, saturated fat, and cholesterol.
4. Choose a diet with plenty of vegetables, fruits, and grain products.
5. Use sugars only in moderation.
6. Use salt and sodium only in moderation.
7. If you drink alcoholic beverages, do so in moderation.

IX. CONCLUSIONS

Nutrition quackery and fraud continues to flourish in the U.S. Consumers are at the mercy of widespread advertising that claims a wide variety of "unfounded" benefits. Governmental regulations are currently inadequate to protect consumers from these companies. The medical community needs to have an active dialogue with patients to help

TABLE 6
Weight Loss Program Summary

| | Satisfaction with overall program in (%) | Satisfaction with weight loss (%) | Satisfaction with maintenance (%) | Percent of weight lost | |
				End of program (%)	6 months after end (%)
Diet programs					
Weight Watchers	78	74	54	8	5
Jenny Craig	62	65	35	11	6
Physicians' Weight Loss	58	65	37	12	7
Diet Center	56	68	38	10	6
Nutri/System	50	63	34	11	7
Liquid-fast programs					
Health Management Resources	68	82	43	20	15
Optifast	42	73	24	20	12
Medifast	40	65	23	15	8

From "Weight Loss Program Summary" Copyright 1993 by Consumers Union of U.S., Inc., Yonkers, NY 10703–1057. Adapted with permission from **CONSUMER REPORTS**, June 1993. Although this material originally appeared in **CONSUMER REPORTS**, the selective adaptation and resulting conclusions presented are those of the author(s) and are not sanctioned or endorsed in any way by Consumers Union, the publisher of **CONSUMER REPORTS**.

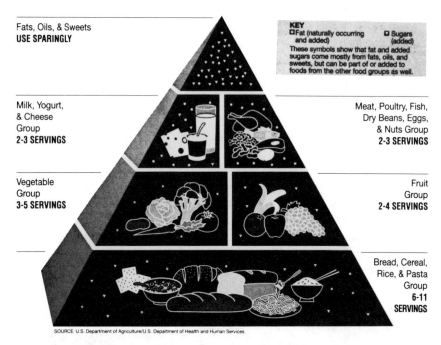

FIGURE 1. The Food Guide Pyramid from U.S. Department of Agriculture. (From The Food Guide Pyramid. Home and Garden Bulletin No. 252, Washington, DC, GPO, 1992, pp 7.)

them choose among medically proven vs. unproven therapies and particularly those which may be dangerous. The federal government needs to take a much more active role in protecting consumers from nutrition fraud and quackery, but until that time it will be an area where it is true that "Let the buyer beware!"

REFERENCES

1. **Eisenberg, DM, Kessler, RC, Foster, C, et al.** Unconventional medicine in the United States: prevalence, costs, and patterns of use. *N Engl J Med,* 328:246–52, 1993.
2. **Nightingale, SL and Snyder, L.** Position paper on health quackery. *Observer,* 9:3–7, 1989.
3. **Oliver, LD, Mehta, R, and Sarles, HE.** Acute renal failure following administration of ethylenediamine-tetraacetatic acid (EDTA). *Tex Med,* 80:40–42,1984.
4. **Starkey, JV and Kirby, DF.** Nutrition and the family. *Pract Gastroenterol,* (in press).
5. **Levine, BS, Wigren, MM, Chapman, DS, et al.** A national survey of attitudes and practices of primary-care physicians relating to nutrition: strategies for enhancing the use of clinical nutrition in medical practice. *Am J Clin Nutr,* 57:115–9, 1993.
6. **Department of Health and Human Services.** "Quackery: The Billion Dollar Miracle Business," Publication no. (FDA) 85–4200. Food and Drug Administration, 5600 Fishers Lane, Rockville, MD 20857.

7. **Beecher, HK.** The powerful placebo. *JAMA,* 159:1602–6, 1955.
8. **Nutrition Headquarters Catalog.** One Nutrition Plaza, Carbondale, IL 62901.
9. **Tyler, VE.** Apricot Pits (Laetrile), In: *The Honest Herbal: A Sensible Guide to Herbs and Related Remedies.* George F. Stickley Company, Philadelphia, 1982, pp 27–28.
10. **Moertel, CG, Fleming, TR, Rubin, J, et al.,** A clinical trial of amygdalin (laetrile) in the treatment of human cancer. *N Engl J Med,* 306:201–6, 1982.
11. **Green, S.** A critique of the rationale for cancer treatment with coffee enemas and diet. *JAMA,* 268:3224–6, 1992.
12. **Ott, M, Lembcke, B, Fischer, H, et al.,** Early changes of body composition in human immunodeficiency virus-infected patients: tetrapolar body impedance analysis indicates significant malnutrition. *Am J Clin Nutr,* 57:15–19, 1993.
13. **Lovejoy, NC, Moran, TA, and Paul, S.** Self-care behaviors and informational needs of seropositive homosexual/bisexual men. *J Acquir Immune Def Syndr,* 1:155–61, 1988.
14. **Beach, RS, Mantero-Atienza, E, Fordyce-Baum, MK.** Dietary supplementation in HIV infection. *FASEB J,* 2:A1435, 1988 (abstract).
15. **Dwyer, JT, Bye, RL, Holt, PL, and Lauze, SR.** Unproven nutrition therapies for AIDS: what is the evidence?, *Nutr Today,* 23:25–33, 1988.
16. **Clark, N.** Protein and performance, In: *Nancy Clark's Sports Nutrition Guidebook.* Champaign, Leisure Press, 1990, pp 157.
17. **Applegate, L.** Performance protein, In: *Power Foods: High-Performance Nutrition for High-Performance People.* Rodale Press, Emmaus, 1991, pp 113.
18. **Hertzman, PA, Blevins, WL, Mayer, J, et al.,** Association of the eosinophilia-myalgia syndrome with the ingestion of tryptophan. *N Engl J Med,* 322:869–73, 1990.
19. **Silver, RM, Heyes, MP, Maize, JC, et al.,** Scleroderma, faciitis, and eosinophilia associated with the ingestion of tryptophan. *N Engl J Med,* 322:874–81, 1990.
20. **Varga, J, Peltonem, J, Uitto, J, and Jimenez, S.** Development of diffuse fasciitis and eosinophilia during L-tryptophan treatment: Demonstration of elevated type I collagen gene expression in affected tissues: a clinicopathologic study of four patients. *Ann Intern Med,* 112:344–51, 1990.
21. **Martin, RW, Duffy, J, Engel, AG, et al.** The clinical spectrum of the eosinophilia-myalgia syndrome associated with L-tryptophan ingestion: clinical features in 20 patients and aspects of pathophysiology. *Ann Intern Med,* 113:124–34, 1990.
22. **Medsger, TA, Jr.** Tryptophan-induced eosinophilia-myalgia syndrome. *N Engl J Med,* 322:926–8, 1990.
23. **Kazura, JW.** Eosinophilia-myalgia syndrome. *Cleveland Clin J Med,* 58:267–70, 1991.
24. **Hedberg, K, Urbach, D, Slutsker, L, et al.** Eosinophilia-myalgia syndrome: natural history in a population-based cohort. *Arch Intern Med,* 152:1889–92, 1992.
25. **Long, P.** The vitamin wars. *Health,* 7:45–54, 1993.
26. **Schaumberg, H, Kaplan, J, Windebank, A, et al.** Sensory neuropathy from pyridoxine abuse: a new megavitamin syndrome. *N Engl J Med,* 309:445–48, 1983.
27. **Berger, A and Schaumberg, H.** More on neuropathy from pyridoxine abuse. *N Engl J Med,* 311:986–987, 1984.
28. **Basu, TK and Schorah, CJ.** Safety considerations on high intake of vitamin C. In: *Vitamin C in Health and Disease.* Basu, TK and Schorah, CJ, Eds., AVI Publishing, Westport, CT. 1982, pp 115–123.
29. **Herbert, V and Barrett, S.** The truth about nutrition. In: *Vitamins & "Health" Foods: The Great American Hustle.* Herbert, V and Barrett, S, Eds., George F. Stickley Company, Philadelphia, 1981, pp 8.
30. **Skerrett, PJ.** Mighty vitamins. *Med World News,* 34:24–32, 1993.
31. **Raiten, DJ.** Nutrition and HIV infection. *Nutr Clin Pract,* 6(Suppl):53S–61S, 1990.
32. **Diplock, AT.** Antioxidant nutrients and disease prevention: an overview. *Am J Clin Nutr,* 53(Suppl.):189S–93S, 1991.
33. **Slater, TF.** Concluding remarks. *Am J Clin Nutr,* 53(Suppl):394S–6S, 1991.
34. **Imaly, JA and Linn, S.** DNA damage and oxygen radical toxicity. *Science,* 240:1302–9, 1988.
35. **Pryor, WA.** The antioxidant nutrients and disease prevention—what do we know and what do we need to find out? *Am J Clin Nutr,* 53(Suppl):391S–3S, 1991.
36. **Weisburger, JH.** Nutritional approach to cancer prevention with emphasis on vitamins, antioxidants, and carotenoids. *Am J Clin Nutr,* 53(Suppl):226S–37S, 1991.
37. **Zeigler, RG.** Vegetables, fruits, and carotenoids and the risk of cancer. *Am J Clin Nutr,* 53(Suppl.):251S–9S, 1991.
38. **Knekt, P, Aromaa, A, Maatela, J, et al.** Vitamin E and cancer prevention. *Am J Clin Nutr,* 53(Suppl.):283S–6S, 1991.

39. **Abreo, K, Adlakha, A, Kilpatrick, S, et al.** The milk-alkali syndrome: a reversible form of acute renal failure. *Arch Intern Med,* 153:1005–10, 1993.

40. **Anon.** Alphabet soup: Nutrients from food and supplements. The American Dietetic Association. (Brochure) 1987.

41. **Weight, LM, Noakes, TD, Labadarios, D, et al.** Vitamin and mineral status of trained atheletes including the effects of supplementation. *Am J Clin Nutr,* 47:186–91, 1988.

42. **Weight, LM, Myburgh, KH, and Noakes, TD.** Vitamin and mineral supplementation: effect on the running performance of trained athletes. *Am J Clin Nutr,* 47:192–5, 1988.

43. **Chandra, RK.** Effect of vitamin and trace-element supplementation on immune responses and infection in elderly subjects. *Lancet,* 340:1124–7, 1992.

44. **Liebman, B.** The ultra mega vita guide. *Nutr Action Healthletter,* 20:7–9, 1993.

45. **Tyler, VE.** Pros and cons. In: *The Honest Herbal: A Sensible Guide to Herbs and Related Remedies.* George F. Stickley Company, Philadelphia, 1982, pp 7.

46. **Huxtable, RJ.** The myth of beneficient nature: the risks of herbal preparations. *Ann Intern Med,* 117:165–6, 1992.

47. **Anon.** Rating the diets. *Consumer Rep,* 58:353–7, 1993.

48. **Bray, GA.** Effect of caloric restriction on energy expenditure in obese patients. *Lancet,* 2:397–8, 1969.

49. **Lammert, O and Hansen, ES.** Effects of excessive caloric intake and caloric restriction on body weight and energy expenditure at rest and light exercise. *Acta Physiol Scand,* 114:134–41, 1982.

50. **Welle, SL, Amatruda, UM, Forbes, GB, et al.** Resting metabolic rate of obese women after rapid weight loss. *J Clin Endocrinol Metab,* 59:41–4, 1984.

51. **Horton, ES.** Metabolic aspects of exercise and weight reduction. *Med Sci Sports Exerc,* 18:10–18, 1986.

52. **Stern, JS, Schultz, C, and Mole, P.** Effect of caloric restriction and exercise on basal metabolism and thyroid hormone. *Nutr Med,* 1:361, 1980.

53. **Stern, JS and Lowney, P.** Obesity: the role of physical activity. In: *Handbook of Eating Disorders: Physiology, Psychology and Treatment of Obesity and Anorexia, and Bulimia.* Brownell, KD and Foreyt, JP, Eds, Basic Books, New York, 1986, pp 145–158.

54. **Phinney, SD.** The metabolic interaction between very low calorie diet and exercise. In: *Management of Obesity by Severe Caloric Restriction.* Blackburn, GL and Bray, GA, Eds, PSG Company, Littleton 1985, pp 99–105.

55. **Foreyt, JP and Goodrick, GK.** *Living Without Dieting.* Harrison, Houston, 1992.

56. **Foreyt, JP and Goodrick, GK.** A non-diet approach to obesity. *Nutr M.D.,* 19:1– 2, May 1993.

57. **U.S. Department of Agriculture.** The Food Guide Pyramid. Home and Garden Bulletin No. 252, Washington, DC GPO, 1992, pp 7.

APPENDIX III

The National Center for Nutrition and Dietetics, established by the American Dietetic Association Foundation, has a consumer nutrition hot line that is staffed with registered dietitians. The hot line is intended to be a resource to provide immediate access to reliable nutrition information.

Callers have three options:

1. Talking directly to a registered dietitian
2. Selecting recorded nutrition messages
3. Locating a registered dietitian in their area

The hot line is staffed from 9:00 AM to 4:00 PM (Central time) Monday through Friday. Nutrition messages are also available in Spanish.

CONSUMER NUTRITION HOT LINE

1–800–366–1655

Chapter 15

AN ETHICAL AND LEGAL ANALYSIS
OF ENTERAL NUTRITION

Karen N. Swisher and Kathy B. Miller

TABLE OF CONTENTS

0-8493-7847-8/94/$0.00+$.50
© 1994 by CRC Press, Inc.

I. INTRODUCTION TO THE PROBLEM

Advances in medical science have allowed physicians to accomplish feats that would have astonished their colleagues of generations past. The aggressive use of antibiotics, mechanical ventilators, resuscitation, and artificial feeding has enabled people to remain biologically alive far after the mental capacity to understand and appreciate these procedures has left. It is now possible to maintain vital bodily functions even in the face of an irreversible underlying process. As the result of this technology, it is estimated that over 10,000 patients diagnosed as "in a persistent vegetative state" (PVS) remain alive in the U.S. today, sustained indefinitely through artificial feeding tubes.

The debate over the long-term benefits of life-prolonging technology is relatively young, spanning barely two decades. Patients, physicians, and health care policy makers differ in their opinions on the long-term benefits of such technology to individual patients and its effect on society in general. The debate over medically assisted nutrition and hydration has been particularly complex. Civilization and prosperity have made the provision of nutrition and hydration a "powerful symbol of concern and compassion."[1] The provision of food and drink to those in need is basic to all human relationships. It crosses all cultures and has played a significant role in Christian and Judaic traditions. In the nursing profession, it represents the giving of comfort care and symbolizes the compassion a nurse has for a patient.

When terminally ill patients are unable to tolerate oral feeding, it signals the onset of the final stages in the dying process. Because food is such a powerful symbol for the living, it is difficult for many to understand that when the dying lose their appetites, it is a part of allowing nature to prepare for death. For the healthy, the thought of starving to death is abhorrent, yet the dying find little physical comfort in eating and drinking and most, if given the choice, will decline food.[2] It is at this juncture between the natural desire of the dying to refuse food and the compassionate urge of the living to provide sustenance that family members may request the utilization of artificial feeding tubes.

Unfortunately, the use of a feeding tube does not improve the quality of life for many patients. For PVS patients, feeding tubes do nothing but promote longevity of biological life. For others, studies have shown that patients on feeding tubes for extended periods of time did not regain their ability to perform activities of daily living.[3] Indeed, the surgical procedure of inserting a feeding tube, and the subsequent care required, carry inherent risks of further medical complications. Tube feeding must be recognized as an invasive procedure "with inherent risks and possible side effects instituted by skilled health providers to compensate for impaired physiological functioning."[4] Sometimes these complications can be extensive, greatly diminishing any benefits of tube feeding. It is not surprising, therefore, that after a period of time, some families and patients want these tubes removed. In reality, 70% of all deaths in this country involve a willful decision to forgo life-sustaining treatment, including feeding tubes.[5] However, physicians fear legal liability for removing a tube which is sustaining life, and these conflicts often end up in litigation.

It is an unfortunate reflection of our own litigious society that these sensitive ethical dilemmas are most often resolved in a court of law. In this inappropriate forum, the legal system resolves medical and ethical issues using a legal framework of rights vs. responsibilities. The legal debate over medically assisted nutrition and hydration has focused on tube feeding rather than total parenteral nutrition. Courts have not discussed ultimate treatment goals or quality of life issues. A judge will seldom consider the ramifications of such decisions on family cohesiveness or family grief. The judiciary is simply not equipped to consider the costs to individuals and society when forcing patients to accept unwanted care.[6]

This debate is far from resolved, and indeed, the implementation of national health care reform will bring the ethical and legal issues of appropriate medical care to the forefront of public attention. However, before one can speculate as to how this debate will resolve, it is first important to see where the debate has been in the past. This chapter will describe the legal and ethical issues involved in artificial feeding. By understanding the interaction between legal and ethical issues, one can better understand how these variables should affect public policy in the provision of medical care for all Americans.

II. A LEGAL FRAMEWORK—INDIVIDUAL RIGHTS VS. STATE RESPONSIBILITY

The past decade has yielded over forty published, and possibly hundreds of unpublished, court decisions involving denial of artificial nutritional support to patients.[7] These judicial opinions form the basis for a legal framework used by courts to analyze artificial support cases.

It is well founded in law that individuals have the right to consent to or refuse any medical treatments. This is the concept of informed consent, which is also recognized as the ethical principle of respect for patient autonomy. However, the right of an individual to accept or refuse medical treatment is sometimes offset by the state's responsibility to protect its citizens. State-imposed limits on individual freedom in the realm of health care is an ancient concept, dating from the writings of Plato.[8]

American courts have affirmed a group of state interests which could supersede a patient's right to choose. These interests include the preservation of life, the prevention of suicide, the protection of innocent third persons, especially children, the preservation of the integrity of the medical profession, and encouraging the charitable and humane care of afflicted persons. The varied nature of the judicial attempts to define such state interests is a reflection of diversified values in a pluralistic American society.[9]

The responsibility of the state to preserve life has been discussed in several cases. One court stated that:

> It is clear that the most significant of the asserted State interests is that of the preservation of human life. Recognition of such an interest, however, does not necessarily resolve the problem where the affliction or disease clearly indicates that life will end soon, and inevitably be extinguished. The interest of the State in prolonging a life must be reconciled with the interest of an individual to reject the traumatic cost of that prolongation. There is a substantial distinction in the State's insistence that human life be saved where the affliction is curable, as opposed to the State interest where the issue is not whether but when, for how long, and at what cost to the individual that life may be briefly extended. . . . The value of life as so perceived is lessened not by a decision to refuse treatment, but by the failure to allow a competent human being the right of a choice.[10]

A. AUTONOMY AND PATIENT COMPETENCE

The concept of autonomy is intimately woven into the special fiduciary relationship all physicians share with their patients. It is a legal relationship with duties and responsibilities as well as an ethical relationship. Immanuel Kant argued that respect for autonomy flows from the recognition that all persons have unconditional worth, each having the capacity to determine his or her own destiny.[11] However, what happens if one's destiny is to kill one's self, to commit suicide? The Case of Elizabeth Bouvia represents conflicting values in medicine and society's valuation of individual worth.

Elizabeth Bouvia initiated one of the first ethical/legal confrontations surrounding nutritional support. It is an interesting case study because it dealt not with the reluctance of an institution to provide or withdraw artificial nutritional support, but rather with the right of a young woman to starve herself to death. Elizabeth received national publicity regarding her refusal of nutrition and her desire to die, and her case began an active debate about methods of suicide. Most importantly, however, her case reflected a struggle between patients' rights and institutional responsibility.

In September of 1983, Elizabeth Bouvia voluntarily admitted herself to a psychiatric hospital to be treated for suicidal tendencies. She was 25 years old. She had been born with cerebral palsy and was in constant pain from severely crippling arthritis. She had little control over her body, but she could use her right hand to operate a battery powered wheelchair. She had control over her facial muscles for chewing, swallowing, and speaking. Her parents divorced when she was ten, and after a few years Elizabeth's mother placed her in a children's home. She married an ex-convict and the couple lived in poverty. Despite her attempts to ask her father for help, he declined to become involved with his daughter at all. Elizabeth's husband finally abandoned her, stating that he could not "accept her disabilities."

While in the hospital, Elizabeth decided not to eat, intending to starve herself to death. "Death is letting go of all burdens," she said. "It is being able to be free of my physical disability and mental struggle to live."[12] Elizabeth's attending physician could not accept her declining caloric intake and ordered her to be force-fed. Elizabeth called the ACLU and a newspaper reporter, making her case into a public spectacle. At the resulting court hearing, Elizabeth's psychiatrist, Donald Fisher, testified that he would not let Ms. Bouvia starve. Fisher felt Elizabeth would eventually change her mind and stated that "the court cannot order me to be a murderer nor to conspire with my staff and employees to murder Elizabeth." Despite the fact that the judge found Elizabeth rational, sincere, and fully competent, he ordered that the hospital be allowed to force-feed her. Elizabeth continued to resist tube feeding. She bit through the plastic feeding tube and was restrained so that liquids could be infused into her stomach.

In reaction to this case, law professor George Annas does not believe that patients who can make their own decisions should ever be force-fed. The treatment team should attempt to persuade the patients to follow an appropriate treatment plan including appropriate nutrition, yet:

> If a court determines, however, that invasive force-feeding is required
> . . . then to avoid hospitals from becoming the most hideous torture
> chambers, some reasonable limit must be placed on this 'treatment'.[13]

Elizabeth eventually checked out of that hospital. She continued to seek outpatient care elsewhere, but soon had to accept inpatient care for her degenerative arthritis. While she did eat voluntarily, it was not enough to suit the hospital. Though Elizabeth was by nature a very slight woman, the hospital began to force-feed her to achieve a more "ideal" weight. Again she petitioned the courts for relief. The judge ruled against Elizabeth, believing that her low weight was evidence of starvation and a desire to terminate her life. She appealed this decision.

The appellate court upheld Elizabeth's right to refuse medical treatment, including nutrition. In a very thoughtful opinion, the court stated:

> [Elizabeth] has been subjected to the forced intrusion of an artificial mechanism into her body against her will. She has a right to refuse the increased dehumanizing aspect of her condition. . . . The right to refuse medical treatment is basic and fundamental. It is recognized as part of the right of privacy protected by both the state and federal constitutions. Its exercise requires no one's approval . . . (if) the right of the patient to self-determination as to his own medical treatment is to have any meaning at all, it must be paramount to the interest of the patient's hospital and doctors. . . . The right of a competent adult patient to refuse medical treatment is a constitutionally guaranteed right which must not be abridged.[14]

While many courts have had clear difficulties reconciling patient rights with the state's interest in preventing suicide, the *Bouvia* court remained focused on Elizabeth's right to self-determination. One judge even commented:

> Elizabeth apparently has made a conscious and informed choice that she prefers death to continued existence in her helpless and, to her, intolerable condition. I believe she has an absolute right to effectuate that decision. . . . The right to die is an integral part of our right to control our own destinies so long as the rights of others are not affected. That right should in my opinion, include the ability to enlist assistance from others, including the medical profession, in making death as painless and quick as possible.[15]

The case is a tragic example of forcing societal values onto individuals without first understanding the reasons behind an individual's choice. While this case narrowly focused on the lengths to which the state can intervene in actually force-feeding patients to prevent suicide, some critics cite *Bouvia* as an example of the rampant social prejudice and indifference toward disabled people.[16]

B. AUTONOMY AND THE INCOMPETENT PATIENT

Elizabeth was conscious, adamant, and persistent in her resistance to forced feeding. However, many patients do not have the capacity to consent to or refuse such treatment. Courts have taken a very different approach in disputes over medical care where capacity is at issue.

Capacity is the ability to understand the elements of informed consent. Incapacity, therefore, is an inability to consent due to mental or physical disability or because the patient is a child. Incapacitated patients can be divided into two categories: those with former capacity and those who have never had capacity. For incompetent adults with prior capacity, courts inquire as to whether these patients have expressed their wishes regarding medical care in the past, either through a living will or through oral statements to family and friends. Few patients have living wills, and those who do seldom state their wishes on particular medical interventions such as artificial feeding. Absent these written documents, physicians look to family members or other surrogates to make decisions on behalf of the incompetent patient. Courts then assess the credibility of the evidence which is said to demonstrate that withdrawing or withholding medical care is what the patient would have wanted.

There does seem to be a consensus that incompetent patients should not be denied the right to refuse medical treatment any more than their competent counterparts. When family members make decisions on behalf of a patient, the courts use the "substituted judgment test." Under this test, the surrogate decision maker must stand in the shoes of the patient and determine what the patient would have wanted. The court:

> [a]ttempts to establish, with as much accuracy as possible, what decision the patient would make if he were competent to do so. Employing this theory, the surrogate first tries to determine if the patient had expressed explicit intent regarding this type of medical treatment prior to becoming incompetent. . . . Where no clear intent exists, the patient's personal value system must guide the surrogate.[17]

It is a logical presumption that family members are in the best position to assume the decision making role under the substituted judgment test. Yet, some courts are hesitant to discontinue life-sustaining care including hydration and nutrition, of a permanently unconscious patient, without a written statement by that patient. The first reported case where a family member asked for the withdrawal of an artificial feeding tube is that of Paul Brophy.

Paul Brophy was in his 40s in April of 1983, when he had to undergo emergency surgery for a ruptured cerebral aneurysm. He never regained consciousness. In June, he was transferred to a convalescent hospital with a diagnosis of PVS.[18] While his wife consented to a "do not resuscitate" order, she also consented to a surgical insertion of a feeding tube into his stomach. He remained in that condition for about a year.

The Brophys were a very close family. Paul, his wife, and five daughters had several discussions about quality of life should one be rendered gravely ill. Long before his illness, Paul had made several comments to his family to "pull the plug" if he should ever be in a coma. Years earlier, he had expressed the same view to his wife while they were discussing the case of Karen Ann Quinlan, the comatose New Jersey woman whose respirator was finally removed by a court order. And just before his aneurysm surgery, Paul told one of his daughters, "If I can't sit up to kiss one of my beautiful daughters, I may as well be six feet under."[19]

Mrs. Brophy eventually decided that she wanted to discontinue the feeding tube and let her husband die. A devout Catholic, she contacted her priest and then an ethicist, John Paris. Paris sent her several articles on the subject and discussed the problem with her in detail. He asked her three questions: Was she convinced her husband's condition was hopeless? Did she believe he would want the feeding tube discontinued? Was the entire family (five grown children, seven siblings, and his mother) in agreement on the cessation of treatment? She replied yes to all questions.

Despite the familial consensus, the doctors at the facility adamantly opposed Mrs. Brophy's request to discontinue feeding and stated they would seek legal intervention. So began the 19 month legal battle Mrs. Brophy endured to carry out her husband's wishes.

The initial trial judge was convinced that Paul Brophy would not have wanted the feeding tube. However, he ruled that tube feeding should be continued against the family's wishes. He stated that "apart from the injury to his brain, Brophy's general state of health is relatively good." He noted that "proper focus should be on the quality of treatment furnished . . . to Brophy, and not on the quality of Brophy's life." He felt that feeding (as opposed to the feeding tube) is a basic, ordinary care which should be distinguished from extraordinary medical care. Finally, the judge was concerned that discontinuing feeding would be the cause of death rather than the underlying disease. "I find that denying a patient food and water . . . will inevitably in each and every instance guarantee and cause the death of the patient.''[20]

The feeding tube remained and Mrs. Brophy was forced to appeal. Three years later, the Massachusetts Supreme Judicial Court held that Brophy's feeding tube could be removed. Basing its decision on the common law right of patients to refuse any unwanted medical care, the majority judges ruled that there is no distinction between starting and stopping treatment. They further ruled that artificially administered hydration and nutrition is just like any other medical care rendered in a hospital.

The court found that it had to examine more than the patient's wishes, however. The court's analysis weighed the wishes of the patient and the patient's right of autonomous choice against the states' responsibility to protect the integrity of the medical profession. The court acknowledged the strong sentiment among Brophy's treating physicians that withdrawing the feeding tube would kill the patient, and that such an event did not constitute death by natural causes.[21] The court realized that it could not force physicians to breach their ethical duties toward their patient by honoring the wishes of the patient or his family.[22] The physicians also feared some unarticulated liability for possible murder if such a feeding tube should be removed. In resolving this impasse, the court held that if one hospital would not honor a patient's wishes, then the hospital has the duty to transfer that patient to another hospital which will withdraw the feeding tube in order to protect the patient's right of choice.

Shortly after the Brophy case was decided, the American Medical Association published its consensus paper on the ethical requirements for physicians discontinuing unwanted medical care. It stated that:

> [i]n deciding whether the administration of potentially life-prolonging medical treatment is in the best interest of the patient who is competent to act in his own behalf, the physician should determine what the possibility is for extending life under humane and comfortable conditions and what the prior expressed wishes of the patient and attitudes of the family or those who have responsibility for the custody of the patient.
>
> Even if death is not imminent but a patient's coma is beyond doubt irreversible and there are adequate safeguards to confirm the accuracy of the diagnosis and with the concurrence of those who have responsibility for the care of the patient, it is not unethical to discontinue all means of life-prolonging medical treatment.
>
> Life-prolonging medical treatment includes medication and artificially or technologically supplied respiration, nutrition, or hydration. In treating a terminally ill or irreversibly comatose patient, the physician should determine whether the benefits of treatment outweigh its burdens.[23]

While this statement may have clarified the treatment options available for physicians to give their patients, it has not had a similar effect on legislation passed since its publication. Most legislation on the subject reflects the determination of state legislators to pursue a course of social policy, not the individual value of autonomy, or medical values of beneficence and nonmaleficence.

III. AN ETHICAL FRAMEWORK—NONMALEFICENCE AND BENEFICENCE

Principles of ethics are an integral foundation of the medical profession. While some analyze medical ethics with judgment regarding what is right or wrong, such an analogy is more appropriate when discussing table manners rather than resolving a difficult medical dilemma. The reason is, principles of right and wrong have meaning only when one places these principles into a particular social structure. What is wrong in one society may be quite appropriate in another. While some believe that medicine is universal in nature, in reality, medicine, and particularly the goals of medicine, are well founded within the value and moral structure of any particular society.[24] Students of medicine bring with them certain sets of values regarding how medicine ought to be provided. Physicians practice medicine within the parameters of government regulation, financial constraints, and the technology available within that country. Using this paradigm, the study of bioethics becomes one of understanding social values and morals, and ethical philosophy becomes a discipline in understanding how moral reasoning is derived.

> Morality expresses society's basic instructions about what people may and may not do. Ethical theory, on the other hand, describes and justifies such traditions. . . . The scientific branch of ethics gathers and reports accurate empirical information about existing moral beliefs, without evaluating the worth of moral judgments in any way. Philosophical ethics moves beyond and either evaluates important moral concepts . . . and moral reasoning from a logical as opposed to a psychological perspective or establishes theoretical justifications for what is right and wrong in human actions.[25]

While respect for patient autonomy has been well founded in the legal principle of informed consent, the medical principles of beneficence (the duty to help others by doing what is best for them) and nonmaleficence (the duty not to inflict harm or risk of harm on others) are not so well understood and articulated in a legal framework. The cases described in this chapter reflect this difficulty that the courts have in translating principles of biomedical ethics into principles of law and justice.

A. NONMALEFICENCE AND THE INCOMPETENT PATIENT

While Brophy was being debated in a New England state court, the family of another PVS patient, this time in Missouri, decided that they wanted their daughter's feeding tube removed. Unlike Brophy, however, the physicians of this patient concurred with the family that tube feeding was futile and only delayed the inevitable dying process. The case of Nancy Cruzan became the first so called "right-to-die" case heard before the United States Supreme Court. Unfortunately, rather than dealing with this case in terms of patient autonomy, or even protecting the integrity of the medical profession, the Court analyzed Cruzan within the abortion rights framework.[26]

Nancy Cruzan was rendered in a PVS as the result of an automobile accident in January 1983. She was maintained in this condition for several years with the aid of an artificial feeding tube. Her parents eventually asked that the feeding tube be removed, and Nancy's physicians concurred. However, the hospital refused to comply. A court order was sought and granted, but the order was immediately appealed by the Attorney General of Missouri, who had been appointed Nancy's official guardian.

The Supreme Court of Missouri would not allow the feeding tube to be removed, stating that there was not enough evidence to indicate that Nancy would have wanted removal. It focused narrowly on the state's legitimate interest in preserving life, at least when continued care does not cause pain and is not particularly burdensome to the patient. Because this state had been so active in the anti-abortion movement, its recurring theme was the state's interest in life, regardless of its quality.

The issue on appeal to the United States Supreme Court was whether a state could require "clear and convincing" evidence of a patient's wishes to withhold or withdraw unwanted life sustaining medical treatments. This Court answered in the affirmative.[27]

There was no question in this case that the family was acting in good faith for their daughter. Nor was there any question that Nancy was not receiving any benefit from the continued treatment other than maintaining her biological life. While physicians stated that such continued treatment would be inhumane and their duty was to prevent further harm to their patient, the Court found such reasoning secondary to a state interest in the preservation of life.

Clearly, the Court ignored the ethical framework within which a physician must function. Nonmaleficence mandates that physicians have a right, perhaps a duty, to stop treatment if life is being preserved only through extraordinary means and the family consents to such withdrawal.[28] While the Court did rule that all patients have a right to refuse unwanted medical care, the ruling did not consider the medical risks and benefits of continued treatments, nor did it consider that the treatment might be causing harm. Because Nancy did not have a living will specifically stating that she would not want artificially administered hydration and nutrition, the assumption was to maintain the status quo and keep her feeding tube intact.

The vast majority of Americans were appalled by the Cruzan family's ordeal.[29] After the United States Supreme Court decision, the Cruzan family appealed the case yet again, this time with additional evidence of statements by Nancy that she would not want to be in this condition. The state of Missouri withdrew any protest, and a state judge allowed Nancy's feeding tube to be removed, stating there was clear and convincing evidence of Nancy's intent.

The Cruzan case was not about withdrawing unwanted medical treatments, patient autonomy, or medical beneficence; rather it was about the power of a state to proscribe social values. The courts of the 1990s reflect real political struggles over control over the way individuals live their lives. "The modern state . . . uses its technological power to homogenize and normalize life, not just through law, but through education, military training, medicine, public health and housing, and other regulatory mechanisms. Constitutions far from protecting against such normalization, were forms that made an essentially normalizing power acceptable."[30]

B. BENEFICENCE AND THE ALWAYS INCOMPETENT PATIENT

For those patients who have severe mental retardation, mental illness, or a physical disability, including infancy, the substituted judgment test simply doesn't work. These patients have never developed capacity to understand the risk and benefits of any medical treatment. These patients seem to present the most difficult legal and ethical dilemma for both courts and health care providers. The majority of courts, however, have allowed family members to discontinue life-prolonging treatment, realizing that such care is futile and represents a symbolic loss of dignity for the patient.

> The real reason why most people would prefer death over permanent unconsciousness, and why courts are willing to allow guardians to make such determinations on behalf of vegetative patients, is that an indefinite insensate limbo constitutes a demeaning and degraded status devoid of human dignity. The total helplessness, dependence, dysfunction and exposure of every aspect of privacy to others—all without any prospect of regaining consciousness—make permanent unconsciousness distasteful and undignified.[31]

It is here that the principle of beneficence becomes most significant. Beneficence requires the provision of benefits which include the prevention and removal of harm and the promotion of the patient's welfare. It also requires the balancing of benefits and harms for patients.[32] Courts are not fully cognizant of these ethical principles, yet attempt to achieve the same beneficial end results nonetheless. An example of such an attempt is the case of ''Jane Doe''.

In 1990, Jane was a 33-year old, profoundly retarded woman diagnosed in a PVS. She had been mentally retarded since birth and suffered from Canavan's disease.[33] She was also afflicted with brain atrophy, cortical blindness, cortical deafness, flaccid quadriparesis with contracture of the upper and lower extremities, seizure disorder dysphagia with external feeding, permanent tracheostomy, chronic urinary tract infections, osteopenia, congenitally dislocated hips, and severe scoliosis. While her physical and mental condition was grim, her parents cared for her at home until age five, at which time her mother became pregnant with a third child and felt it necessary to place Jane in a state school. At the state school, a nasoduodenal tube was placed without the family's knowledge or consent. For the next 7 years, Jane was fed through this tube as her condition continued to deteriorate. After she was diagnosed in as PVS, the mother requested that the feeding be discontinued and the physicians agreed.

The state Department of Mental Retardation, while supporting the decision, asked that a legal guardian be appointed for Jane to make all medical decisions. The parents declined to be the legal guardians, stating that they could ''foresee the day when they would be confronted by this situation in which their opposing viewpoints (from that of the department's social workers) would lead to a long and painful court fight for which the parents did not have the emotional strength.''[34]

During the initial hearing, the judge ordered termination of the feeding tube. Counsel for Doe appealed. The decision to withdraw the feeding tube was upheld by the Supreme Court of Massachusetts. The court realized that the traditional ''substituted judgment'' test to determine what Jane would have wanted for herself was not valid, and that such a decision should be based on other criteria. These criteria included the impact of such a decision on other family members, the probability of adverse side effects, and the prognosis with and without treatment. The judges found that Jane's family was acting in Jane's best interests.

The case is significant for many reasons. The majority of the judges were very interested in the welfare of the family, family unity, and family values. The judges also gave deference to the medical profession by acknowledging that medicine is as much an art as a science. By all medical accounts, Doe's prognosis was grave and her disease process, with or without a feeding tube, would steadily and quickly have led to an inevitable death.

More courts are concluding that when patients have never had autonomous choice, the judiciary should weigh the risks of treatment against the benefits of such treatment. For example, in a court case dealing with a terminally ill, comatose cancer patient, the court looked at a number of factors in deciding whether continued blood transfusions and chemotherapy should be continued. These factors included: (1) the fact that most people elect chemotherapy, (2) the chance of a longer life, (3) the patient's advanced age, (4) the adverse side effects of treatment, (5) the low chance of producing remission, (6) the certainty that treatment would cause immediate suffering, and (7) the fact that the patient would not be cooperative to such treatment.[35]

Other courts, in attempting to develop a more realistic test for determining what to do for patients who have never had autonomous choice, have stated that:

> The net burdens of the patient's life with the treatment should clearly and markedly outweigh the benefits that the patient derives from life. Further, the recurring, unavoidable and severe pain of the patient's life with the treatment should be such that the effect of administering life-sustaining treatment would be inhumane.[36]

The responsibility of families to care for and make medical decisions on behalf of an incompetent patient is an onerous one. That burden is often unrecognized by courts, but it is at the heart of every family's dilemma. As one court noted "in the case of a comatose individual there is no pain and suffering. [I]t would seem to follow that the direct beneficiary of the request (to terminate treatment) is the family of the patient and that the benefits are financial savings and cessation of the emotional drain occasioned by awaiting the medico-legal death of a loved one."[37]

It has become standard medical practice to seek consent from family members when patients are incapable of giving their own consent. Physicians have always had a role in determining whether or not family members are acting in good faith while making these difficult decisions. So popular is this concept that many states have enacted "family consent" laws that authorize statutorily designative family members to make health care decisions when the patient is unable to do so. In 1983, the President's Commission on Deciding to Forego Life-Sustaining Treatment, suggested deference to family members for the following reasons:

1. The family is generally the most concerned about the good of the patient.
2. The family will also usually be most knowledgeable about the patient's goals, preferences, and values.
3. The family deserves recognition as an important social unit that ought to be treated, within limits, as a responsible decision maker in matters that intimately affect its members.
4. Especially in a society in which many other traditional forms of community have eroded, participation in a family is often an important dimension of personal fulfillment.
5. Since a protected sphere of privacy and autonomy is required for the flourishing of this interpersonal union, institution and the state should be reluctant to intrude, particularly regarding matters that are personal and on which there is a wide range of opinion in society.[38]

IV. CONCLUSION

If any good arose from the Supreme Court's decision in *Cruzan,* it was the heightened public awareness of the futility of some medical treatments. Shortly after this decision, the federal government passed the Patient Self-Determination Act of 1991. This act requires all health care facilities, including hospitals, nursing homes, HMOs, psychiatric facilities and others, to provide written information to all incoming patients regarding their rights under state laws to create a living will and a durable power of attorney for health care.[39] While the act is laudable, it should not be used as a substitute for the health care provider's responsibility to discuss the risks, benefits and alternatives to life-sustaining treatments.

Several problems are already apparent with the new law, many arising from interaction with state law. State laws vary considerably, some giving patients more involvement with treatment decisions than others.[40] For example, only a minority of states provide statutory guidance for incompetent patients. Some statutes specifically exclude certain treatments, such as artificial hydration and nutrition, from the choices that patients may make. The law does not require hospitals to actually help patients execute living wills. Despite the good intentions of Congress, few patients do have living wills, and even fewer patients can truly understand the significance of these laws on their own medical circumstances.[41]

In addition to the many logistical problems in carrying out the intent of such a sweeping law, the law itself is not without controversy. Shortly after its enactment, the National Right to Life organization published its alternative to the living will called "a Will to Live." In describing its Will to Live form, the organization states that one should sign a Will to Live because in many states the living will really means:

> [y]ou will be starved and dehydrated if you cannot swallow on your own . . . you will be denied lifesaving medical treatment even if you could live indefinitely if you have disabilities a doctor or court think make your life not worth living. The Will to Live will protect you from being denied lifesaving medical treatment (and even food and water) in these circumstances.[42]

Clearly, the ethical debate about appropriate medical care for patients is still unresolved. The debate will only intensify with the advent of health care reform. Health policy makers are already debating the ethics of appropriate care with its impact on disabled persons.[43]

The court cases cited in this chapter are just some of the examples of how poorly the legal system deals with bioethical issues. Ethical dilemmas involved in providing, withholding, or withdrawing nutrition support are decisions best made at the bedside and not in the courtroom. For the time being, however, there are many things that providers of nutrition support can do to help their patients achieve the maximum benefit from medical treatments and reduce the chances of conflict or ethical dilemma.

1. **Develop a treatment plan**—The foundation of all treatment choices rests within a framework of the treatment plan. Providers must ask "What is the purpose of particular interventions?" Is it to save life, restore health, or alleviate suffering?
2. **Provide informed consent**—Feeding tubes are medical interventions, and therefore require informed consent from the patient or the surrogate. This requires a thoughtful discussion of the risks and benefits of feedings tubes, alternatives to feeding tubes such as oral intake, and the long-term effects of artificial feeding. Patients and families don't always understand that feeding tubes may present risks. Patients may be noncompliant or combative. More importantly, depending on the patient's condition, the feeding tube may provide little long-term benefit other than to prolong a dying process.
3. **Educate patients on living wills**—By giving all adult patients information on the meaning of living wills, you can help them formalize their values regarding quality of life, the dying process and their preferences should a traumatic event occur. This in turn encourages patients to discuss these values with their family members and may very well avoid ethical dilemmas.
4. **Evaluate the treatment plan on a regular basis**—Legally, there is no significant difference between withdrawing, withholding, or initiating feeding tubes. It's a clinical decision based on the patient's condition. Informed consent is the key to any of these decisions.
5. **Remember there is no ethical or legal duty to provide futile treatments**—Offering futile treatments to patients gives false and unrealistic expectations regarding such treatment. Feeding tubes, resuscitation techniques, and mechanical ventilators all have their place for some patients, but are futile for other patients. Discuss which treatments will improve quality of life outcomes and emphasize those treatments instead.

6. **Encourage patients to have a durable power of attorney for health care—** Patients often have several family members interested in making medical decisions. A durable power of attorney for health care will clarify who will make medical decisions for the patient should the patient be incapacitated. It can also specify what types of decisions can be made.
7. **Develop an ethics committee and ethics consultations service for your facility—** When ethical conflict occurs, these resources can be most beneficial in mediating to consensus and developing alternative plans. They are a far better mechanism than resorting to the legal system. However, there may be an occasion when the legal system will be an alternative. Understand the ramifications of any of these mechanisms for resolving disputes.
8. **Know the difference between curing and caring—**Terminally ill patients rarely complain of hunger or thirst. What they need more than any medical intervention is compassion. They can usually be kept comfortable by continuing to offer sips of liquid or spoon feedings. Lubricants can be used to soothe dry mouth and lips. Above all, modifying or eliminating dietary restrictions should be considered. This would have the additional benefit of allowing family members to participate in the symbolism of the feeding process.

The Committee for Pro-Life Activities of the National Conference of Catholic Bishops in 1992 stated that "current debates about life-sustaining treatment suggest that our society's moral reflection is having difficulty keeping pace with its technological progress."[44] For terminally ill patients, the desire of medicine to cure must not supersede the capacity of the medical profession to care. The ethics of caring for those in medical need will become the foundation for providing appropriate medical care for all Americans.

ANNOTATED REFERENCES

1. **Koshuta, M.A., Schmitz, P.J., and Lynn, J.,** Development of an institutional policy on artificial hydration and nutrition, *Kennedy Institute of Ethics Journal,* 133, 1991.
2. **Koshuta, M.A., Schmitz, P.J., and Lynn, J.,** Development of an institutional policy on artificial hydration and nutrition, *Kennedy Institute of Ethics Journal,* 133, 1991.
3. **Wilson, D.M.,** Ethical concerns in a long-term tube feeding study, *Image: Journal of Nursing Scholarship,* 24, 195, 1992.
4. **Capron, A.M.,** The implications of the Cruzan decision for clinical nutrition teams, *Nutr. Clin. Pract.,* 6, 89, 1991.
5. **Koshuta, M.A., Schmitz, P.J., and Lynn, J.,** Development of an institutional policy on artificial hydration and nutrition, *Kennedy Institute of Ethics Journal,* 133, 1991.
   The long-term efficacy of continued nutritional support for some patients is now under scrutiny within the medical profession. In 1983, Joanne Lynn, M.D., a nutritional expert, and James Childress, Ph.D., a bioethicist, wrote a thought provoking and progressive article for its time, "Must Patients Always Be Given Food and Water?" In this article, the authors stated that there "is now widespread consensus that sometimes a patient is best served by not undertaking or continuing certain treatments that would sustain life, especially if these entail substantial suffering." They suggested that specialized nutrition support may be withheld or withdrawn if (1) the treatment is unlikely to improve nutritional status and is considered futile, (2) even if nutritional status improves, but will provide no benefit to the patient; and (3) if the burdens of the treatment outweigh the benefits.

6. **Craig, P.,** Comment: The Supreme Court faces the quest of withdrawal of hydration and nutrition: Cruzan v. Missouri Department of Health, *Health Hospital Law,* 22(12), 375, 1989.

    It was recently estimated that the cost of keeping a patient in the persistent vegetative state alive to be around $110,000 a year. Multiply that by the number of patients in this condition, and the cost of this diagnosis alive reaches over 11 billion annually. Compound this figure with the fact that these patients can live for years in this condition, one can see a staggering price for the cost of (for some at least) unwanted and futile medical treatment.

7. **Lynn, J. and Glover, J.,** Ethical decision-making in enteral nutrition, *Clinical Nutrition: Enteral & Tube Feeding,* 2nd ed., Rombeau, J.L., and Coldwell, M.D., Eds., W. B. Saunders, Philadelphia, 1990, chap. 30.

8. **Plato,** in *The Republic,* used the practice of Asclepians to explore the limits of autonomy: ''But they would have nothing to do with unhealthy and intemperate subjects, whose lives were of no use to themselves or others; the art of medicine was not designed for their good, and though they were rich as Midas, the sons of Asclepius would have declined to attend them.''

9. **Swisher, K.N. and Ayres, S.M.,** Who decides when care is futile?, *Critical Care Digest,* 11(4), 59, 1992.

10. *Belchertown v Saikewicz,* 373 Mass. 728, 370 N.E.2d 417 (1977).

11. **Kant, I.,** *Groundwork of the Metaphysics of Morals,* trans. H.J. Paton (New York: Harper & Row, 1964); *The Doctrine of Virtue, Part II of the ''Metaphysics of Morals,''* trans. Mary Gregor (New York: Harper & Row, 1964).

12. **Pence, G.E.,** Elizabeth Bouvia and voluntary death, in *Classic Cases in Medical Ethics,* McGraw-Hill, New York, 1990, chap. 2.

13. **Annas, G.J.,** When suicide prevention becomes brutality: the case of Elizabeth Bouvia,'' *Hastings Center Rep.,* 14(2) 20, 1984.

14. *Bouvia v. Superior Court,* 179 Cal. App.3d 1127, 225 Cal. Rptr. 297 (1986).

15. *Bouvia v. Superior Court,* 179 Cal. App.3d 1127, 225 Cal. Rptr. 297 (1986).

16. **Pence, G.E.,** Elizabeth Bouvia and voluntary death, in *Classic Cases in Medical Ethics,* McGraw-Hill, New York, 1990, 25.

    As Pence states:

> Some critics of autonomy see Bouvia's case initially as a failure of community, as a failure of caring where Ms. Bouvia ''slipped through the cracks'' of an impersonal American system. . . . Moreover, to cast this case as a simple issue of whether a right to die exists, or a right to ''assisted suicide'' exists, is to miss the heart of the issue. What made Elizabeth want to die was the cumulative effect of centuries of prejudice against the physically disabled. The new virulent form of this attitude is expressed in our culture's narcissistic idealization of youth, athleticism, sex, beauty, and fitness as the only values making life worthwhile.

17. *In re Estate of Longeway,* 133 Ill.2d 33, 549 N.E.2d 292, 299 (1989).

18. The pathology of patients in the PVS invariably entails massive bilateral hemispheric damage with a spared and intact brainstem. Preservation of the primitive brainstem activating system permits behavioral arousal and sleep/wake cycles, but existence is devoid of cognition. A sufficient period of observation is necessary before making a confident diagnosis of PVS. For older patients, those over 40, the chances of any recovery from this condition are nil. For more information, see AMA Council on Scientific Affairs, AMA Council on Ethical and Judicial Affairs, Persistent vegetative state and the decision to withdraw or withhold life support, *JAMA,* 263:426–430, 1990; Position of the American Academy of Neurology on certain aspects of the care and management of the persistent vegetative state patient, *Neurology,* 39:125–126, 1989.

19. **Annas, G.J.,** Do feeding tubes have more rights than patients?, *Hastings Center Rep.,* 16(1), 26, 1986.

20. **Annas, G.J.,** Do feeding tubes have more rights than patients?, *Hastings Center Rep.,* 16(1), 26, 1986.

21. As one commentator stated: ''We cause the death of a patient who cannot feed himself when we don't feed him, but the patient's infection causes the patient's death when it remains untreated.'' Brody, Response to Reader's Letter, *Hastings Center Rep.,* 48–49, 1988.

22. **Steinbrook and Bernard,** Artificial feeding-solid ground, not a slippery slope, *N. Engl. J. Med.,* 318(5) 287, 1988.

Writing for the New England Journal of Medicine, Steinbrook and Bernard state:

> The court acknowledges that ''there is substantial disagreement in the medical community over the appropriate medical action'' in such cases. Brophy's physicians and the hospital could not be forced to withhold artificial feeding from him . . . if such action ran contrary to their view of the ethical duty toward their patient.

The logic here is disconcerting. While physicians cannot be forced to withdraw unwanted medical treatments, if such treatments are against their ethical values, patients on the other hand, are forced to endure unwanted medical treatments against their ethical values to protect the integrity of the medical profession.

23. AMA Council on ethical and judicial affairs, *Current Opinions,* 13, 2.20 (1989); The A.M.A. statement on tube feeding: an ethical analysis, *America,* 321 (Nov. 22, 1986).

24. **Arras, J.H.,** Ethical theory in the medical context, in *Biomedical Ethics,* 3rd ed. Arras J. and Rhoden, N., Eds., 1989, 6.

25. **Gibson J.,** Thinking about the ''ethics'' in bioethics, in *Bioethics: Health Care Law and Ethics,* 2nd ed., Furrow, B.R., Johnson S.H., Jost T.S., and Schwartz R.L., Eds., West Publishing, St. Paul, MN, 1991, chap. 1.

26. **Arras, J.H. and Rhoden, N.,** *Biomedical Ethics,* 3rd ed., as reprinted in Furrow, B., Johnson, S., Jost, T., and Schwartz, R., *Bioethics: Health Care Law and Ethics,* West Publishing Co., St. Paul, MN, 1991. As Professor Arras states in his *Standard of Care,* ''the Court continued to recreate America's legal landscape by transferring traditional rights from its citizens to state legislatures and other government officials.''

27. **Forte F.F.,** The role of the clear and convincing standard of proof in right to die cases, *Issues in Law & Medicine,* 8(2) 183, 1992.

28. **Beauchamp T.L. and Childress J.F.,** *Principles of Biomedical Ethics,* 3rd ed., Oxford University Press, New York, 1989, 137.

29. In one survey prior to the U.S. Supreme Court's decision, 88% of the public thought the family should decide on treatment, 8% thought the doctors should decide, 1% the court, and no one selected the state. Coyle, How Americans view the high court, *Nat LJ,* 1, 36, 1990.

30. **Foucault, M.,** *The History of Sexuality: An Introduction,* Vol. 1, Random House, New York, 1990, 135.

31. **Cantor, N.L.,** The permanently unconscious patient, non-feeding and euthanasia, *Am. J. Law Med.,* 15(4), 381, 1989.

32. **Beauchamp T.L. and Childress J.F.,** *Principles of Biomedical Ethics,* 3rd ed., Oxford University Press, New York, 1989, chap. 4.

33. This is a genetic disorder that causes atonia of the neck muscles, hypertension of the legs and flexion of the arms, blindness, severe mental defects and megalocephaly.

34. *Guardianship of Doe,* 583 N.E.2d 1263, 1265 (Mass. 1992).

35. *Superintendent of Belchertown State School v. Saikewicz,* 370 N.E.2d 417 (Mass. 1977).

36. *In Re Conroy,* 98 N.J. 321, 486 A.2d 1209 at 1232 (1985).

37. *John F. Kennedy Memorial Hospital v Bludworth,* 432 So.2d 611, 615 (Fla. App. 1983).

38. **President's Commission,** Deciding to Forego Life-Sustaining Treatment, 127, 1983.

39. Patient Self-Determination Act, in the Omnibus Budget Reconciliation Act of 1990, P.L. 101–508, sections 4206, 4751, enacted November 5, 1990.

40. **Teno J.M. Sabatine, C., Parisier, L., Rouse, F.,** and **Lynn, J.,** The impact of the patient self-determination act's requirement that states describe law concerning patients' rights, *J. Law Med. Ethics,* 21(1), 102, 1993.

41. **Lynn J. and Teno J.M.,** After the patient self-determination act: the need for empirical research on formal advance directives, *Hastings Center Rep.,* 23(1), 34, 1993.

42. Will to Live and Accompanying Suggestions, as approved by the National Right to Life Committee Board of Directors, January 26, 1992.

43. **Avila, D.A.,** Medical treatment right of older persons and persons with disabilities: 1991–92 developments, *Issues in Law & Medicine,* 8(4), 429, 1993.

44. Committee for Pro-Life Activities, National Conference of Catholic Bishops, Nutrition and hydration: moral and pastoral reflections, *Issues in Law & Medicine,* 8, 387, 1192.

Chapter 16

FOODS OF THE FUTURE: WHAT WILL WE BE EATING IN THE NEXT CENTURY?

Joseph F. Borzelleca

TABLE OF CONTENTS

We may live without poetry, music and art;
We may live without conscience, and live without heart;
We may live without friends; we may live without books;
But civilized man cannot live without cooks.
He may live without books—what is knowledge but grieving?
He may live without hope—what is hope but deceiving?
He may live without love—what is passion but pining?
But where is the man that can live without dining?

Edward R. Bulwer

I. INTRODUCTION

These are exciting and challenging times! We are conquering space and uncovering the mysteries of our solar system. We are rediscovering wind, water, and the sun as energy sources that are not destructive to natural resources. We are mapping the human genome and have identified the genetic basis for some diseases and are thus able to manipulate the very essence of life. By manipulating human and bacterial genes, diseases heretofore untreatable are now being successfully managed. By using sophisticated molecular biological techniques, we are able to modify food-producing animals and plants. The composition of such foods produced naturally can be altered to meet any requirement. The potential for highly varied and nutritionally-sound foods is almost infinite. Will we recognize these new foods and will they be affordable? Will they taste good and be safe for us? Will we have fish products that look and taste like steak, and hot dogs that are fat free, highly nutritious and taste like "real" hot dogs? Will we be able to cook dinner in the car on the way home from work? Will fast-food restaurants serve fat-free foods that taste like the "real stuff"? Will highly perishable foods like tomatoes and strawberries keep fresh for weeks? Will we have a wide variety of foods year round? Will we have fat-free and sugar-free ice cream that tastes like Ben and Jerry's®? Will we be able to eat food packages like we do ice cream cones—the perfect food container? Will we have soft drinks that are highly nutritious but taste like Classic Coke®, and microwaved foods that look and taste like oven-cooked foods? Will the microwave then completely replace the oven? Will cooking become a lost art?

II. BASIC CONSIDERATIONS

What is food, why do we eat it, and what is the basis for food selection? Food is anything we eat or drink to help keep us alive; it usually consists of carbohydrates, fats and/or proteins. It is either unprocessed such as fruits and vegetables, or processed, which means it has been altered in some way, and will provide energy and sustain growth, repair, and other bodily functions. So almost anything we put into our mouths could be classified as food.

Why do we eat? We eat primarily for self-preservation; we are hungry and want to stay healthy and alive. The other reasons include eating for the sheer pleasure of it (hedonic basis) and eating out of boredom, frustration, depression, or other altered emotional states (psychological basis).

What determines our food choices? Why do we eat certain foods and not others? This is a very complex issue. The basis for selecting foods include: nutritional content (not usually the main reason); hedonic value [how the food or drink looks, smells, tastes and feels in the mouth (mouthfeel)]; religious and cultural influences such as kosher or vegetarian; physiological status (e.g., the presence of disease, fever); environmental factors such as temperature or humidity; economic factors, which include availability and affordability; personal or idiosyncratic needs; and for pharmacological effects. Usually, food is consumed for its hedonic value. Nutritive value, or any other value, cannot be appreciated unless the food leaves the plate! Therefore, the food industry is expected to provide food that is nutritious, appealing, satisfying, and safe—an awesome challenge.

However, the consuming public, those who have an adequate, varied, and affordable food supply, wants food to be more than tasty and nutritious. Current and future expectations are that food should also prevent or treat disease. Such foods are called chemopreventive or physiologically functional if they prevent disease and are called nutraceutical or pharmafood if they are used to treat disease. For example, garlic may be consumed not just for its flavor but for its effects on platelets (prevent aggregation), as a preventive for cancer or for its antibacterial and antiviral effects. Because calcium is involved in preventing osteoporosis and may be a critical factor in the etiology of cancer and cardiovascular disease, dairy foods and other foods rich in calcium may be ingested in large quantities or the public may demand that more foods, including beverages, be fortified with calcium. Protein is essential for growth and development and the maintenance of health. The public perceives that protein-enriched foods must be better for health and the food processing industry is responding to this by increasing the ''natural content of proteins'' by protein supplementation (e.g., dairy products). Those foods fortified with micronutrients are perceived to be ''better for you'' than non-fortified foods such as iron-enriched and vitamin-supplemented baked goods. Processed foods can be readily fortified with almost any ingredient, thereby giving consumers ''more for their money'' but the impact of these fortified foods on health must be critically evaluated. This trend for ''health'' foods and fortified foods continues to gain momentum as the public begins to look to plants and foods in nature for solutions to its health problems because traditional medicine may be too costly.

Whether it is friends or food, variety is still the spice of life. This presents a challenge to the grower and to the processor. New and novel natural foods are being discovered in other cultures and countries (e.g., the kiwi fruit) and introduced to the U.S. primarily by immigrants who bring with them their ideas about food that will enhance our food supply. Unfortunately, acceptance may be slow because these foods ''look different''. Food growers may experiment with plant breeding to produce new varieties of items already available or new ''natural'' foods. This is a slow process and the outcome is not always guaranteed. By using modern molecular biological techniques (biotechnology), highly specific traits can be introduced into plants (e.g., controlled ripening as in the Flavr Savr® tomato) and animals (e.g., increased milk production by using BST). These new molecular biological methods are highly specific, reliable, reproducible, rapid, and safe. Food processors are also responding by developing ingenious new products. Some are finding new uses for old foods and/or food chemicals whose safety has been established for some time such as gums used in frozen desserts. Still others are using new physical forms of existing food substances like microparticulated egg white and casein as a fat-substitute for frozen desserts. Some are using heretofore unused food sources to form highly nutritious and acceptable foods, ''simulated foods'' such as simulated shellfish from surimi, which is prepared from bottom trash fish that until now had no commercial value. New food chemicals are also being developed and used by food processors; these include new and intense flavors and colors, texturizing agents, macronutrient substitutes, and preservatives. Some of these new materials are natural, some are nature-identical, and others are synthetic. The public appears to find some comfort in the natural source of a chemical as opposed to a totally synthetic source. However, available data do not support greater safety of natural products. For example, synthetic chemicals can be consistently produced to established specifications and with known purity, whereas the composition of natural products varies with location, climatic conditions, growing and harvesting conditions, and seasons. One thing is certain, the food industry will respond to the consumer's wishes and fancies. It is essential to recognize that the nutritional value and safety of new foods must be assured before the product is introduced into the marketplace.

III. ISSUES AND CONCERNS FOR THE NEXT CENTURY

What are some of the issues, concerns, or needs of the consuming public as we move into the next century, and how are these being addressed by the food industry? The nutritional needs of each segment of the population must be clearly established. These requirements should be based on age, sex, occupation, climate/environment, physical activities, and state of health. Will these basic requirements change as we move into the next century? Our occupations are changing and becoming less energy-intensive and thereby requiring fewer calories. However, some enjoy eating. For these people, the food industry will prepare foods that are tasty and bulky and have low nutrient density. There will be increased use of macronutrient substitutes, which include non-nutritive sweeteners and fat substitutes, to decrease the caloric content of foods. For the elderly who cannot or do not prepare food for themselves, high density foods will be available in convenient forms that have long shelf lives, are tasty, and affordable. Will the only change be in caloric requirements or will there be specific nutrient changes? For example, for those living in heavily polluted areas, will there be a need for greater intakes of antioxidants? As newer types of drugs are introduced, will there be more nutrient-drug interactions necessitating increased nutrient intakes?

IV. MACRONUTRIENT SUBSTITUTES

Reduced-calorie substances used to replace organoleptic and/or functional properties of fats and sugars in the diet are termed macronutrient substitutes. Fat reduction is essential in weight control and the public's interest in reduced-fat foods continues to grow. The estimated market for reduced-fat food products is already nearly $30 billion. Fat replacements include: alternative fats such as Olestra®, a non-absorbable liquid fat, and synthetic chemicals; older food materials such as gums, starches, and cellulosic products, formerly used as thickeners and emulsifiers; and protein-based replacers such as casein and albumin. The latter two categories are often called fat mimetics. It is very difficult to replace all the attributes of fat such as texture, lubricity, viscosity and structural stability, flavor, appearance, and reactivity.

A. CARBOHYDRATES AS FAT-REPLACERS

Fats contribute 9 cal/g whereas carbohydrates such as starches or dextrins contribute 4 cal/g. Cellulose, a polysaccharide, does not contribute calories because it is neither absorbed from the gastrointestinal tract nor metabolized by the body. Starches, when mixed with water, form gels which mimic the bulk and texture of fat. When used to replace fat, these mixtures provide 1 cal/g or less because they are mostly water. They can replace up to 100% of the fat in food, but they cannot be used for frying, which is still a major source of dietary fat. Some examples of starch and modified starch fat replacers include: N-Lite® products from corn and other starches, examples of which are N-Lite B® for baked goods, N-Lite F® for frostings, and N-Lite D® for dairy foods; Sta-Slim® from potato and tapioca starches; Maltrin® from cornstarch maltodextrin; Paselli-SA2® from potato starch maltodextrin; and Oatrim® from oat flour and oat bran. Hydrocolloids and carbohydrate gums also retain water and are essentially noncaloric. These may be used alone or with other gums to completely replace fat or be combined with it to yield a reduced-fat product. Included in this group are xanthan gum, guar gum, locust bean gum, gum arabic, tara gum, pectins (e.g., Slendid® from citrus peel) and carrageenan (e.g., Nutricol®, for use in meat products). Microcrystalline cellulose is widely used as an excipient in drug formulations but mostly as a replacement for fat in salad dressings, baked goods, and frozen desserts; it is not metabolized and is therefore noncaloric. Polydextrose, previously used as a replacement for sugar and as a bulking agent, is now used as a replacement for fat.

B. PROTEIN-BASED FAT SUBSTITUTES

Protein-based fat substitutes contribute about 4 cal/g. The pleasant mouthfeel of fat, the creaminess in yogurt, ice cream, etc., is due to the presence of small particles (0.1 to 0.3 μm), fat globules. To simulate the feel of fat, it is necessary to prepare a product with globules of the same size to fool the taste buds and other receptors in the mouth. Two such products, Simplesse® from Nutrasweet® and Trailblazer® from Kraft General Foods, have been prepared using casein from skim milk and egg white (albumin). These proteins are microparticulated to yield a creamy product. Whey protein has also been used by Nutrasweet® and Simplesse® was marketed as a frozen dessert, Simple Pleasures®. Still under development is Lita, a microparticulated zein, a protein from corn, which provides less than 2 cal/g.

C. ALTERNATIVE FATS

There are several forms of alternative fats, each of which provides less calories than fat, but may have different properties. Olestra®, a sucrose-polyester, is derived from corn or soy oil and can be used for baking and frying. It is not absorbed from the gastrointestinal tract and therefore does not contribute calories, thus completely replacing fat. Caprenin® is a reduced-calorie fat substitute for cocoa butter and primarily yields about 5 cal/g. Esterified propoxylated glycerols (EPGs) are chemically modified natural fats and oils that are only slightly metabolized or not metabolized at all and can be used for frying and food formulations. Dialkyl dihexadecylmalonate (DDM), a fatty alcohol ester of malonic and alkylmalonic acids, is noncaloric and is designed for high temperature applications, and tricarballylic acid esterified with fatty alcohols (TATCA) is also noncaloric and can be used as an oil substitute in margarine and mayonnaise-type products.

D. ALTERNATIVE SWEETENERS

Low calorie, high-intensity (10 to 1000 times sweeter than sucrose), non-nutritive sweeteners had their beginning with the use of saccharin for diabetics around the turn of the century. The wide-spread use of non-nutritive sweeteners began after World War II when the consumption of carbonated beverages began to increase substantially. The public wanted sweetened beverages that had few calories and the search began for substitutes for saccharin. It should be noted that the only public health problem associated with sucrose, table sugar, is development of caries in the presence of poor oral hygiene. Of course, it yields 4 calories per gram and this concerns a diet-conscious public. Cyclamate® was the first of the new high-intensity sweeteners. It is used in most countries, including Mexico and Canada. It is inexpensive, has no after-taste, is acid- and heat-stable and is compatible with most foods. Unfortunately, it was banned by the U.S. FDA because of the high intake by children and concerns about potential adverse health effects, but there were no toxicological data to support this concern. The U.S. FDA is considering its return to the U.S. marketplace. Aspartame (Nutrasweet®) is a peptide sweetener prepared from aspartic acid, phenylalanine, and methyl alcohol that is not very acid- or heat-stable. Acesulfame-K (Sunette®), the potassium salt of 6-methyl-1,2,3-oxathiazin-4(3H)-one 2,2 dioxide; Alitame®, an amino-acid based sweetener; and sucralose, a chlorinated sucrose which is acid- and heat-stable, are new and highly effective sweeteners. Some potentially new sweeteners from natural sources include: dihydrochalcones from citrus bioflavonoids, stevioside from the stevia plant found in South America, glycyrrhizin from licorice root, and thaumatin (proteins) from a West African fruit. A unique new family of sweeteners may be the L-sugars ("left-handed sugars"); these have all the desirable properties of the D-sugars but are not caloric since they are not absorbed. The search continues for the ideal non-nutritive and high-intensity sweetener that is acid- and heat-stable, has no after-taste, is cheap and is safe for all age groups. Until the ideal substance is found, the materials available are effective and safe and will continue to be used.

V. BIOTECHNOLOGY IN THE NEXT CENTURY

In the next century our food supply will be more varied, more nutritious, organoleptically appealing, with longer shelf life and less expensive as a result of molecular biological manipulations (biotechnology). This will require a concerted effort on the parts of the food industry, the government, and especially the media to educate the public and the "consumer advocates" who believe that molecular biological manipulations are intrinsically evil and pose a health threat to the general public. The safety of food chemicals and new foods is assured by the extensive testing conducted by the food and chemical industries with the approval and supervision of the Food and Drug Administration. Manipulation of plants by conventional plant breeding techniques is an age-old agricultural practice which does not appear to concern consumers. But the word "biotechnology" conjures up horrible visions of harmless and useful microorganisms mutating into highly pathogenic organisms that infect humans and cause untreatable and deadly diseases. This is highly unlikely when proper precautions and techniques are used. The only difference between traditional plant breeding techniques and the newer biotechnology is that the newer techniques are specific, faster, and cheaper. It is not a "shotgun" approach. Safety will be assured using the most sensitive toxicological techniques available. Approved biotechnologically-derived foods will not pose a risk to public health. The use of these techniques will result in an expanded and exciting food supply. Some of the benefits of biotechnology on the food supply are listed below.

- A greater variety of foods that are more nutritious and have a longer shelf life.
- The more efficient use of animals. For example, BST used to increase milk production, increase lean-to-fat ratio in meat, lower-fat milk, and lower cholesterol in eggs.
- The significant reduction or elimination in spoilage and potentially pathogenic organisms such salmonella, listeria, and botulinum.
- More hypoallergenic foods achieved by desensitization of allergens in foods and dealing with T-cell epitopes.
- Plants that have controlled ripening, high solids content, resistance to insects and pathogens, resistance to chemicals (pesticides), improved nutrition, lower content of alkaloids and other pharmacologically active chemicals, and are stable in temperature extremes.
- Plants that are used for specific pharmacological/therapeutic effects. For example, garlic and rosemary eaten as cancer preventives.

- New and novel plant food sources such as algae (including marine macroalgae) and mycoproteins being used.
- Plants that will produce plastics, food chemicals, and drugs.
- Animals that will produce products with desired pharmacological activity such as anti-diarrheal antibodies in cow's milk, and naturally occurring antibiotics in cow's milk.
- The use of newer sources of animal protein such as fish and shellfish farming.

Biotechnology will also be used to develop food packaging that is organoleptically acceptable to consumers and environmentally friendly. Some of these contributions are summarized below.

- Environmentally acceptable consumable packages consisting of edible film or foam packaging. The ice cream cone is the perfect food package—it is consumed during or after the product it delivers is consumed.
- Aseptic, active packaging that preserves the contents; for example, plastic film that contains a microbicide, thereby eliminating/minimizing the need for preservatives. Controlled atmosphere packaging that, for example, replaces oxygen with an inert gas.
- More use of sous vide packaging; uncooked food is packaged in a vacuum bag, then the food is cooked and chilled.
- Packaging that will also cook or cool foods. For example, a self-chilling beverage can by the use of an activator tab.
- The development of tamper-evident packaging.
- Although not biotechnology, the irradiation of food is the most efficient method known to preserve food: no chemicals are added, no radiation is retained, and no radiolytic products are formed.

There are exciting new possibilities in the area of food preparation and processing that biotechnology and advanced engineering promise. These should result in less time in food preparation and more time for other purposes, as listed below.

- Computerized cooking by the use probes and pots that are connected to the stove and are programmed to cook at various temperatures for specified times; temperature can be raised and/or lowered, thus resulting in "perfectly prepared meals".
- Better, more, and cheaper cordless appliances for preparing foods, some of which will never need recharging.
- Computerized vending machines into which a person can type in requests and the food will be assembled for home cooking or will be cooked to order.
- Microchips imbedded in foods that will tell ovens when to turn on and off, thereby insuring proper preparation.
- More robotics in fast-food and other restaurants to minimize contamination and expedite service.
- Greater and greater need for convenience foods as the population finds "better" use of its time.
- Simulated foods such as textured vegetable protein to prepare bacon, sausage, and other cuts of meat; poor cuts of meat and fish made to look like the "real thing".
- Hydroponics emerging as a significant source of vegetables and fruits.
- Use of enzyme-synthesizing processes such as honey and milk produced without bees and cows.

- Foods prepared by categories for special age groups such as infant, pediatric and geriatric, which would have more flavor and be fortified.
- Greater use of nutritional substances as ergogenic aids that would enhance athletic performance without the use of drugs.
- The use of foods with improved nutritional profiles containing increased nutrients and decreased anti-nutrients.
- Foods that have enhanced organoleptic properties such as improved flavor, color, and texture.
- More food chemicals produced "naturally" such as bacterial, fungal, or yeast production of flavors, enzymes, and sweeteners.
- More foods that are microwavable.
- Foods that have longer half-lives because of chemical preservatives, irradiation, shrink-wrap packaging (reduces need for refrigeration), sous vide technique and the use of biocides in packaging materials.

Despite the excellent record in the U.S., there are always concerns about the safety of our food supply. These concerns are often based on ignorance from a misinformed media. Efforts to enhance food safety will continue and newer and more sensitive methods will be used, examples of which are listed below.

- Use of immunochemical methods, DNA probes, and monoclonal antibodies for example, to rapidly detect the presence of pathogens, pesticides, and drugs.
- Use of a sensitive marker, such as a dot that appears or changes color, on packaging for perishable foods to indicate when the food is unfit for human consumption.
- Similar to new drugs, human testing of new foods prior to marketing.
- International harmonization of food safety requirements.

The public must be educated to take better care of itself. Considerable effort has to be expended to better educate the public as to nutrition and health, with preventive medicine as the key issue. This will be expensive but is cheap when compared to treating those with nutritionally induced disorders, which include obesity, osteoporosis and possibly cancer and birth defects. Some of the health and education issues are detailed below.

- Greater use of nutraceuticals or pharmafoods, which are foods with desirable pharmacological properties, to prevent or treat disease.
- Drugs to reset the metabolic rate ("the ideal anorexigenic agent").
- Appropriate patient monitoring to be established as part of routine physical examinations, as well as individualized nutrient requirements determined by the appropriate analysis of blood and/or other body fluid.
- Improved prenatal nutrition to decrease the incidence of impaired development and protect against disease.
- Greater and more effective health education in elementary through professional or graduate school, resulting in a better informed public. This assumes that the media will cooperate, and also encourage a greater use of television and product packaging to teach nutrition.
- Consumer-friendly labeling that will include complete compositional and nutritional analysis, absolute amounts and percentages of recommended daily requirements, and health claims. For example, specific indications such as the prevention of osteoporosis.

VI. CONCLUSION

In the next century foods will be somewhat different from foods presently consumed. They may have different shapes, colors, flavors, nutritional and pharmacological profiles, and longer shelf-lives. Although the foods of the future may be unusual, they will not be bizarre (e.g., green bread), and they will be more intense in flavor and natural or nature-identical. They will be more nutrient dense, have increased concentration of desirable chemicals, decreased concentration of undesirable chemicals, and have extended shelf-lives due primarily to irradiation since nothing is added to foods during this process. Some foods will be new and novel, the only limitation being the imagination of the food technologist. Simulated foods (look, smell, taste, and feel like the "real thing") will increase in popularity because they will be healthier and cheaper. Beverages will be nutritionally fortified so that they provide more than just pleasure and calories. The greatest change in the area of foods and nutrition will be the heightened awareness of the role of nutrition in disease prevention and cure by both the general public and by the medical profession. But how far will we have really advanced? Hippocrates, in the 4th century B.C., taught that the role of the physician in the healing process is to assist nature by increasing nature's healing forces. That was true then and is now; it is best accomplished by proper diet, rest, and exercise.

ACKNOWLEDGMENT

The author thanks Sheryl L. Miller for her literary and secretarial skills that were utilized while preparing this chapter.

REFERENCES

1. **Advisory Committee on Novel Foods and Processes.** Department of Health Guidelines on the Assessment of Novel Foods and Processes Rep. 38, 1991.
2. **American Academy of Allergy and Immunology.** Adverse Reactions to Foods, Brochure, 1984.
3. **Anon.** Cancer prevention: focus on foods urged, *Food Chem News*, 35, 7– 11, 1993.
4. **Archer, DE and Kessler, DA.** Foodborne illnesses in the 1900s. *JAMA*, 269:2737– 2738, 1993.
5. **Baumgardt, BR and Martin, MA.** Agricultural Biotechnology: Issues and Choices, Information for Decision Makers. Purdue University Agr Exp St, West Lafayette, IN, 1992.
6. **Behrens, L.** Smart drinks pour on the brain power. *Chicago Tribune*, January 26, 1992.
7. **Borzelleca, JF.** Macronutrient substitutes: safety evaluation. *Reg Tox Pharm*, 16:253–264, 1992.
8. **Cliver, DO.** Eating Safely: Avoiding Foodborne Illnesses. American Council on Science and Health, NY, Brochure, 1993.
9. **Clydesdale, FM and Gorgatti-Netto, A.** Present and future of food science and technology in industrialized and developing countries. *Food Technol*, 43:134–168, 1989.
10. **Expert Panel on Food Safety and Nutrition of the Institute of Food Technologists.** Potential mechanisms for food-related carcinogens and anticarcinogens, *Food Technol*, 47:105–118, 1993.
11. **Gerber, J.** How the aging explosion will create new food trends. *Food Technol*, 43:134, 135, 150, 1989.
12. **Glanz, J.** Diffraction physics redefines biosensors. *Res Devel*, March, 1993
13. **Goldblith SA.** The legacy of Columbus, with particular reference to foods. *Food Technol*, 46:62–85, 1992.
14. **Harlander, SK.** Biotechnology—a means for improving our food supply. *Food Technol*, 46:84–95, 1991

15. **Harlander, SK.** Engineering the foods of the future cereal foods. *Cereal World,* 35:1106–1109, 1990.

16. **Harper, AE.** Diet and behaviour: an assessment of knowledge. *Food Technol Australia,* 89(Special suppl.):ii-xi, 1987.

17. **Howards, SS and Peterson HB.** Foods of the future: the new biotechnology and FDA regulation. *JAMA,* 269:910–914, 1993.

18. **Institute of Medicine of the National Academy of Sciences.** Estimating consumer exposure to food additives and monitoring trends in use. *Nat Acad Press,* Washington, DC, 1992.

19. **Kirschman, J.** Priority food safety issues for the Year 2000. *Reg Tox Pharm,* 17:1–2, 1993.

20. **Lachance, PA.** Nutritional responsibilities of food companies in the next century. *Food Technol,* 43:144–150, 1989.

21. **Lee, K.** Food neophobia: major causes and treatments. *Food Technol,* 43:62–72, 1989.

22. **Long, P.** Unreal meals. *Health,* July/August, 55–60, 1992.

23. **Lepkowski, W.** Food research. *Chem Eng News,* 71:3, 1993.

24. **Liddle, RA, Goldstein, RB, and Saxton, J.** Gallstone formation during weight-reduction dieting. *Arch Intern Med,* 149:1750–1753, 1989.

25. **Mermelstein, NH.** Food flavors. *Food Technol,* 43:99–106, 1989.

26. **Mermelstein, NH.** A guide to the new nutrition labeling proposals. *Food Technol,* 46:56–62, 1992.

27. **Mermelstein, NH.** Safety issues: foods of new biotechnology vs. traditional products. *Food Technol,* 46:99–120, 1992.

28. **Mermelstein, NH.** Religious and philosophical bases of food choices. *Food Technol,* 46:91–126, 1992.

29. **Mermelstein, NH.** Potential mechanisms for food-related carcinogens and anticarcinogens. *Food Technol,* 47:105–118, 1993.

30. **Miller, GA and Frier, HI.** Lifestyle-driven foods and ingredients required for their development. *Food Technol,* 43:136–143, 1989.

31. **National Agricultural Biotechnology Council.** Report 1. Biotechnology and sustainable agriculture: policy alternatives. 1989; Report 2. Agricultural biotechnology, food safety and nutritional quality for the consumer. 1990; Report 3. Agricultural biotechnology at the crossroads: biological, social and institutional concerns. 1991; Report 4. Animal biotechnology: opportunities and challenges. 1992.

32. **Regenstein, JN and Kilara, A.** Religious and philosophical bases of food choices. *Food Technol,* 46:91–126, 1992.

33. **Research Committee of the Institute of Food Technologists.** America's food research needs: into the 21st Century. *Food Technol,* 47:1S-40S, 1993.

34. **Rosenberg, IH.** Symposium on nutrition and aging. *Nutr Rev,* 50:347–502, 1992.

35. **Sampson, HA, Mendelson L, and Rosen, JP.** Fatal and near-fatal anaphylactic reactions to food in children and adolescents. *N Engl J Med,* 327:380–384, 1992.

36. **Setser, CS and Racette, WL.** Macromolecule replacers in food products. *Rev Food Sci Nutr,* 32:275–297, 1992.

37. **Sills-Levy, E.** U.S. food trends leading to the year 2000. *Food Technol,* 43:128–132, 1989.

38. **Taylor, S and Sumner, SS.** Risks and benefits of foods and food additives. In: *Food Additives,* Branen, LA, Davidson, MP, Salmen, S, Eds., Marcel Dekker, New York, 1990.

39. **Thayer, AM.** Food additives. *Chem Eng News* 70:26–44, 1992.

40. **Vanderveen, JE and Glinsmann, WH.** Fat substitutes: a regulatory perspective. *Ann Rev Nutr,* 12:473–487, 1992.

41. **Whelan, EM.** Food label folly. *Wall Street Journal,* December 9, 1992.

42. **Williams, MH.** Nutritional ergogenic aids and athletic performance. *Nutr Today,* 24:7–14, 1989.

INDEX

H

T

TATCA, see Tricarballylic acid esterified with fatty alcohols
Taurine, 208
TBK, see Total body potassium
TBN, see Total body nitrogen
T-cells, 23, 24, 67, 68, 70–73
    functions of, 73, 75, 76
    proliferation of, 73
    surgery and, 166
Tetrapolar impedance, 248
TGF, see Transforming growth factor
Thermogenesis, 35
Thromboxanes, 66, 75
Thrompocytopenia, 26
Thyroid cancer, 230
Tinitus, 250
TLC, see Total lymphocyte count
TNF, see Tumor necrosis factor
TOBEC, see Total body electrical conductivity
Total body albumin, 199
Total body electrical conductivity (TOBEC), 11, 12
Total body fat, 2
Total body neutron activation, 10
Total body nitrogen (TBN), 10
Total body potassium (TBK), 9, 10, 34
Total body water, 9, 34
Total body weight, 2, 8
Total lymphocyte count (TLC), 7
Total parenteral nutrition (TPN), 52, 135–161
    administration of, 153–154
    care management development and, 186, 188
    complications of, 154–156
    fistulas and, 60
    formulation and composition of solution in, 149–150
    future of, 156–161
    hepatic disease and, 57
    history of, 136–141
    immune system and, 76–78
    indications for, 146–147
    inflammatory bowel disease and, 54
    monitoring of, 153–154
    nutritional assessment and, 147–149
    pancreatitis and, 55, 56
    renal disease and, 209, 210
    short-bowel syndrome and, 53, 54, 219, 221
    surgery and, 167–173, 176, 177
    techniques of administration of, 151–153
TPN, see Total parenteral nutrition
Traditional medical care delivery failure, 184–187
Transfer dysphagia, 126
Transferrin, 7, 16, 170, 201
Transforming growth factor (TGF), 71
Transminases, 25
Trauma, 77, 78, 123, 127, 166
TREE, see True resting energy expenditure
Tricarballylic acid esterified with fatty alcohols (TATCA), 283
Triceps skinfolds (TSF), 6, 201

Triene/tetraene ratios, 154, 222
Triglycerides, 2, 3, 25, 38, 51, see also specific types
    cancer prevention and, 230
    excess, 200
    immune system and, 75
    long-chain, 154, 156, 209
    medium-chain, 122, 124, 154, 156, 209, 221, 222
    removal of, 200
    secretion of, 200
    short-bowel syndrome and, 221
    short-chain, 156, 221, 222
Tritium, 9
True resting energy expenditure (TREE), 13
Tryptophan, 250
TSF, see Triceps skinfolds
Tube enterostomy, 93–101
Tuberculosis, 169
Tuberculous enteritis, 147
Tumor necrosis factor (TNF), 22–24, 69

U

UBW, see Usual body weight
Ulcerative colitis, 54, 147, 168
Ulcer diets, 57, 58
Ulcers, 147
Ultrasonography, 12, 223
UNA, see Urea nitrogen appearance
Unsaturated fatty acids, 232
Uracil, 76
Urea, 199
Urea nitrogen appearance (UNA), 202, 203
Uremia, 202
Urinary measurements, 7
Usual body weight (UBW), 5, 201
Uterine cancer, 234

V

Valine, 173, 204
Vascular disorders, 169, see also specific types
Vasoactive intestinal polypeptide (VIP), 218
Very low-energy diet, 40, 41
Villous hypertrophy, 217
Vinegar, 138
VIP, see Vasoactive intestinal polypeptide
Vitamin A, 51, 52, 56
    cancer prevention and, 235, 236
    deficiency of, 167
    immune system and, 73, 78
    quackery and, 252
    renal disease and, 200, 210
    total parenteral nutrition and, 144
Vitamin B, 50, 52, 54, 56, 58, 171, 217
    cancer prevention and, 235
    deficiency of, 167
    immune system and, 73
    quackery and, 251, 252
    renal disease and, 210
    short-bowel syndrome and, 218, 221, 222
    total parenteral nutrition and, 144

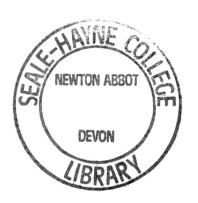